Classics In
Child Development

Classics In
Child Development

Advisory Editors

JUDITH KRIEGER GARDNER
HOWARD GARDNER

Editorial Board

Wayne Dennis
Jerome Kagan
Sheldon White

The Child: His Nature and His Needs

Prepared under the Editorial Supervision of

M. V. O'SHEA

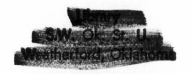

ARNO PRESS

A New York Times Company

New York – 1975

Reprint Edition 1975 by Arno Press Inc.

Classics in Child Development
ISBN for complete set: 0-405-06450-0
See last pages of this volume for titles

Manufactured in the United States of America

Library of Congress Cataloging in Publication Data

O'Shea, Michael Vincent, 1866-1932, ed.
  The child, his nature and his needs.

  (Classics in child development)
  Reprint of the ed. published by Children's Foundation,
New York.
  Bibliography: p.
  Includes index.
  1. Child study. 2. Children--Care and hygiene.
3. Education of children. I. Children's Foundation.
II. Title. III. Series.
LB1115.O7 1975   155.4   74-21424
ISBN 0-405-06473-X

THE CHILD: HIS NATURE
AND HIS NEEDS

The Child: His Nature and His Needs

A Survey of Present-Day Knowledge
Concerning Child Nature and the
Promotion of the Well-Being
and Education of the Young

Prepared under the Editorial Supervision of

M. V. O'SHEA

Professor of Education, The University of Wisconsin

A CONTRIBUTION

of

THE CHILDRENS FOUNDATION

NEW YORK · VALPARAISO · CHICAGO

PREFACE

THE Childrens Foundation has for its objects the study of the child and the dissemination of knowledge promotive of the well-being of children. It came into existence at Valparaiso, Indiana, late in 1921, when a charter was granted to it by the State of Indiana as a corporation not for profit, and a gift was made available to its Trustees for effecting its organization and developing its program of work.

The Foundation has first undertaken the task of appraising present-day knowledge relating to the nature, well-being, and education of children, and through this volume, "The Child: His Nature and His Needs," it seeks to make this knowledge available for practical use everywhere by those who are in immediate contact with children, fashioning their intellect, moulding their character and influencing their physical development.

Special acknowledgment is due Professor M. V. O'Shea of the University of Wisconsin, and the staff of eminent students in the field of child life who have collaborated with him in the preparation of this work.

The second contribution of the Foundation will appear late in the year 1925. It will deal comprehensively with the problems arising out of the changing, economic and social conditions as they affect the well-being of childhood and youth in the American home.

The Trustees invite the counsel and desire to enlist in the work of the Foundation the coöperation, good will, and efforts of individuals, associations, institutions, or enterprises, having directly or indirectly for their objects the well-being of the childhood of the human race, or having at their command the facilities or instrumentalities desirable to be employed for arousing individual and public interest in, and disseminating knowledge about, the well-being of children.

LEWIS E. MYERS

Valparaiso, Indiana
April, 1924

What the best and wisest parent wants for his own child, that must the community want for all its children.

—*John Dewey*

CONTENTS

PART I

Present Status of Our Knowledge of Child Nature

CONTENTS

PART II

Present Status of Our Knowledge of Child Well-Being

CONTENTS

PART III

Present Status of Our Knowledge of Education

INTRODUCTION

BOOKS, pamphlets, and articles relating to child nature and ways and means of improving the mental and physical condition of childhood and youth have increased enormously in number and variety during the last eight or ten years. Legislation designed to promote the welfare and training of the young has also increased greatly during this period. Of course, men and women in all times have been interested in the well-being of children, but in most countries this has been the chief concern of only a small minority. Until very recently, the care and culture of the young have been assigned almost entirely to parents, governesses, and teachers. But this is not the case to-day. In some countries, particularly in our own, statesmen are coming to see that the stability and prosperity of a nation depend mainly in the long run upon the mental poise and acumen, and the social understanding and good will of the rising generation, which values can be secured only by a proper regimen of bodily, mental, and social training. Those who are studying the requirements of national welfare as well as those who are charged with the conduct of governmental affairs, at home as well as abroad, are turning their attention to-day, very much more generally and acutely than they did formerly, to the promotion of the physical, intellectual, and social well-being of the rising generation. Our own country has led in this new movement, but all progressive countries have shown, or are now showing, that they regard the careful investigation of the nature and the needs of childhood and youth and the dissemination of knowledge relating to education and child welfare as of supreme importance.

One of the most significant phases of the awakening
of interest on the part of all our people in childhood and
youth relates to the shifting of emphasis in the activities
of psychologists. A few years back, most American
psychologists and all the psychological laboratories in
our country were devoted to the analytical or experimental
study of the mature mind. One of the most distinguished
of these psychologists said two decades ago that he could
see no reason for studying the mind of the child as distinguished from the mind of the adult; if we could find out
how the mature mind was constituted and how it functioned, we would know how the child mind was constituted and how it functioned, because the latter was
simply a miniature copy of the former. He and his psychological and philosophical colleagues did not take seriously those who were beginning to say that in the
development of the human mind from birth to maturity
changes occur which make it different, not only in strength
or range or power but also in other important respects, in
the adult stage from what it is in infancy, childhood, or
youth. But every psychologist of any standing agrees
to this view to-day. A majority of the psychologists who
were formerly indifferent to the study of mental development as distinguished from the analytical and experimental study of the mature mind are now devoting a part
of and some of them all their time and energy to the study
of one or another aspect of the mind of the child or the
youth. The psychological laboratories of our country are
being utilized in considerable measure everywhere, and
almost completely in many places, for the investigation
of problems connected with the maturing processes of the
human mind. Numerous clinics have been established
during the past ten years especially for the investigation
of child development, alike in its normal and in its
abnormal manifestations. It would probably be within
bounds to say that there is at least ten times as much

intelligent attention being given now to a study of the physical, intellectual, social, and moral development and well-being of childhood and youth as was the case two decades ago in our country.

As it happens in respect to every movement of this character, individuals and institutions have been concerned in their investigations and in their service with special aspects of the development and well-being of childhood and youth.. There has been little attempt thus far at coördination of the results of investigations and the outcome of various efforts to promote the well-being and education of the young. Each student of mental development has confined his attention to some particular phase of child nature or child training, so that he could go farther in exploring it than anyone had done before him. Every investigator understands that if he attacks a very complex problem he is not likely to go a great way with it unless he breaks it up into subordinate problems and selects the one that he is equipped to investigate with some degree of success. The individual student depends upon others to combine the results of his particular investigation with the results of the work of his colleagues who are studying related problems. He does not consider it to be a part of his task to show how the results he secures are related to the results secured by those who are investigating different problems from his own. It is essential to the development of any science that the individual investigator should not be concerned so much with the science as a whole as with the particular problem with which he is wrestling, even though this problem has to do, in the case of human development, with but a very small section of the nature and needs of a child or a youth.

The Individual Investigator or Agency is Concerned with but a Special Phase of the Nature or Needs of the Young

The Childrens Foundation, as Mr. Myers, its founder, has pointed out in the Preface to this volume, is seeking to be of service in performing the task of coördinating, interpreting, and applying the results of investigations

The Task of The Childrens Foundation

3

relating to the development of childhood and youth which have been made in recent years, and also the outcome of experiments in promoting the well-being and education of the young. In the present volume it has been the aim to sum up and apply what is known regarding the nature and the physical, intellectual, social, and moral needs of childhood and youth. It has not been possible, of course, to treat all aspects of child nature and every requirement for the well-being and education of the young; only the more general aspects have received attention. It is anticipated that in due course other volumes will be published in which it will be possible to deal in much detail with the well-being and education of childhood and youth in the home, in the school, and in society. It is expected that when this program shall have been completed, it will have been possible to present a coördinated view of the nature and needs of childhood and youth under all the conditions and all the situations of contemporary American life.

Bridging the Gulf Between Knowledge and Practice Anyone who has become aware of the gulf that exists between our knowledge of the nature and needs of the young, and our practice in the care, training, and education of children, will appreciate the importance of a program designed to organize, interpret, and apply what has been or is being established regarding the requirements for sound physical, intellectual, social, and moral development. In Chapter I, Professor Baldwin has shown the need of bridging the gap between our knowledge of childhood and youth and our practice in the training of the young. Probably few persons will question the statement that we have gone much farther in our investigation of child psychology and child development than we have gone in adapting our training to the nature and needs of children. As a matter of fact, those who have been charged with the care and culture of the young have not been in close touch with those who have been busy in

4

the study of childhood and youth. The investigator and the practitioner have not been walking side by side; in fact, they have had little or no communication with one another. The investigator has been saying: "It is not my duty to see that the truths I have been establishing are recognized and taken advantage of by parents, teachers, and social workers. I have all I can do to ferret out truths, and I must let somebody else apply them. If no one who is training the young, or looking after their physical development and their health, hears about the facts I am establishing, why I am blameless in the matter. I cannot be an investigator and a trainer at the same time. It is not my duty even to present my results in a form so that they can be understood by the practitioner. He must grow up to my position if he wishes to understand what I am doing. I cannot do justice to my scientific work if I cannot employ terms and modes of expression which will accurately and adequately convey the truth as I find it, whether or not the practitioner can comprehend these terms and understand the modes."

On the other hand the practitioners, i.e., the parent, the teacher, and the social worker, have been saying: "We are too busy with practical matters to spend time and energy in trying to understand technical material pertaining to the nature and needs of childhood and youth. We are confronted by actual problems that have to be solved from moment to moment; at least, something has to be done in regard to them, and we cannot take time off to speculate about scientific matters. We must treat children the best we know how until someone shows us, in an intelligible and practical way, that we can employ better methods than we have been employing."

Too Busy with Practical Matters

As a consequence of the attitude of practitioners and investigators toward one another's work, the care and the training of the young have not been greatly influenced

by all the investigation of child nature and child development that has been going on in our country and to some
extent in other countries during the past decade. Not only
has Professor Baldwin shown in Chapter I, but Professor
Goddard has shown in Chapter VIII, and Commissioner
Tigert in Chapter XVI that a gulf exists between what
we know about the nature and needs of childhood and
youth and what we are actually doing to promote the
physical, intellectual, social, and moral well-being and
development of the young. The home is probably farther
behind than the school in taking advantage of established
knowledge regarding childhood and youth; but society
is farther behind than either of them. They are all a
long distance in the rear of our knowledge of child nature
and the most effective methods of promoting the well-
being and education of the young.

For the Performance of the Task   As suggested above, The Childrens Foundation has
addressed itself to the task of bridging the gulf between
knowledge and practice in respect to the care and culture
of childhood and youth. For the performance of this
task, men and women have been selected who are familiar
with what has been established regarding the problems
which they have discussed, and they are also familiar with
the practical needs of the parent, the teacher, and the
social worker. Each contributor to this volume has been,
and is, an investigator in the department which has been
assigned to him. He has also been, and now is, a student
of ways and means of making the knowledge in his
department available to practitioners.

It was said to each contributor at the outset: "It is
expected that you will make a survey of what is known in
your special department, and will present this knowledge
in such phrases and in such form that it can be readily
understood and its importance appreciated by those who
are actually in contact with childhood and youth. It is
expected further that you will show how the knowledge

6

which you present relates concretely and practically to the every-day problems of dealing with the young. It is not desired that you should attempt to apply this knowledge in every possible way in which it can be applied, but only that you should go far enough to show the parent, the teacher, and the social worker that the knowledge in question has a vital relation to the actual task of rearing the young so that they may gain physical, intellectual, social, and moral stability and efficiency. Neither the trustees of The Childrens Foundation nor the Editor of this volume will impose any particular views upon you in the treatment of your theme. You will have a free hand, only so that you conform to the general aims of The Childrens Foundation and the objects of this volume." It is believed that each contributor has performed his task efficiently, and has gone as far as space limitations would permit in presenting knowledge in his particular field and suggesting how it can be applied in practice.

With a view to assisting the reader to become familiar with the contents of each chapter and of the volume as a whole most readily and with the least expenditure of time and energy, each important point discussed is indicated marginally at the proper place in the text. The essential points developed in each chapter are summarized and phrased simply; and the analytical Index will assist the reader to locate easily any topic he is interested in and which is treated in this volume. A list of the most helpful books and articles in the fields covered is given in the Bibliographies. Finally, biographical data concerning each contributor are given in the Appendix, so that any reader who is interested may become familiar with the principal facts regarding the interests and achievements of any author whose views and suggestions seem to him to be of value.

Aids for the Reader

The Editor desires to express his gratitude to various persons, in addition to the contributors to this volume, who have been of service to him in the performance of his editorial duties. Without the advice as well as the material assistance rendered by Mr. Lewis E. Myers, Founder of the Childrens Foundation and president of the board of trustees, the completion of THE CHILD: HIS NATURE AND HIS NEEDS would have been impossible. He read all the manuscripts contributed to this volume and made very helpful suggestions relating to the arrangement, content, and style of each chapter and of the volume as a whole. His profound interest in promoting child well-being and his experience as an educator as well as a man of affairs have made his counsel and constant encouragement and support of exceptional value.

Mr. Lorne W. Barclay, vice president of the Childrens Foundation, formerly Director of Education of the Boy Scouts of America, has brought to the task of putting this volume through the press an extensive knowledge alike of child life and of the most effective methods of making scientific knowledge intelligible and helpful to those who are charged with the care and culture of the young. His expert knowledge of the problems involved and his enthusiasm and skill in solving them are reflected in the final form and character of this book and its mechanical features.

The thanks of The Childrens Foundation and of the Editor of this book are due to a number of persons who coöperated in securing effective photographic illustrations. Mention should be made in particular of the service rendered by the following: The Playground Association of America; the Visual Education Bureau of the Board of Education of Chicago; Woman's Home Companion; D. Appleton and Company; Professor C. G. Sargent of the State Agricultural College at Ft. Collins, Colorado; Mr. J. F. Abel, specialist in rural education, the United States Bureau of Education; Mr. O. H. Greist, superintendent of schools in Randolph County, Indiana; Mr. Raymond W. Osborne, the Francis W. Parker School, Chicago; Miss Estaline Wilson, assistant superintendent of schools, Toledo, Ohio; Miss Mary O. Pottinger, supervisor of elementary schools, Springfield, Mass.; Mr. Charles L. Spain, deputy superintendent of schools, Detroit, Michigan; and Mr. H. A. Riebe of the Department of Education of the University of Wisconsin. The Editor secured from these sources a large number of photographs, many of them made especially for this volume, from which those that appear herein have been selected.

When the plans for this book were made it was decided that an account should be given of the aims and achievements of all the foundations, agencies, or institutions in our country devoted to the study of child nature or the promotion of the well-being of the young. This program was carried through, with the result that stories of the aims and achievements of a large number of foundations and welfare institutions have been secured. It has been found, however, that the volume would be far too large if all this material should be included, so it has been decided to issue it some time in the near future as a separate monograph. The Editor desires to express his appreciation of the coöperation of all these foundations and institutions in preparing accurate and readable accounts of their purposes, plans of organization, and the work which they have already achieved.

M. V. O'SHEA

The University of Wisconsin
  Madison, April 1924.

PART I

PRESENT STATUS OF OUR KNOWLEDGE OF CHILD NATURE

There is really no clue by which we can tread our way through the mazes of culture and the distractions of modern life save by knowing the true and natural needs of childhood and adolescence. Childhood is thus our pillar of cloud by day and fire by night. Other oracles may grow dim but this one will never fail.

—*G. Stanley Hall*

I

BRIDGING THE GAP BETWEEN OUR KNOWLEDGE OF CHILD NATURE AND THE TRAINING OF CHILDREN

THE development of scientific principles and the practical application of scientific laws are frequently independent lines of human effort and originality. Some investigators are chiefly interested in extending the theoretical boundaries of their science, while others are absorbed in extending the applications of their science to human welfare. In the field of physics, for example, on the one side we find Einstein and Michaelson working during a life-time on the theoretical aspects of the law of gravitation and the nature of the atom; on the other side, Edison absorbed in applying the theoretical principles discovered by others to their practical use in the electric light, the phonograph, and other devices, and Ford furnishing cheap automobiles. The same is true of the science of child welfare. Occasionally a scientist combines the theoretical with the practical, but such persons are rare. To-day we have sixty national organizations to promote child welfare and thousands of persons engaged in this praiseworthy activity, but the number of organizations devoted to research in this field is limited to very few. Consequently much of the welfare work is misdirected propaganda, inefficient effort, and inaccurate application of the fundamental principles of child development.

Application of Scientific Knowledge to the Enrichment of Child Life

In child psychology and in child training many workers are advancing their own special fields. In some lines, the theoretical scientific work is going far ahead of the practical; in other lines, the practical scientific is clearing the

13

way for the theoretical. Those of us who are most interested in the study of children believe that we are just beginning to find the basic problems of child development and child training. At no period in history have the science and the practice of child development been more intimately associated than at the present time, when the study of the child is the center of interest in home, in school, and in social and religious organizations.

The Aim of this Chapter The aim of this chapter is to present in a brief way some of the outstanding examples of how scientific knowledge is being applied to the enrichment of child life. This will be done by presenting a few of the contributions which child psychology has made to educational practice in the application of the principles of child development to school training; the outstanding books that combine the best theory and practice of to-day; the application of the principles of individual development to school promotion; the application of psychology to education; the development of laboratory schools for the study and training of children; the application of psychology to the growth of normal and superior children; and the application of the principles of mental and physical growth to the promotion of superior children in school.

The Gap Between Theory and Practice of Long Standing The gap between the theory and practice of child psychology has extended throughout the history of education. In some instances these two aspects of the science of child development have run parallel for long periods of time with little or nothing in common. On the other hand, child psychologists and some great teachers have consciously or unconsciously fused theory and practice into a unified attitude toward children. Herbart's psychology and methods of teaching in the nineteenth century furnish an illustration of theory and practice running parallel, but almost independently. His theoretical psychology with its intricate and arbitrary mathematical symbols was obsolete before his methods of

14

teaching became assimilated into educational practice. The same condition may be said to hold true in a less marked degree of English education of to-day, where little or no relation exists between English child psychology and English educational practice. But in France, and particularly in America, the science of *educational psychology* with its vast amount of data and its systematic methods has in a very large measure determined educational practice and administration.

The outstanding contributions of recent years that have most successfully combined theory and practice in child development are those of James, Dewey, Hall, Thorndike, Binet, Stern, Bagley, and Terman. William James, in his *Talks to Teachers*, 1894, produced the first distinctive book in educational psychology in this country. It is as interesting as a first-class novel and the chapters on the laws of habit and will, and on what makes life significant, are classics in this field. John Dewey's *School and Society*, 1900, brought the earlier cultural epoch theory of Herbart, Ziller, and Rein in Germany, and the new philosophy of pragmatism directly into schoolroom practice so that pupils were taught to "make" knowledge in accordance with the theory of following the order of development of the race. This book is a description of the University of Chicago Laboratory School of the earlier days. G. Stanley Hall's *Youth*, 1916, gives a multiplicity of applications of the value of instinctive development in child life. E. L. Thorndike's *Principles of Teaching*, 1906, was the first successful attempt to bridge the wide gap that had existed between the subject matter and methods of instruction on the one hand and the development of the child on the other, with particular reference to native and acquired characteristics of children. There is a rich mingling of theory and practice on every page. Alfred Binet's *The Development of Intelligence in Children*, 1916, first published in

Outstanding Books of Modern Times

the form of scales for the measure of intellectual level of children, 1905, 1908, and 1911, is the greatest single contribution to the application of psychology to the problem of measuring mental development. William Stern's *Psychological Methods of Testing Intelligence*, 1914, has fused theory and practice into an applied psychology. William C. Bagley's *Educative Process*, 1905, combined most effectively the general problems of child development and the processes involved in training and school work. It was the beginning of the present-day movement that takes child psychology into the schoolroom. Following Binet's development of a scale for measuring the intelligence of children and elaborating upon Stern's concept of an intelligence quotient for designating children of different degrees of intelligence for the same chronological age, Lewis M. Terman's *Measurement of Intelligence*, 1916, is the outstanding book that successfully combines intelligence testing with schoolroom practice and schoolroom administration.

In the field of child psychology a series of books has contributed to specific phases of child growth from both the theoretical and practical points of view. Among the most used books are those by J. M. Baldwin, Claparéde, Colvin, Freeman, Gates, Judd, Kirkpatrick, McCall, Norsworthy and Whitley, O'Shea, Pintner, Pyle, and Whipple.

In the field of mental deficiency, Binet, Goddard, L. S. Hollingworth, Kuhlmann, Wallin, and Fernald have combined theory and practice in public school and institutional training. In juvenile delinquency, Healy and Bronner carried the principles and the practice of child psychology side by side from the laboratory into the courts of Chicago and Boston.

During the last twenty years, several school systems have attempted to concentrate on a particular plan or theory of educational training. Frequently portions of such plans have been taken over by other school systems and in this way the educational work of the country at large has been modified and frequently greatly improved. As a general rule, changes from theory to practice are slow and often result in many modifications and compromises before an effective practice is worked out. A few years ago it was generally conceded that private schools were more likely to carry out experimental investigations and practice than public schools, but this is no longer true. To-day most of the extensive experiments in education, aside from those in laboratory schools of the types mentioned, are being carried out in public school systems. A few of the best organized plans for relating some of the basic principles of child development to the methods of school administration and teaching are cited as type illustrations:

Application of the Principles of Individual Development to School Promotion

The Dalton plan provides for the various phases of individual development. This plan treats the school as a sociological laboratory and provides for free activity, individual needs, and different rates of speed. Instead of classrooms there are subject laboratories, each under the charge of a teacher, where the children go as they feel the need, working by themselves or in groups and asking for aid as they require it. Half of the day is free time used as the child wishes; the rest of the day is taken up with conferences, assembly, art, athletics, manual training, and such subjects. This type of organization was first tried by Helen Parkhurst at Dalton, Mass. It is being used in several hundred schools in England and in an increasing number in this country.

The Dalton Plan

The Batavia plan is the outgrowth of over-crowded schoolrooms. The plan requires, in addition to the regular teacher, a teacher who devotes her time to giving the laggards individual help as needed. It is another attempt to provide more individual instruction through the course of study and the recitation. The Batavia

The Batavia Plan

17

plan grew, in the main, from a congested schoolroom situation and later led to the study of individual differences. This is a good illustration of practice preceding theory.

The Winnetka Plan The Winnetka system is somewhat similar to the others in the method of assignment and provision for individual differences, but it does not provide for separate subject teachers. There are some group activities. The checking up of work is by diagnostic tests.

The Mannheim Plan The Mannheim system is based on class distinctions. This plan, which was started in Germany in 1889, provides for children of varying ability by offering different types of education. It provides the regular eight grades for normal children; six grades for furthering classes; and four grades for defective children, in auxiliary schools, and special language classes for the gifted children. Here we have an application of the more general principles of the theory that children mentally fall into three or four distinct classes, with social distinctions more or less parallel. It also recognizes the inability of the schools to hold their pupils for equal periods of years.

The Platoon Plan The Platoon school provides for supplementary work. This type of school, while making sure that the "tool subjects" receive necessary attention, aims to provide ample time and opportunity for physical training, for cultural subjects such as music, art, and literature, for shop work, and for other special subjects, and also to provide socializing and Americanizing activities in the auditorium. It combines social participation and theory. The pupils are divided into two platoons. Each spends a half day in the home room and the other half day in auditorium, gymnasium, library, shop, and in domestic science rooms, music, art, and special classrooms. The platoons change places at the middle of the forenoons and afternoons. The plan was introduced in Detroit and is being tried in Pittsburgh, Akron, and Newark.

Other school systems somewhat on the same plan as those just mentioned are the two or three track systems. In Santa Barbara three courses—minimum, average, and enriched—are provided. In this plan the assumption is made that the normal child of one year is not the normal child of another year, and therefore a "concentric method" of repeating the same subjects on different levels of attainment is followed. The Cambridge plan begins at the fourth grade with two parallel courses; in one the work is done in four years, in the other the same amount is done in six years. At LeMars this division begins at the first grade and provides one six-year and one nine-year course of elementary school work with two transfer points.

The Two and Three Track Plans

A detailed study of any one or all of these illustrative plans of child training will show that the problems of school promotion not only involve, but also furnish, many of the fundamental principles of child development and child training.

In order to develop sound fundamental principles and norms, educational psychology needs to be characterized by painstaking detail in scientific procedure, investigation, and experimentation. It is the scientific attitude and method, which acquire a multitude of organized facts for analysis, description, and explanation, that will give us principles for our new science. No science is isolated; all sciences work into each other and are interdependent, especially during the earlier stages of their standardization. No science can appropriate the results of other sciences and become a new science. The allied sciences are not adequate to furnish and explain all the principles involved in education, since they are necessarily incomplete; and, what is equally important, education has its own data, its own point of view, its own problems and situations, its own history, and its own practices and opportunities for

Application of Psychology to Education

experimentation. While education will develop proportionally with its most closely allied sciences, during the next decade we must look, in the main, to experimental education and educational practice as the chief sources for the discovery and formulation of new principles.

Educational psychology is rapidly becoming an empirical science with its own data, its own point of view, its own problems and situations, its own history, and its own practices and opportunities for experimentation. It is largely through scientific experimentation that principles are established and "tried out," as indicated by the types of school training and experimentation that have been mentioned.

In our experimental work we need not only aggressive scientific analysis, but consecutive studies through a long course of years, giving full, accurate, and systematic accounts of problems in school administration, methods of teaching special subjects, and the accompanying changes in the progress of learning. As in all sciences, it is essentially the point of view and the methods of attack which this new phase of educational psychology takes that characterize it as a science and distinguishes it from the history of education, methods of teaching, and school administration. The purpose of educational psychology is to analyze, classify, describe, explain, and evaluate educational processes in the child in order to discover principles of child development and to bring the child into situations which will stimulate and foster good mental and physical growth.

Development of Laboratory Schools for the Study of Children

One of the best means for the discovery and application of principles of education is to control, direct, and modify the scholastic life of the child on an experimental basis, aiming to "try out" definitely conceived theories on a limited number of children, to verify observable principles from miscellaneous school practices, and to discover new principles that may be further tested. This is what Pestalozzi attempted and what Froebel did most successfully, although the followers of each have, in many instances, stereotyped the principles into dogmas or changed them into petty devices. Experimental schools like those of Pestalozzi and Froebel isolated and intensified certain principles that were not apparent in more complex situations. In the one, these centered in the main around sense perceptions; in the other, around self-activity. There have been several similar schools, and the number is rapidly increasing. In Germany, Rein's "Uebungschule" in Jena and Francke's "Stiftung" in Halle are examples; in France, Binet's Laboratory School at 36 Rue Grande aux Belles, Paris; in Italy and Switzerland, the Montessori schools; and in England, the Fielden Demonstration School in Manchester.

In this country, aside from several progressive preparatory schools which are attempting reform movements in education, we have in Chicago the Francis W. Parker School, which emphasizes community life and claims that the formation of character, and not the acquisition of knowledge as an end in itself, is the chief purpose of the school. It therefore discourages all artificial incentives such as grades and prizes. The University of Chicago Elementary and High Schools, and the Lincoln and Horace Mann Schools, of Columbia University, and the University of Iowa Observation Schools and Pre-School Laboratories have become great working laboratories for educators and psychologists throughout North America. There are also schools at the universities of California, Illinois, Indiana, Minnesota, Missouri, Nebraska, North Dakota, Utah, Wyoming, and Wisconsin, and at Bryn Mawr College, as well as at other state and private institutions. These and other laboratory schools are centers of research where the gaps between the theoretical and experimental knowledge of child development and child training are constantly being bridged and new chasms are constantly being brought to light for further study.

Coöperative Research and Training To-day the science of child psychology has developed to such an extent and the field of education is so changing and so complex in its various aspects that no one student can conceive a complete laboratory school which will meet the requirements of an adequate educational theory, a constructive system of training, and a complete psychology of the child. Consequently our laboratory schools of to-day are based on the principles of coöperative research and coöperative training. In these schools, specialists are in charge of special subjects, such as reading, writing, and spelling. Other specialists are in charge of the pre-school, the elementary, or the high school children, the psychological examination of the children, the course of study, and the administration of the school. In short, a group of specialists direct the various phases of the child's training and development.

Need and Value of the Study of Physical Development The dependence of health upon physical well-being, the large percentage of physically defective children in our public schools, the relation between physical growth and school progress, and the relation between mental and physical development, all point to the need of widespread information in regard to physical growth and development of school children. A knowledge of a child's stage of physical development is an important factor in placing him in the grade where he can do his best work, in prescribing the amount of school work he should be expected to do, in promoting him, in providing suitable schoolroom equipment, in directing his physical training and choice of games and sports, and in interpreting his stage of social maturity. With school children of the upper grades, who are about to enter the industrial world, physical status must be considered when advising them as to the type of occupation they should enter.

Although many early investigations had been made of the height, weight, and other physical measurements of large numbers of children of various school ages, it is only within recent years that consecutive measurements of the same groups of children have been carried on in order to find out *how* children grow physically. The earlier method measured groups of different children for each age and attempted to standardize, on the basis of the results of these measurements, heights, and weights that should be attained by each child of a given chronological age. This method is inadequate and inaccurate for studying the growth of individual children and for predicting a child's probable measurements at a later age. The method of individual growth curves of a child's development is used by the writer (Chart 1, p. 26.)

Methods of Determining Physical Development

For parents and teachers, the weight-height-age relationship is the most practical index of the physical status of the child, as normal growth in weight and height is probably the best single index of good health and good nutrition during childhood. Teachers, health workers, and parents should understand that the weight tables supplement and contribute directly to physical examinations. They are not supposed to take the place of a medical examination, which should be given every child at least once a year.

Use and Abuse of Weight-Height-Age Tables

The weight-height-age table in the hands of the uncritical examiner may be grossly abused. The abuses of the table are due to lack of standardization of instruments, methods of measuring and recording, and, especially, to wrong interpretation of data. Every effort should be made for a consistent, careful, and intelligent use of weight-height-age indices of growth (Tables 1 and 2, pages 24 and 25).

The use of the table is illustrated at top of page 26.

THE CHILDRENS FOUNDATION

TABLE I

WEIGHT-HEIGHT-AGE TABLE FOR GIRLS OF SCHOOL AGE

BY

DR. BIRD T. BALDWIN and DR. THOMAS D. WOOD

Ht. Ins.	5 yrs	6 yrs	7 yrs	8 yrs	9 yrs	10 yrs	11 yrs	12 yrs	13 yrs	14 yrs	15 yrs	16 yrs	17 yrs	18 yrs	Ht. Ins.
38	33	33													38
39	34	34													39
40	36	36	36												40
41	37	37	37												41
42	39	39	39												42
43	41	41	41	41											43
44	42	42	42	42											44
45	45	45	45	45	45										45
46	47	47	48	48											46
47	49	50	50	50	50	50									47
48		52	52	52	53	53	56								48
49		54	54	55	55	56	56								49
50		56	56	57	58	59	61	62							50
51			59	60	61	63	65								51
52			63	64	64	65	67								52
53			66	67	68	69	71	71	73						53
54				69	70	70	71	71	73						54
55				72	74	74	74	75	77	78					55
56					76	78	78	79	81	83					56
57					80	82	82	82	84	88	92				57
58						84	86	86	88	93	96	101			58
59						87	90	90	92	96	100	103	104		59
60						91	95	95	97	101	105	108	109	111	60
61							99	100	101	105	108	112	113	116	61
62							104	105	106	109	113	115	117	118	62
63								110	110	112	116	117	119	120	63
64								114	115	117	119	120	122	123	64
65								118	120	121	122	123	125	126	65
66									124	124	125	128	129	130	66
67									128	130	131	133	133	135	67
68									131	133	135	136	138	138	68
69										135	137	138	140	142	69
70										136	138	140	142	144	70
71										138	140	142	144	145	71

Age—years		6	7	8	9	10	11	12	13	14	15	16	17	18	
Average Height, Inches	Short	43	45	47	49	50	52	54	57	59	60	61	61	61	
	Medium	45	47	50	52	54	56	58	60	62	63	64	64	64	
	Tall	47	50	53	55	57	59	62	64	66	66	67	67	67	
Average Annual Gain, Pounds	Short	4	4	4	5	6	6	10	13	10	7	2	1		
	Medium	5	5	6	7	8	10	13	10	6	4	3	1		
	Tall	6	8	8	9	11	13	9	8	4	4	1	1		

Age is taken at the nearest birthday; height at the nearest inch; and weight at the nearest pound. A girl is considered 6 years old at any time between 5½ and 6½ years.

The following percentage of net weight has been added for clothing (shoes and sweaters are not included)·

For weights from 35 to 65 pounds—3.0%.

For weights from 66 to 82 pounds—2.5%.

For weights from 83 pounds and over—2.0% of net weight is added.

Printed by the Iowa Child Welfare Research Station, State University of Iowa, Iowa City, Iowa.

TABLE II

WEIGHT-HEIGHT-AGE TABLE FOR BOYS OF SCHOOL AGE

BY

DR. BIRD T. BALDWIN and DR. THOMAS D. WOOD

Ht. Ins.	5 yrs	6 yrs	7 yrs	8 yrs	9 yrs	10 yrs	11 yrs	12 yrs	13 yrs	14 yrs	15 yrs	16 yrs	17 yrs	18 yrs	19 yrs	Ht. Ins.
38	34	34														38
39	35	35														39
40	36	36														40
41	38	38	38													41
42	39	39	39	39												42
43	41	41	41	41												43
44	44	44	44	44												44
45	46	46	46	46	46											45
46	47	48	48	48	48											46
47	49	50	50	50	50	50										47
48		52	53	53	53	53										48
49		55	55	55	55	55	55									49
50		57	58	58	58	58	58	58								50
51			61	61	61	61	61	61								51
52			63	64	64	64	64	64	64							52
53			66	67	67	67	67	68	68							53
54				70	70	70	70	71	71	72						54
55				72	72	73	73	74	74	74						55
56				75	76	77	77	77	78	78	80					56
57					79	80	81	81	82	83	83					57
58					83	84	84	85	85	86	87					58
59					87	88	88	89	89	90	90	90				59
60						91	92	92	93	94	95	96				60
61							95	96	97	99	100	103	106			61
62							100	101	102	103	104	107	111	116		62
63							105	106	107	108	110	113	118	123	127	63
64								109	111	113	115	117	121	126	130	64
65								114	117	118	120	122	127	131	154	65
66									119	122	125	128	132	136	139	66
67									124	128	130	134	136	139	142	67
68										134	134	137	141	143	147	68
69										137	139	143	146	149	152	69
70										143	144	145	148	151	155	70
71										148	150	151	152	154	159	71
72											153	155	156	158	163	72
73											157	160	162	164	167	73
74											160	164	168	170	171	74

Age—years		6	7	8	9	10	11	12	13	14	15	16	17	18	19	
Average Height, Inches	Short	43	45	47	49	51	53	54	56	58	60	62	64	65	65	
	Medium	46	48	50	52	54	56	58	60	63	65	67	68	69	69	
	Tall	49	51	53	55	57	59	61	64	67	70	72	72	73	73	
Average Annual Gain, Pounds	Short	3	4	5	5	5	4	8	9	11	14	13	7	3		
	Medium	4	5	6	6	6	7	9	11	15	11	8	4	3		
	Tall	5	7	7	7	7	8	12	16	11	9	7	3	4		

Age is taken at the nearest birthday; height at the nearest inch; and weight at the nearest pound. A boy is considered 6 years old at any time between 5½ and 6½ years.

The following percentage of net weight has been added for clothing (shoes, coats, and sweaters are not included):
For weights from 35 to 63 pounds—3.5%.
For weights 64 pounds and over—4.0%.

Printed by the Iowa Child Welfare Research Station, State University of Iowa, Iowa City, Iowa.

Take, for example, a boy whose height is 60 inches. On the boys' table find 60 in the first column and follow this line horizontally across. As shown in the age columns, the weight is 91 pounds for 10 years of age, 92 pounds for 11 years of age, and so on up to 16 years of age, when the weight is 96 pounds. The weights are estimated for the few children who may be too tall or two short for this table.

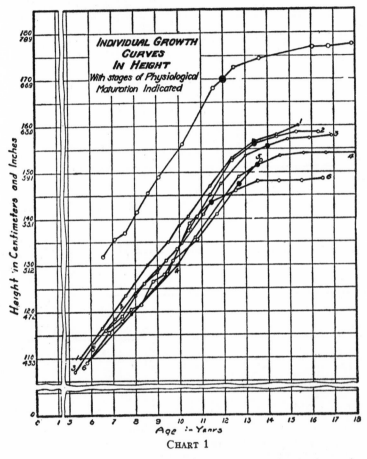

CHART 1

Physiological Ages of Children The normal child not only has a chronological age in years, months, and days, but also a physiological age indicative of its physical development and its stages of physiological maturity. There are several ways to compare the physiological maturity and chronological age: the teeth of the physiologically older child are usually further developed and more in number, the height is greater (Chart 1), and the change in voice takes place earlier than in the physiologically younger child.

Adolescent boys and girls mature at varying chronological ages. Some girls mature at eleven years of age and others not until sixteen or seventeen years of age. Some boys mature at twelve years of age and others not until sixteen or seventeen years of age. As a general rule, tall boys and tall girls mature earlier than short ones. That is, tall, well-developed children are older physiologically than short children at any age during childhood.

Physiological age is directly correlated with stages of mental development. The physiologically more mature child has different attitudes, different types of emotions, different interests from the child of younger physiological development, although of the same chronological age. Physiological age has a direct bearing on pedagogical age, or ability to do school work, as many of our schools are beginning to realize. The larger and more physiologically mature child may be able to do certain types of school work better, although of inferior ability in specific traits which have been greatly emphasized by the school curricula. No child should be promoted or demoted without consideration of his or her physiological age. Girls may be expected to progress more rapidly through the grades than boys.

The writer's results show that tall, heavy boys and girls are older physiologically and further along in their stages toward mental maturity, as evidenced by school progress, than short, light boys and girls. Studies of boys and girls in the Horace Mann School of Teachers College, Columbia University, the Francis W. Parker

Relation of Mental to Physical Growth

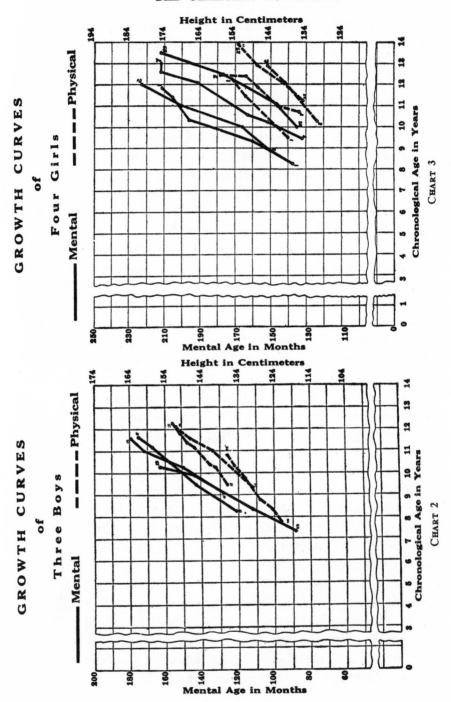

GROWTH CURVES

of

Four Girls

Mental ■ ■ ■ Physical

Height in Centimeters

Chronological Age in Years

CHART 3

Mental Age in Months

GROWTH CURVES

of

Three Boys

Mental ■ ■ ■ Physical

Height in Centimeters

Chronological Age in Years

CHART 2

Mental Age in Months

School in Chicago, the Johns Hopkins Demonstration School, the University of Iowa Observation Elementary and High Schools, and a special group of mentally superior children in California show that, as a general rule, good mental development accompanies good physical growth during childhood (Charts 2 and 3, page 28).

The writer is carrying out an investigation in Cleveland, Ohio, where representative schools in each of the five districts have been selected, to provide practical school methods for promoting or advancing pupils in accordance with the basic laws of child development and with a view to giving each child opportunities and training for the highest degree of efficiency which his capacity and stage of maturity affords. A thorough analysis of the pupil is made physically, mentally, socially, and educationally.

The Application of the Principles of Mental and Physical Growth to the Promotion of Children in School

Basing the practical school problem on the experimental data presented, it is recommended that pupils who are physiologically accelerated (those children who are relatively large for their chronological age, sex, race, and social status) be promoted as rapidly as thoroughness and educational accomplishment will permit. It is believed that the superior children may safely be permitted to advance two, three, or perhaps four grades beyond their chronological age if their health is good and their mental and educational maturity corresponds with their physiological acceleration, as is usually the case.

The children of superior ability (advanced mental age) can complete the course at an early chronological age with superior knowledge and training on account of their superior ability and advanced maturity.

The physically accelerated pupils of normal or average ability can complete with average training the school course at an early age chronologically.

Pupils who are physiologically young (children who

are relatively small for their chronological age, sex, race, and social status) are not hurried through school, even though they be of superior mentality. Such superior children are advanced in the horizontal direction of the course by means of enrichment of the course of study through some type of grade sectioning, by adding extra subjects, by allowing for elective work in special fields, by encouraging elementary research work, by supplementary training through excursions, or by other types of supplementary work. The average or retarded pupils may safely be permitted to continue in the normal grade in average or lower sections. Many of these pupils may safely be permitted to continue in a grade below their average chronological age. The pupils of superior ability can complete the course at the normal age or later with greatly enriched information, enriched attitudes, enriched training in approaching problems and in taking part in extra-school activities. They will have many educational assets, without the great liability of immaturity for college, for society, or for their life's work.

Summary To recapitulate: The development of scientific principles and the application of scientific laws are frequently independent lines of human effort and originality. The science and practice of child development and training are more intimately associated to-day than ever before in the history of psychology and education. This is shown by the many excellent available books in educational psychology, by the numerous schools and school systems based on the principles of the individual development of the pupils, by the present status of educational psychology as a science, by the establishment of laboratory schools for studying children, by the application of the laws of physical growth to the practical problems of health education, mental development, and the promotion of normal and superior children in school.

II

THE CHILD'S INSTINCTS AND IMPULSES

O F LATE there has been much controversy as to what constitutes an instinct, indeed as to whether anything properly called instinct even exists. Without entering upon what would probably prove a boring and unprofitable discussion, let us explain that our study is to be of the sorts of spontaneous behavior we may expect from the great majority of children, in contrast to the actions they have been deliberately taught to perform. Certain trends to behavior are found so universally, and are, so many of them, recognizable in the lower animals apart from direct education, that it seems simple to explain them by saying they are due to original nature, however modified they may become by the particular life experiences of any one child. Moreover, many characteristic ways of behaving appear at similar successive periods in the life history of so many children that it is fair to conclude that some inner law of growth determines their development in this customary sequence.

For some of these behavior trends we use names such as curiosity, jealousy, suggesting primarily the emotions felt. For others we use abstract terms such as ownership, gregariousness. For the simpler, more definite modes of behavior we describe the act itself, such as crying, sucking, walking. Thorndike would prefer us to give in detail the acts observed and the immediately provoking cause, such as "dodging the head" when "seeing a blow aimed at us," rather than to be led astray in interpretation by any term such as "the instinct of self-preservation."

Our chief task in this section of this volume is to consider the commonly observed ways in which children behave, and the likes and dislikes they reveal, so that we may differentiate normal from unusual behavior and thus be guided in our dealings with children. Whether normal or unusual, these tendencies must all be evaluated as desirable or undesirable for the children's best ultimate adjustment to the physical and social world in which they live. If desirable we shall want to perpetuate them; if undesirable we may need to eliminate them but surely to redirect them. We will sketch first these three methods of dealing with tendencies, and then take up four or five of the most fundamental manifestations of original nature.

Perpetuation of Original Tendencies: Satisfaction or Reward

If an instinct or impulse leads to desirable results we wish to strengthen and encourage it. This is effected in one of two ways. *First*, we may associate some *satisfaction* in the child's mind from having acted in the desired manner. Since it is a fundamental law of our nature to repeat an action that brings pleasure as a result, this method of reward is an obvious one to utilize in perpetuating an instinct. Thus, we praise a child's efforts at construction in wood or textiles; we show appreciation when he manifests sympathy; we smile at the child who obeys a generous impulse. Many actions bring their own reward without any emphasis by the adult on the pleasant effect. Thus, the desire to make a noise brings joy to the ears of the small drum beater and horn tooter, whatever it does to the ears of those not actively producing the noise themselves. The baby's impulse to grab food finds a reward in the satisfaction of hunger, and the more immediate pleasant taste in the mouth.

The second method of encouraging instincts is that to which we resort when a child seems to be slow in responding, or when the environment offers little opportunity for the tendency to find expression. It is called the method of *stimulation, or use,* and represents some effort on our part to supply the deficiencies of the environment, or to make certain aspects of it more attractive. Thus, the adolescent who is slow in adjusting socially is provided with extra opportunities to meet varied social groups. A sluggish appetite is coaxed by special dainties. The collecting instinct is stimulated by the example of other children.

Two warnings are necessary here. One is to see that these methods of reward and stimulation are applied to the truly desirable, not to the undesirable tendencies. Bad training would stimulate the fear instinct by shutting a child up alone in the dark; it would stimulate the fighting response by grasping him and shaking him when he was inattentive. Bad training rewards the disposition to whine, cry, and complain, by favoring the child on the occasion of such behavior and letting him gain what he wants.

The other warning is that the reward must be connected *in the child's mind* with the desirable action, not given vaguely because of good behavior. To this end, the younger the child, the sooner must the pleasant effect come after the act, since the memory for time intervals is poor. Also the pleasantness should preferably be a natural result of the deed, not some artificial pleasure in no way logically linked with the action.

If an impulse leads to undesirable results we may wish to get rid of it. This, too, is effected in two ways, each of them the opposite of the two already described.

First, we associate *dissatisfaction* in the child's mind with the wrong response, using the law of human nature

Strengthen the Right Impulses

Elimination of Original Tendencies: Dissatisfaction

that a tendency is weakened when the effect is unpleasant. Thus, when a boy is jeered at for cringing and showing fear he is less likely to play the coward in just that way again. A bad tasting substance will check the impulse to cram things undiscriminatingly into the mouth.

Disuse   The second method of elimination is called *disuse*, meaning simply removing every favorable stimulus to the action so that it will not occur. Thus we take precautions to avoid alarming children. We keep knives, matches, and other harmful things out of the baby's reach.

Again some warnings are necessary. First, disuse can be merely a temporary method of treatment, suitable only for the very youngest children, or those below par physically or mentally. Second, as in the case of rewards, the pains and penalties must be associated in the child's mind with the deed, not with the person who administers them. For the smaller children retribution must be swift, if not immediate. In all cases the logical outcome of the action is preferable to an artificial punishment. Herein lies one value of self government in a group, where the penalty imposed represents no one person's temper, no caprice, but the collective judgment of one's mates.

A third warning is that neither disuse nor punishment is sufficient to eliminate a very strong tendency; all it does is to check that particular manifestation of it. Either method is but negative, and should be followed up by a positive way of dealing with undesirable instincts.

Ways of Redirecting Tendencies: Substitution   What we need chiefly to consider is how to modify the less desirable behavior, how to find another and a better outlet for the impulse than the one the child happens to be using. Here again we have two ways. The simplest is known as *substitution*. To take small bites rather than to cram the mouth full, to stroke the cat's head rather than to pull its tail are substitutions for the two-year-old. To wash and dry the hands rather than rub the stickiness off on the clothing, to lead the gang on a nature study treasure hunt instead of on a pilfering expedition, are substitutions for older children. Good form and movement in dancing rather than holds and gestures that are objectionable are substitutions for the adolescent.

The other method, known as *sublimation*, usually involves changing the ideas and the emotional attitudes, so that the action is consistently modified, or is forthcoming on a different occasion. Thus, to fight, not just in self-defence, or in personal rivalry, but in defence and rescue of another, or for a cause, is sublimation. So also is giving up desired food in order to feed someone else. Still further, the action may be completely transformed, as when a boy fights, not physically, but through a committee or by writing in the school paper. **Sublimation**

Other illustrations of all these six methods, reward, stimulation, punishment, disuse, substitution, sublimation, will be given in connection with special tendencies that will now be discussed.

John B. Watson, from his intensive work with young infants, tells us there are just *three* typical modes of behavior indicating *instinctive emotions*. These we may name *rage*, *love*, and *fear;* and since the distinctive reactions are observable from birth we may well call them fundamental trends. **How Children's Tempers May be Spoiled**

The first, *anger*, is excited by hampering the baby's movements. Even gentle restraint of the head or limbs with no attendant pain suffices to produce the anger responses. Later, any thwarting of movement, any failure to make physical objects move at wish, any foiling in a purpose, any obstruction in carrying out a plan serves to arouse anger. What wonder then that we find nervous children of two to three years old who frequently fly into a rage. Consider the stimulations to anger they receive all day long. Their bodies are pulled, twisted, held, restrained in so many of the exigencies of being taken for a walk in busy streets, of being lifted in and out of cars, of being dressed. They tug at heavy furniture, fail to manipulate fine mechanisms, are constantly disappointed in going where they wish to go, and doing and getting what they desire. They are hurried, when they are all set to stop and examine.

The first undirected slashing movements and easily recognizable cry of temper of the infant grow into attacks on objects or people, plus a bellowing roar. A child may throw himself down, kick and fight any would-be assistant, or even pound and hurt himself. Extreme glandular changes affect the circulation and respiration to the point of physical exhaustion when the fit is over. Older children cry less and fight more. Crying, as Woodworth points out, is an expression of baffled helplessness and inefficient self pity. Once a child finds more efficient outlets for his impulses he need no longer cry.

Aids in Control of Anger

How shall we deal with anger? Prevention is of course desirable, in that a little thoughtful care may avoid many of the constant, daily provocations to wrath. Check in the early stages if possible, for often when the flames are well started the fire has to burn itself out. Before that uncontrollable stage, however, there are various helps. One is the physical cooling off by cold water, and plenty of it, inside and out. Another is violent muscular activity to work off the rage, a race up and down stairs for instance. Another is substituting another emotion, even fear—"Look out, you'll fall!" Then there is the proverbial "soft answer," which indicates no malevolence on the part of the person who is doing the thwarting. Humor, from gentle amusement to a good laugh with the revelation of comradely fun, is the best solvent of disagreeable tempers, and is perhaps one of the most constructive ways of helping a child to acquire the habit of self-control. To this we can add reasonable explanation of the necessity of thwarting, if such exists; or we can help the child to find a better way of overcoming the obstacle if there is no reason to be baffled.

Rage, like fear, can be conquered by finding ways to control the opposing circumstances. Like fear, too, it can be developed into veritable obsessions and abhorrences, real perversions in the adult. Like fear, too, if aroused by one person chiefly it can mar a child's development, and warp and twist the young growth into a mental deformity later on.

The second fundamental group of emotional reactions **Love Manifestations** has to do with what we call *love*, or sex in the Freudian sense. This impulse involves phenomena in two distinct realms. One is purely physiological and includes the specific sensations, the muscular reflexes, and the glandular secretions occurring in normal sexual excitement, which are called *detumescence*. The other is mental, and includes the thoughts of romance, the imagination, the complex of motives and behavior that accompany being in love, which together are called *contrectation*.

During the first few years, from birth to at least **Three Periods in the Sexual Life of a Child: The Neutral Period** three years old, more commonly five, and sometimes seven or eight, a child is in the neutral period, so named because gratification may result from stimulating almost any part of the body. The infant expresses pleasure when he is laid face down over someone's knee, when he is patted or stroked. Later, intense gratification is derived from sucking the thumb or some form of "pacifier." Apart from the danger to the thumb and the mouth it is an undesirable habit for a child, since it functions as an abnormal source of sex pleasure. To break it, we must remember that it is the mouth, not the hands, that should experience unpleasantness; that neither punishing the hands, nor disuse by restraint of the hands will be likely to set in motion the natural inhibitions by which a child learns self-control. Extreme delight in being tickled is another early phase of sex pleasure, and should be avoided unless we care to bring about premature stimulation.

In general, proper hygienic care, seeing that the genitals are kept clean, that the evacuation processes are regular, that there is no friction from rough or ill-fitting clothing will serve to keep little children developing normally.

The contrectation phenomena show chiefly in that the young child's affections go out to anyone who feeds him, cuddles him, plays with him, acting the part of nurse or mother. If one parent does this entirely while the other is mainly associated in the child's mind with thwartings and stimuli to fear, he will fixate on one and feel repelled by the other, an early bent which may very considerably influence the character of his sexual development later.

The Un-differentiated Period The undifferentiated period succeeds the neutral period, beginning at any one of the above ages, depending on the particular child, and lasting till the onset of puberty. Detumescent phenomena are still incomplete since the body is immature; but specific sensations of pleasure become gradually localized in the sex organs. Curiosity is early directed to them, and we need to be on the watch to prevent any bad sex habits or any dirty tricks such as children sometimes perform together in toilet and bath rooms. Later perversions of exhibitionism and other revolting acts may originate in bad practices in this childhood period. We must not forget that bedroom and bathroom manners need as direct and graded teaching as do table and parlor manners;

and that the right mental attitude is immensely more important in this case.

Contrectation impulses find expression in the strong attachments a child may feel for another child, or for a grown-up, or even for an animal. There is generally a fairly continuous sequence of these attachments, and therein lies a better chance for normal development than if there is fixation for long on one person. The attraction may involve great desire to be with the loved one, to exchange caresses, to kiss and fondle the person. This desire may extend to objects worn, used or touched by the one beloved. Sometimes there is a longing to be ill-treated, to suffer at the hands of the beloved; sometimes there is a pleasure in causing them pain. In these tendencies originate adult perversions of fetichism, masochism, and sadism respectively; they therefore surely need re-direction into more normal lines. The emotions of so-called shame or modesty, and of jealousy, may be felt very keenly in this childhood period, needing sympathetic guidance.

In the third, or developmental, period, since the body matures at any age from eleven on, the two sides *The Developmental Period* of the sex impulse come together, and the detumescent processes are complete for the first time. Any one of four types of stimuli may arouse them. (1) direct excitation, as in sexual intercourse; (2) indirect physical means, from local irritation or stimulation of other parts of the body. Thus, trouble in the bladder and rectum, too warm a bed, masturbation, climbing a pole, or riding a bicycle may serve to cause detumescence. The other types of stimuli are psychic: (3) violent emotions of dread, anger, horror, as well as the emotions natural to sex desire; (4) imagination dwelling on romantic thoughts or on sexual acts may bring about detumescence.

There are three possible phases in this coming

together. One is that of complete association, as in full and final development; another is of complete dissociation, each set of processes working independently as to occasion, and not understood by the adolescent as in any way related. There is a third possibility, that contrectation and detumescence may occur at the same time, but that their inter-relationship may not be appreciated by the boy or girl. Thus, in the first flush of worshipful romance, when occupied with pure and adoring thoughts of the beloved, an involuntary orgasm may prove overwhelmingly horrifying for the half-informed adolescent, though fortunately this experience is rare.

The hygiene of this period is to be treated in a later chapter. Let us consider some of the emotional phases.

Emotional Phases of the Developmental Period

For awhile, from ten or eleven on to fourteen or more, boys and girls develop an aversion for each other's society, an impatience and lack of sympathy with the group aims and interests of the opposite sex. They do not frequently play together, boys will not read girls' books, and so on. They have plenty of slighting remarks for the personal appearance and habits of the other sex, and joyful derision for the kissing and embracing they see portrayed in moving pictures. Chums and friends are of their own sex, though occasional idolizing of some one much older is found. Then, one day, the fifteen-year-old finds him or herself no longer indifferent to, but strangely interested in some one. Physical characteristics are discovered as beautiful, mannerisms are found fascinating, and lo, the youth or maiden is "in love," and weaves a most disguising halo round the loved one's head. For the next few years there is probably a succession of these attachments. When enquiring of the eighteen-year-old boy after his best girl it might be more tactful not to give her name; for the chances are she is not the same individual as the one you heard of six months ago. Besides being boy or girl crazy, as the case may be, an adolescent frequently includes among the transient loves some member of the same sex, and people far removed in age, and quite unsuitable as possible mates. Thus we have the "crush" on a teacher, the worship of the matinée idol, the boy of sixteen to nineteen willing to marry a woman three times his age, the girl longing for a heart-to-heart talk with the middle-aged doctor or spiritual adviser. The emotions are more keen than in the undifferentiated period so that they are liable to lead to more pronounced behavior.

Manifestly, this instinct calls for guidance. Too strong to be inhibited, ignorant attempts at suppression may simply force individuals to find outlets which may or may not be desirable. In fact, numberless maladjustments, psychoses, "complexes," erratic ways of thinking and behaving are traceable to repressed sex instinct. Substitution and sublimation are emphatically the methods to be used in directing these impulses. From the earliest questionings of children as to the functions of their own bodies, as to where babies come from, as to animal matings they may observe, we may give the scientific truth with all the atmosphere of interest in the true and the beautiful. Children get information anyway—it is the parents' privilege to see that they get the right kind in the right way, instead of from questionable sources with a morbid, even obscene emotional coloring. Biological facts are taught in nature study and hygiene courses, love episodes are dwelt on in literature and the drama, but they may not be connected in the adolescent's mind with the chivalric ideals that should function in matters of dress, of dancing, of desirable etiquette.

Direction of Sex Instinct

The physical restlessness may find substitutions in hard work and in athletics. The disturbing thoughts and emotions need sublimation in some form of creative work. It is here that talents in art, in music, in craftsmanship, in writing may be helpfully developed, also the ability to organize and direct others, to be of service to groups of one's fellows.

Much more of this will be suggested in the chapter on adolescence. We will pass to a study of the third fundamental emotion, that of *fear*.

Children's Fears

In an elaborate study of *children's fears* made by Dr. G. Stanley Hall, numberless things are listed of which people confessed they have been afraid. Watson assures us that we have *learned* to fear these, that originally only two causes of fear behavior are found, these being a sudden, loud sound, and the removal of support (fear of falling). Strike a piece of metal loudly behind an infant, or twitch and jerk the blanket on which he is lying, and, immediately, fear reactions are induced. How does he become afraid of so many other things, then? Because on some occasion one of these causes occurs simultaneously with some other stimulus—say a barking dog approaches—henceforward the fright at loud sounds may be shown at the mere sight of an animal, even though he is quiet and friendly. Then the fear of the sight of a dog may be transferred to the feel of his coat, thence to fur, and so on in long sequence. Or a child is wakened by some loud sound and by the violence of his muscular reaction perhaps rolls off his pillow.

"Hush, Don't Wake the Baby!"

Two original causes of fear now unite to terrify him. If he is in the dark, fear is quickly transferred to darkness itself. If it is light, the transfer may be to the sight of his sleeping place, so that thereafter he screams when laid down, awake, in it. If he is alone, the transfer may be to the feeling of solitude; though darkness and solitude, as Thorndike points out, are conditions which always enhance fears of any kind. Since terrified screams ordinarily bring prompt help and relief, a baby soon links crying with summoning people for any whim. Here, then, we see development in two lines, one an endless chain of associated fears, the other a bad habit from an original impulse.

Fears are much more easily induced than they are cured. It would seem advisable to apply the method of disuse so far as possible, and prevent children from becoming frightened, especially in the extreme degrees of alarm. Paroxysms of terror are as dangerously potent for the psychic life as are the bacilli of tuberculosis for the physical life. Like them, these terrors may be walled up, so to speak, for years; but let a weakened nervous condition ensue in later life and they may become active with deadly effect, just as the germs will issue from their segregated sac when disease weakens the lung tissue. Thus the obsessions, phobias, horrors of "nervous" adults are almost always traceable to some early childhood experience, forgotten but not lost as a factor for abnormal behavior.

Fright in Childhood a Source of of Mal-adjustment

Granted that disuse is often out of the question, the problem is how to deal with fears that do exist. Fear is a very real experience in child life, and our task is to dispel useless fears and train children to fear the right things and to act efficiently. Warning shouts and the loud honk of the automobile serve their purpose only if they incite to suitable action. Fear of falling must teach improved motor control. We might well substitute fear of germs, with measures to combat them, for senseless behavior at fear of mice.

Fears must be met in the open and conquered, rather than suppressed. There are two main ways of laying them. One is by the example of others. A little child soon takes his cue in emotions from those around; so that if in the doubtful situation of a new experience he hesitates, then is the opportune time to express some other emotion, interest, enjoyment, amusement or what

Aids In Control of Fear

not, and encourage him to share our point of view. The other way is that of better knowledge, and control of the situation. Superstitions vanish when we investigate scientifically. Dread of the unknown disappears when mastery is assured. The imaginative child need not fear witches, goblins, giants, etc., for we can help him to see the difference between fact and fancy. He himself can create such beings to talk about at pleasure; but never can he see, feel or hear them, nor can they touch him.

An illustration of overcoming fear of the dark, so long a hindrance in children's thoughts, is given, combining the force of example, the change of emotion, the definite association of pleasure, and the element of control.

"We can make it dark when we choose by shutting our eyes. Blind people have it dark all the time; how do they manage? By feeling and listening. Let us see what we can find out that way. Let us both shut our eyes and walk round the room. You touch something and tell me what it is. Now I'll do something and you listen and tell me what I did. . . . Now we'll count how many steps from the door to the big chair. Now you go out of the room; I'll stay here and turn off the light. You come in when I call, and find if I'm in the chair. . . . Now we'll both go out. You go in again while it is dark, and see if you can take just the right number of steps to the chair. If it is a book I have left there you may bring it here. If it is a candy you may eat it. . . . Now see how quickly you can go upstairs. Now try again with your eyes shut; do you know how many steps before the turn? . . . Now I'll blindfold you; try again, and be quicker. . . . Now this time I'll lift you and put you part way up. Find out by your feet when you get to the turn, and see how quiet you can be. . . . "

There seems to be a very deep-seated tendency in the human race to hoard. In common with the magpie, the squirrel and the bear, children manifest a proclivity to help themselves to attractive, portable articles, to store them away, and later to visit the repository, contemplate, manipulate and enjoy the contents. Undirected, this tendency may become dissipated in harmless and useless ways; misdirected, it may become a social nuisance; wisely directed it may serve to further scientific knowledge and to bring aesthetic pleasure to thousands.

Collecting

At first, developing from noticing and grasping, a young child simply picks up an attractive object and finds delight in holding it, or keeping it near by till his attention is distracted. By the time he is four years old, there is a joy in having a special, definite place in which to keep the treasures, and the further joy of turning over the collection, examining and handling it. Until the age of seven or eight, the objects collected are quite miscellaneous and of a trivial nature. The material easily found in the environment will determine what particular things are amassed. Pebbles, hen feathers, buttons, marbles, scrap pictures, bits of metal, pieces of ribbon are all welcomed if available.

Age Changes in Collecting Interests

After the age of six or seven the social elements of imitation and competition begin to affect the collecting craze. A fashion may set in for shells, or paper dolls, or cigar bands, or little pictures. The child whom the others envy is the one who has the largest collection. From eight to twelve the fever seems to be at its height, over ninety per cent of children collecting something or other then, and frequently acquiring great stores of more than one kind of thing. Burk, in a study of California children's collections, points out age periods of greatest interest, such as marbles from six to thirteen, but chiefly at eight and nine. Birds' eggs are interesting from nine

45

on, but mostly between twelve and fourteen. Stamps hold the field from nine to fourteen or fifteen, after which the bored adolescent may present the too-little-appreciative small sister or brother with a well-filled stamp album. In the teens the sentimental factor is more dominant. Then it is that personal souvenirs are sought for—autographs, friendship symbols, dance programs, anything to remind the collector of the good times experienced or the personalities admired. The accompanying diagram shows the general age of waxing, height of attractiveness, and waning of several different interests:

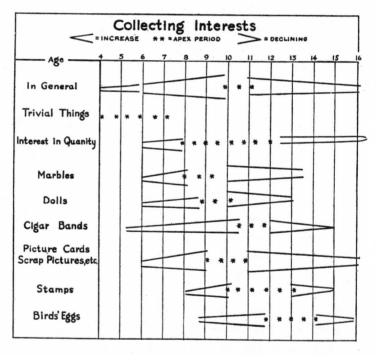

Sex Differences in Collecting Interests — Boys and girls show characteristic differences both in the type of things desired and in the manner of acquiring them. More boys than girls collect scraps of metal, marbles, birds' eggs, stamps and cigar bands. More girls than boys collect buttons, picture cards, colored

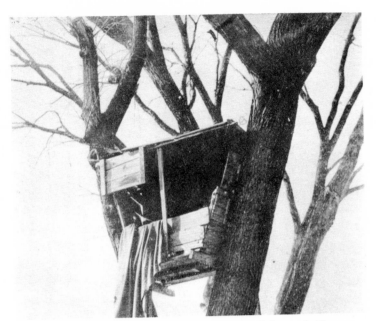

These tree dwellers have no fear, for they draw their rope ladder up after them.

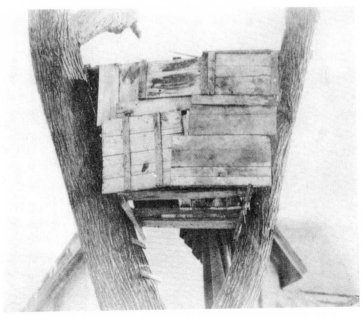

Boys will be boys.

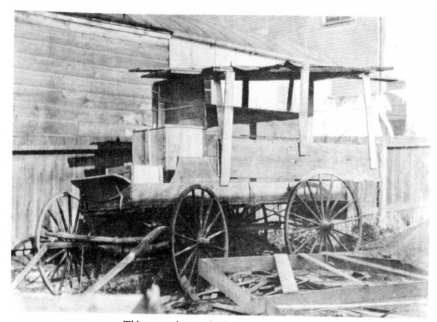

This gang changes its headquarters at will.

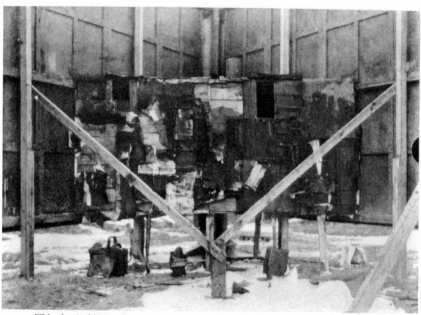

This shack, hidden from view, is the favorite resort of the neighborhood gang.

glass and pottery chips, scraps of textiles. In nature study material boys' tastes run to animals' teeth, claws, legs and other parts, not to mention live frogs, insects, lizards and the like. Girls' tastes run to leaves, mosses, seaweed, butterflies and other colorful things. Both boys and girls value small samples of food products, though it is scarcely likely that they remain for long on exhibition; but it is the girls who appreciate samples of soap, perfume, and other toilet articles. Both sexes enjoy finding or active hunting for treasures, but boys show more initiative in buying and in driving hard bargains with each other in a brisk trade.

Seldom is any but a crude attempt at classification evident. At eight or nine some arrangement by size or color may obtain; while after eleven some basis such as price, shape, or, in the case of girls, artistic effect, may be chosen; but before thirteen it is rare to find any kind of genuine organization of permanent worth. Obviously, here is the great opportunity to direct this instinct, substituting emulation for quality rather than for mere quantity at the nine-year level, and leading on to the idea of the "best" being the most complete and representative collection. We can suggest better values, either aesthetic or scientific, for the type of thing collected, and coöperate for arrangement of the material on a worthwhile basis.

The instinctive desire to acquire and own things arises in close connection with the interest in food. The first object a little child claims as his own are those which help to satisfy hunger. Soon the sense of possession includes articles which minister to other bodily needs. Thus it is *my* bottle, *my* spoon, *my* little chair, *my* crib, *my* place by mother. Toys and clothing are recognized and treated as special belongings, too, and thus the child is well on the way to developing what proves to be one of the strongest motives in our life

Ownership: Me and Mine

endeavors. To gain or retain possession of anything—lands, education, friends, health, goods—we will dare and do almost anything. Wisely directed, then, this is a tremendous force towards achievement; undirected, it may go to waste; misdirected, it may work untold misery.

The sense of ownership is bound up with a child's sense of self and with the extent of his group consciousness, and is therefore both an index of and a factor in his moral growth as he changes from a self-centered little individualist to a more socialized citizen. Let us list the various reasons a child feels as valid to prove ownership.

The First Basis of Valid Ownership

One reason is the amount of *effort expended* in acquisition. A young child counts effort to attain as the equivalent of the right to possess. With the baby this is physical effort to reach and grasp something attractive —notice how strenuously he objects if the coveted object is removed. The older child hunts, or risks himself physically. The child of ten or eleven feels the truth of "first come, first served," "findings is keepings." J. Johnson in his studies among the boys on the McDonough Farm noted that they acknowledged as owner any child who would mark his find, much as we respect the staking claim of a miner, or the right of the first comer who has marked his seat in the car.

Other Bases of Valid Ownership

Another reason for the feeling of ownership is that of *labor expended.* Thus, in the orphans' home the door handles are Annie's because she cleaned them. At home they are Fred's chickens because he looks after them, though the parents pay for the food and shelter required. *Constructive work* gives a specially clear sense of ownership. Though it be father's tools and materials yet the bird-house Harold made is unquestionably his. The effort may be less direct, as in *choice and purchase;* if the money for the purchase has been difficult to amass then the sense of possession is the more keen. Lastly, an object *bestowed* upon a child is regarded as his own, somewhat in proportion as the child likes the donor, and partly as he previously desired the object.

In all these cases children not only lay claim themselves to things but recognize the claims of others as just. If they know that another child has worked for, made, bought or been given something, they look upon it as his, and would sympathize with him in its loss, or in any accident to it.

A child does not distinguish individual ownership when goods are bestowed in bulk, or are held in common by a group, or are acquired in routine fashion. The groceries on the pantry shelf belong to whom? To the family? To mother who bought them? To father whose money paid for them? Or to any child who is hungry? But food once served on individual plates at a meal is unhesitatingly claimed as one's own. Not a few squabbles arise from the necessity of determining whether articles are held in common indiscriminatingly for any would-be owner, or belong to one member of the group. More arise from the need to prove priority rights in treasure trove, or in the claim renewed first after an interval. Marshall races after supper to the coveted corner of the couch with his book; it is his for the next half hour because he got there first. He is called away on an errand and Elsie slips into it meanwhile—thereby inevitably setting the stage for a quarrel.

Complicated Problems of Ownership

Until the adolescent's group sense is widened beyond the limits of the gang, or his class in school, or his school, he is unlikely to feel ownership for fixtures in the streets, for trees and bushes in the parks. But once the group spends labor, or constructive effort, or its own cash on public grounds the attitude is completely changed.

Mine and Ours

The two to three year old's experience that older

children object violently, tends to check his first impulse to grab indiscriminately what he wants. The fact that the others explain their objections by such reasons as "It is mine, I found it first," "Mama gave it to me," help him differentiate between mine and thine. His own first all-sufficient reason for claim, "I want it," has to be replaced by reasons which others will respect. When called upon to give up something he is using, or to prove that it is his, a further appreciation of socially acceptable criteria for ownership is developed.

Responsibility in ownership comes partly through sympathy, but may be trained by utilizing the suggestions given above. Working with mother to clean and polish the bath-room fixtures, or the furniture, will beget a feeling which will oppose wanton treatment thereof. The job of sweeping the porch will help prevent the careless tracking in of dirt. The club's interest in decorating the room where they meet will lead to better understanding of property rights. Lastly, in the abstract sense, we not only work for the cause because it is ours, but feel it is ours because we have spent effort and labor upon it.

Summary

What children feel impelled to do may or may not be desirable from the social standpoint. Some tendencies may be perpetuated by seeing that they bring satisfaction, or by stimulating children to act in the required way. Undesirable tendencies may be eliminated by seeing that dissatisfaction results, or by preventing any opportunities for their exercise. Most tendencies need redirection, by substituting different modes of action, or changing the thoughts and emotions in connection with the tendency.

Three types of emotional response are shown in early infancy. Anger is aroused by thwarting. Wise guidance is necessary if self-control is to be gained over rage, temper, sullenness. Love impulses have two aspects, each meriting study of its characteristic phases in each of three periods of childhood. Normal development in the third period is helped by careful training in the first two. The adolescents' love emotions may be intense and lead to erratic behavior; they need a sympathetic understanding. Most fears are induced, not original. They require intelligent coöperation for their cure. All these emotions need control and sublimation, rather than suppression and repression, if children are to develop into normal adults.

Collecting is a dominant interest for many years, with characteristic age changes. Unguided, the tendency may be useless and wasteful; guided, it has great educative value. The feeling of ownership is an index to a child's sense of self and of his social relationships. Conditions are pointed out which do, and do not promote the growth of this feeling. As a motive, it may be perverted to criminal uses; trained, it develops responsibility.

III

The Active Nature and Needs of Childhood

IS IT necessary for Ann to make such a clatter as she goes up and down stairs? Do all children bang doors at this age or that? Is John being babied because he is helped with his buttons and has his face washed? Does it need special training to enable children to turn corners without bumping, and to keep their hands off the wall at the turn of the stairs? Is Mary below par because she does not carry a well filled cup and saucer without spilling? Why does this youth appear so disjointed, whether walking, sitting, or standing?

No Scale of Normal Motor Abilities Yet How much we should appreciate standardized scales of motor abilities in ordinary life tasks, so that we could get a rating for performance just as we do for reading ability or for general intelligence! Most of the norms that are available, however, are for tests such as strength of grip, rapidity of tapping, steadiness in fine movements of aiming at a mark or tracing a line. From the thousands of measures taken on such tests we know—what we probably guessed before—that boys are stronger than girls, on the average, at every age; and that strength and speed increase with age. Over 86% of children are right handed, while dull children are more likely to be left handed than bright children.

Observation of infants reveals that the first use of the limbs is in simultaneous, parallel fashion. Nerve coördination has developed by the sixth month so that deliberate alternate movement is possible. Grasping is stimulated at first by the sense of being touched; but during the fourth month reaching and grasping follow upon seeing an attractive object. In the earliest grasping, thumb and fingers act together, making the hand a simple hook. By the twelfth week the thumb is opposed to the fingers. For a considerable period in taking hold of an object proffered, say a book, the overhand grasp is preferred (thumb under, fingers over) in distinction from the older, adult underhand hold (fingers under, thumb over). For smaller objects, such as a spoon, the overhand grasp will be retained till the wrist motion of turning at the right time to permit safe conveyance of the contents of the spoon to the mouth is coördinated. That is to about three years old.

By courtesy of Miss R. Andrus, whose intensive observation work with young children is yet unpublished, a few selected norms of performance are here given. Beyond the age of four we have little as yet but vague generalizations from the experience of gymnasium directors, psychologists, doctors and health clinics. **Capabilities From Two to Four**

Children can use a cup by the handle by two years and a half. They can carry cups from two and a half to three, and carry a small pitcher of water easily by three. By three also they can assist in laying plates, spoons, etc., on the table, and by four should be able to fold their table napkins. They can wash their hands, palms and backs, by three years old, and dry their hands, too. Shoes and rubbers can be put on unaided from two and a half to three, and fastened by buttons or lacing by three and a half. The stockings should be put on at this age also. In learning to go upstairs, they hold on and go both feet on one step at first, then with the feet the same way but without holding, till two and a half. Then, using the feet as we do but with hand assistance till three or more; between three and a half and four they can progress as we do.

Children can use a dust pan and brush by three and a half. In playing ball, it is after three before it is usual to catch a ball of tennis size, though it may be successfully thrown forward a distance of seven feet between two and a half and three. Bouncing a ball straight is a feat for the four-year-old.

Therefore some few of the queries above for Ann, John, Mary and the rest can be answered. Much of the bumping, clattering, spilling, dependence on assistance is an unnecessary retention of an earlier habit, and is an evidence of lack of good training.

Large, Simple Movements First

How is control gained? Movements of the larger muscles, those older in point of developmental history, and nearer the trunk, are controlled before movements in the smaller, accessory muscles. Thus, a baby is able to bend, to roll over, sit up, hitch along, before it can stand or walk. It can use the tongue for efficient eating before the adjustments for speech sounds are possible. The fine adjustments for the dentals, d, t, th, and for r, l, and s are learned last of all. The nerve strain of focusing the eyes and steadying the hands to thread a needle and string small beads is too much for the four-year-old. Fine technique of violin and piano work is not to be demanded of five-year-olds' fingers, nor delicate wrist play in fencing from the eight-year-olds. But running, balancing, climbing, jumping rope, tossing balls, dancing, are helpful activities, in graded series of difficulties.

Tyler points out three stages of growth for every organ in the body. First is mere enlargement, when exercise is unnecessary, second is growth requiring much exercise for healthy development, third is the approach to full maturity, when severe training looking towards endurance of strain is possible. The restlessness and quick tiring of young children indicates a need for plentiful free exercise which is not continued for long at a time. The ten-year-old could well go for an eight-mile hike which the five-year-old could not do; though the five-

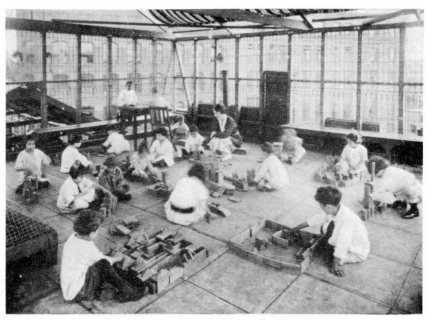

Every normal child loves to be busy building things.

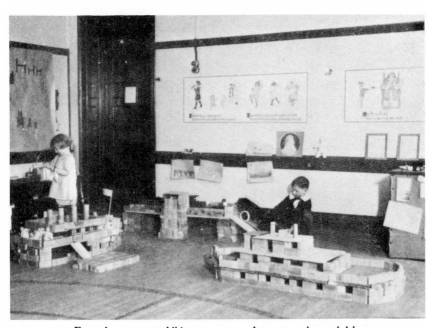

Even the youngest children can engage in constructive activities.

year-old may easily walk that far in the course of the day's ordinary activities.

Three things about the facts of growth are important to remember because of their bearing on motor ability. One is that increase is not uniform, but that there are periods of spurt, and periods of comparative rest. Another is that all parts of the body, bones, muscles, limbs, trunk, the various organs, follow a law of growth of their own, also marked by these accelerations and retardations. The third is, that rapid enlargement of one part may coincide with a resting period for another part. The legs increase in length more than the trunk between nine and fourteen, which taxes the internal organs to supply heat and growth material to the limbs. Plenty of nourishing food and fresh air and exercise is obviously necessary. When bones are lengthening more rapidly than the muscles which act as their levers, the stretch on the latter may give rise to crampy "growing pains." When the muscles increase disproportionately a resulting flabby weakness is evident. This means that children are continually obliged to readjust their mechanisms of control. Awkwardness in sitting down, and in gait, may be lack of habituation to the changing hip and pelvic bones as well as to the extra length of limb to be managed. "Nervous" movements may indicate imperfect adjustment due to irregularity in growth. *Growth and Motor Ability*

Persistent practice is the only way to acquire all the series of habits. The hunger for climbing, balancing, doing stunts is a sign of the great need of the constantly changing body. Certainly up to fifteen children should be freely encouraged in all that tends towards graceful coördination. Later, feats of strength and endurance are welcomed.

If we were to sum up comprehensively, yet briefly, how to understand children's active nature, we would say—Watch them at play. Play is, truly, their chief *Children's Activities* business in life. In its many varied forms we may see revealed the possibilities for the development it affords, the dominant interests at different age levels, some distinctive characteristics of boys and girls, and get the clues as to the needs of childhood.

We will deal with these in reverse order.

Children's Needs in Play: "No Place to Play"

A crying need in many homes is sufficient *space*. Though the children's room, the attic, the barn, to say nothing of the great out-doors, wait with friendly mien for the small-town or country-bred child, yet probably one-third of our child population live under conditions of urban life which preclude much play. The congestion in our cities, from the nine people in three rooms of the tenement, to the family of three in the expensive two-room-and-bath hotel apartment, is hard alike on children and on adults from the standpoint of normal child activity. Nor are our streets a desirable playground from any point of view. True, our social conscience is stirring itself to provide more parks, playgrounds, and recreation centers, and to divert traffic from particular streets during a certain few hours, and also to recognize the rights of other people's children to a place in which to play; but much remains to be done in providing facilities for play.

No Time to Play

A second need of active children is *time*. This may sound ridiculous when we think of the long "golden days of childhood," so free in retrospect from the pressure of care and the rush of work of which we are now so conscious. Yet the fact remains that the "poor little rich girl," as well as her fellow citizen of the slums, already a victim of child labor, may have no free time in which to play, since she is so constantly supervised, so hurried from study to social engagement.

No One to Play With

A third need is that of *playmates*, preferably of a like age, but not imperatively so in the first two or three years of life. Our sympathy goes out to the only child,

56

and the child widely separated in age from others in the family. Even though such may have school friends with whom they pass hours in play, they miss a good deal in their continuous family relationships.

A fourth need, apt to occur instantly to an adult mind, is that of *equipment*. What would the playground be without its swings, basket-ball stands, sand-box and other apparatus? The recreation park suggests at once various ball fields, the tennis nets, wading pool and lake with boats. The play room implies playthings; a gift to a child calls to mind a long array of bats, balls, kites, tops, dolls, boats, puzzles and the like—in fact the bewildering variety offered to our gaze in such profusion at the holiday season. Here is a real problem.

Nothing to Play With

A toy, as Woodworth points out, is primarily something a child can make move in some way. The more he can do with it, the more he can find new possibilities of bending it to his will, of making it carry out some purpose, the greater the enjoyment from that toy. The movement may bring enjoyment to the senses, such as noise, or the feeling of swift motion, or pleasing spatial arrangement. Herein lies the fascination of toy drums, fire crackers, swings, roller skates, a box of paints, and pattern making with colored cardboard.

How to Choose Toys for Children: No Fun Unless It Moves

Then again, the movement may be of his own body, gaining skill, or gaining power at a distance. Balls, bows and arrows, slingshot, bicycles, radio sets, give this sort of joy. The movement may be due to manipulation by which the child creates shapes to his fancy. Clay, damp sand, snow, fire, water, building blocks, illustrate this sort of plaything. The movement may be attractive because it appears to defy gravity; hence the pleasure in kites, soap-bubbles, tops. Lastly, the movement may be chiefly in the child's imagination, and the toy that stimulates it is loved because it is a diminutive edition of things adults use. Dolls and their manifold appurtenances, boats, miniature animals, toy railways, farm scenes and a host of models of all kinds will readily be recognized by adults and children alike as fit toys.

From this standpoint, daddy's foot is a toy when the wee child gets a ride on it; likewise the high-powered racing car with which his older brother defies the speed laws. Both bring the sensory enjoyment of unusual and rapid motion.

Get a "Do-With" Toy What of the mechanical toy that is wound up and does one thing only, and does it all by itself? Children soon tire of it, and no wonder. After the first novelty of its movements has worn off, if no further developments can be expected, and if no manipulation brings any change except to destroy the mechanism, the interest is lost. Obviously, then, in selecting toys one consideration should be what the children *can "do with"* them. Very often the simpler the toy the richer it will be in possibility of manipulation or imagination, and therefore the more stimulating. It is the joy in activity that is the essence of play, not mere passive admiration of a technical perfection. Better the box of clothespins from which people and log houses can be constructed, than the most accomplished, and therefore finished, limited, mechanical doll.

Another guiding consideration in selecting playthings is of course the age of the child. While motor coördination is poor, no complex, small objects requiring fine muscular adjustments are suitable. A wagon or car rather than a bicycle for the three-year-old; three simple light-weight tools rather than the complete carpenter's kit for the seven-year-old. Mechanical instruments requiring precise control at eleven rather than at eight; and fine sewing materials and implements later still.

A fifth need is that of *intelligent suggestion* of plays and occupations that will open up new vistas to the child and prevent his remaining bored on a low level of achievement when he is ready for something further. With a child who lacks initiative, this method of stimulation is very helpful; and for many groups, wise guidance will provide opportunities for enjoyment and progress which they would be unlikely to discover for themselves. It is in this sense that we teach or supervise play. Such teaching must fulfil its function of leading and encouraging along the path of adventure, and avoid the fatal mistake of driving and commanding along the track of slavery. For children most emphatically do not want to be "bossed" in their games continually. To be told what to do, and how and when to do it at every step is no fun, since one essential in play is freedom of choice.

One thing the play teacher should know is what games are appropriate to the mental and physical developmental level at each age period. Another thing is the relative values of different games, as well as, obviously, a great variety of games. The first two points will be discussed below. For directions as to how to help children construct their own toys and find new occupations the following books will be found of value, as also some given in the Bibliographies.

Bancroft, J. H.: *Games for the Playground, Home, School and Gymnasium.*

Forbush, W. B.: *The Manual of Play.*

Grey, Marion: *Two Hundred Indoor and Outdoor Games.*

Keys, A.: A series, with titles such as *When Mother Lets Us*— (*Cook, Cut Out*, etc.).

Lucas, E. V., and Elizabeth: *Three Hundred Games and Pastimes*, or *What Shall We Do Now?*

Read, Mary L.: *Mother Craft Manual.*

White, Mary: *The Child's Rainy Day Book.*

An instinct that may be seen functioning in many kinds of play is that of habitation. The wee toddler discovers delightful niches and cubby holes into which he will crawl with manifest pleasure. By three or four, children may see the value of forming an enclosure with chairs, and show every evidence of contentment at sitting safely esconced within. The tent of the pendant tablecloth, the shelter of rugs or sheets hung on the laundry line, the empty crate, the dog kennel, have irresistible charms for the smaller children. After five or six, the boys are more active in constructing their habitation. As observed in the kindergarten, about four boys to one girl will work persistently in erecting a play house. Problems of openings for doorways and windows, even of hoists and elevators engross the men of the future, while the women wait aloof. When all is finished, however, it is the latter who will promptly move in with their doll family, and realize the need for cook-stoves, beds, and curtains at the windows.

This difference in interest is maintained during the next few years. It is the girls who modify the boys' effects by decorative ventures in roof line and color scheme. After the age of eight or so, each sex follows its respective bent separately, unless it be for very temporary purposes in the hay mow, the sand heap, the snow fort, or the wood pile. Little girls' outdoor retreats are frequently simply a secluded spot under the bushes, in the area way, in an angle of the rocks. On a bare surface sometimes the walls are merely marked out by lines, and the edifice left to the imagination; but furnishings will somehow be found, and perhaps a "garden" will be added, made with stones, leaves, colored fragments of glass and china. Boys will prefer to build, using any material handy. In the woods a wigwam will make its appearance; on the hillside a scooped-out cave. On the city lot old tins hammered out flat, odds and ends of tar paper, linoleum, matting and of course barrels and boxboards can all be utilized. By ten or eleven, the shelter is a stronghold or hang-out for the group whose password identifies them, and who share many joys there together, from simple cooking to thrilling narrative. After twelve or thirteen, children lose interest in this make-believe house and begin to take pride in their real club quarters. Girls soon, and boys later, wish to transform their own private rooms at home. By seventeen or so, a keen rapture may come from re-furnishing and decorating the adolescent's room according to his or her own tastes.

Already at five or six years of age, we may note some differences between boys and girls in their *choice of playthings* and play activities. For instance, more girls than boys choose painting and crayon work, and are content with that occupation longer. More girls draw flowers, while boys draw ships and engines. This greater interest of girls in *aesthetic spacing* and in color shows also in their large constructive work. It is they who attempt decorative effects outside and inside the houses, the building of which may have been a project for a mixed group of boys and girls. It is the girls, again, who care about an artistic arrangement of their collection of leaves or pebbles, who delight in ornamenting their handwork and sewing, and who thrill to the beauties of the sunset, or the mountain view. Meantime their more practical-minded brothers have enjoyed carpentering, and many, even at six, have glimpsed some of the mechanics' problems involved in their construction work. It is they who find it so absorbing to watch industrial processes such as concrete mixing and glass blowing; it is they who gravitate as naturally as do the older men to where excavating or street paving is going on. It is they, too, who acquire prodigious stores of information anent the makes of cars, or the details of railroad administration; and it is they who find out how to set up a wireless receiving set.

Boys' Play and Girls' Play

Another sex difference in play interest is that the *joy of violent running about,* of scrimmage and crowd fight, wanes considerably for girls as they pass out of middle childhood; but it waxes, if anything, for boys who at nineteen find nothing too hazardous or too arduous, and who welcome even extreme fatigue in pursuit of pleasure.

A third difference, more apparent in the adolescent period than earlier, is that girls retain their interest in a wide variety of games, whereas boys run rather to a specialty and to a narrower range of continued play activity. Adolescent girls are more attracted to card and table games than are boys, and seem more addicted to games of chance.

A fourth difference is of course the greater and more permanent interest of girls in *dolls.* Round them a whole imaginative life is built up, whether they are big dolls, doll-house size or the two dimensional paper doll. Boys, on the other hand, seldom care much for toy animals or toy people after six or seven years old, with the possible exception of tin soldiers and the puppet show. Even so, it is the maneuvers of the battle or the manipulation of the puppets that is the most attractive part of the play.

A fifth difference is the greater frequency with which boys go tramping, fishing and hunting, fashioning weapons for the chase, slingshot, rod and line, or—joy of joys—managing to handle a real gun. Girls roam about less, and apparently are not impelled to the hunter's life so urgently.

Certain Age Changes in Play Interests The fantastic fancy of the pre-school-age child shows in the frequent creation of an imaginary companion, as well as in his enjoyment of pretending he is a horse, a squirrel, or a jumping frog. At eight or nine the dramatization of pirates and bandits requires far more realistic stage properties and costumes. By eleven the language the characters use assumes a special importance; by fifteen the plot's the thing, with incipient appreciation of character drawing as such.

Doll play reflects these changes in imagination, too. **Doll Play**
The smaller children copy what they have seen their
elders do. The dolls are talked to, scolded, dressed, put
to bed, fed, rolled in a baby carriage, and fondled. By
eight or nine, when the doll interest is at its height, the
accessories of tea sets, laundry equipment, furniture in
the dolls' houses have assumed great importance. The
more the miniature article faithfully imitates the real
one the more the little girls are pleased. By ten, doll
dressmaking may show no little constructive skill and
aesthetic interest. Now, too, is the time for more complex forms of dramatic procedure in which the dolls may
take part. Between eleven and twelve, the interest in
dolls is rapidly lessening and after twelve, most girls cease
to care for them, though occasionally we find sporadic
cases of interest lingering for another year or two.

Traditional plays with a semi-dramatic element are
enjoyed in the seven-to-twelve-year period. It is difficult
to say whether the fun in the contest involved does not
obscure the original significance of phrases used in such
games as old witch, fox and geese, and hare and
hounds.

Curiosity, the love of puzzles, and language interest **Guessing**
find satisfaction in numerous guessing games. Some of **Games**
these turn on descriptions of objects, such as "twenty
questions," "person and thing"; others involve puns and
conundrums. Some demand language building such as
"my ship comes home," "I go to the grocer," "how,
when and where," and word and spelling competitions.
Many of them are beyond the powers of the seven or
eight-year-old, but are increasingly absorbing as mental
development and school achievement proceed.

C. E. Johnson points out as the most prominent **The Most**
feature in each age period, for the child under three, **Prominent Feature in**
sensory and motor control plays; until six, imaginative **Each Age**
play, with crude construction work; until nine, traditional **Period**

games, doll play, games of chasing, guessing games; until twelve, competition, skill, some little coöperation; until fifteen, games involving much physical activity. The accompanying diagrams present a few of the findings of McGhee and Croswell. They are based on answers they received from nearly eighteen thousand children naming play activities they preferred. The activities were

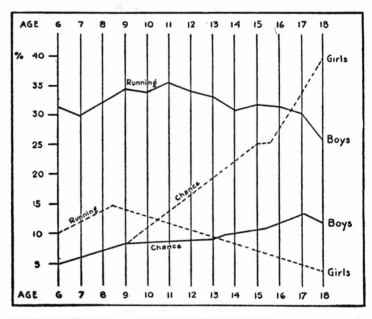

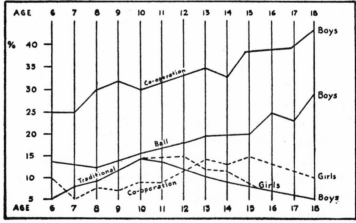

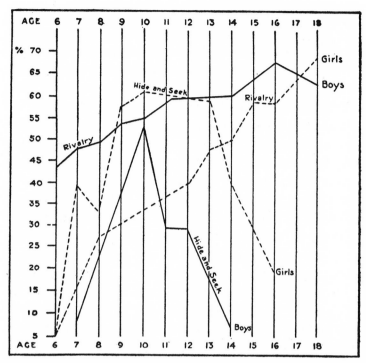

analyzed for the elements contained. The figures on the left represent the percentage of boys (heavy line) and girls (dotted line) mentioning a play in which the element in question is prominent. Not only age differences, but sex differences also are well brought out in these diagrams.

The gradual development of group consciousness is reflected very well in the social type of play in which children engage at different ages. At first the play is exclusively *individualistic*,—child, toy, and spectator, or simply child, toy, and imagination, being all that is needed. This is followed by the play of several children together with similar toys. The *group is small but indefinite in number;* moreover, the play is not a game in the sense of an activity with fixed rules, limited participation, a deliberate goal, and an ending point. Imagination plays a great part in directing the play of the group. The life occupations which children have seen, such as those of the

Age Differences in Group Consciousness: Social Types of Play

65

fireman, the motorman, the mother, the doctor, are acted out with great fidelity at this stage. Characters from stories are also portrayed, though not at so early an age as those from real life. Very little in the way of stage properties is required, the transformation taking place chiefly in the child's own fancy.

Rhythmic movement and singing games are enjoyed in group formation, and here we note the transition to the next form of social consciousness as the group begins to divide, and opposition commences to be part of the game itself rather than a hindrance to it. Thus, in "cat and mouse," or "drop the handkerchief," the pursuer and pursued are in opposition at least, while those in the ring may present obstacles to either successful flight or capture. From this point the element of competition enters increasingly and develops by way of such games as "London Bridge," with its final tug of war between the two completed sides, into the *double group* game proper. There, sides are chosen at the beginning, and the group as such acts against the maneuvers of the opposite group. "Hare and hounds," "prisoner's base," most forms of relay races, exhibit this growing group solidarity, as well as group rivalry.

Coincident with the double group the game for two or four develops. Here the game is very definitely a contest, the aim being to win over one's opponent. "Naughts and crosses" is an early form of this, checkers a later form, both of a quiet nature, just as tennis is a more violently active form of this *pair or double pair type*. In any case the game has very definite rules, whether few or many, and has a method of scoring which marks its close.

The Regular Team Game These elements of definiteness carry forward into the next type, that of the regular *team game*, the most highly developed of all from the standpoint of social consciousness. It is like the third type in that two groups are contending, but unlike it and more advanced in that each group is organized. The numbers on each side are limited, and each member of the team has special duties and special positions on the field. Because of this, individual interests and desires to star must constantly be controlled by the relationship of the individual's activity to the good of the team as a whole—a consideration that enters very scantily into the mere double group type of game. It is seldom that we find a genuine team game before the teen age. It is true that in imitation of admired heroes of the diamond, the small boys' gang will play at baseball; but a careful spectator, or perhaps auditor, will see and hear undoubted evidences of lack of genuine coöperation and an abundance of individual striving for honor. The group is an aggregate of units rather than an organism with differentiated functions.

Now, in this progression from the individualistic play of the little child to the team game of the near-adult the pleasure of the earlier forms is not lost. The eighteen-year-old and the adult may enjoy all five forms of play, but the four-year-old may enjoy only the first. Picture the summer hotel amusements. The smallest children pick up the quoits, stand anywhere, throw anyhow, in no order, just for the fun of throwing. At six or seven a small group of them will be taking turns in pitching. Then come arguments as to how far off to stand, and how to count the score, and whose turn it is to pitch. By ten or eleven, a larger group will have evolved more rules, and are likely to pick sides before beginning, and to count, not each individual's score, but the total of each opposing group. The adolescents are almost sure to do this, and to go on to arrange for a tournament. This particular game hardly lends itself to development into the real fifth type; but there will be shown a consciousness of the value of handicaps, of a scorekeeper, and of an umpire. The well-meaning adult who would insist upon the rules of scoring for the little children, or the tournament for the nine-year-olds, would be forcing growth into adult standards prematurely.

Educative Value: Learning Through Play

Since "we learn by doing" it would seem that the more passive a child is in his play the less he is likely to learn. So again the fact is emphasized that the plaything *at* which he is amused, but which does not stimulate him by further action *with* it, is not the best choice. Again, endless unvarying repetition of the same activity after skill has been acquired is not educative. Therefore, unless it is enjoyed as a hygienic relaxation for muscles, or provides an emotional outlet for harassed nerves, we might be justified in seeking to introduce some form of play more conducive to progress.

However, passivity must not be confused with bodily quiet. Outwardly a child may be passive when he is watching moving pictures or reading a book; but the activity of the mind may be very great, and therein, of course, lies the educative value.

In brief, any play through which a child is led to acquire information, to develop skill, to exercise aesthetic judgment or to gain practice in solving problems may be said to be educative—to the degree that the facts learned, or the power produced, have values in themselves.

Moral Values: Taking Turns

Let us consider the opportunity for learning moral lessons in play. The five-year-old's biggest social problem is that of adapting himself to the necessity of taking turns. This has two aspects, first, that of waiting for his own turn, second, that of quitting a pleasant occupation so that someone else may have a turn. If these enormously important lessons are not well learned at the start there will be endless trouble in the next five or six years, to say nothing of a possible twist in the wrong direction all through life. When difficulties arise, adult suggestion is of greater help than reprimand or a sudden interference. When a veritable hair-pulling contest occurs as two small people simultaneously desire to use the same toy, it is easy to see how ineffective a mere authoritative judgment may be. It only introduces a third angle into the situation instead of helping the mutual adjustment of the two combatants. Consequently, the solution is many times simply deferred, while resentment smoulders, or a sly child watches for a chance to obtain what he wants by a trick. The friendly coöperation of the adult is what is needed, in order to find the reasonable way to act when personal desires conflict.

Another type of moral lesson comes when the eight-year-old finds his friends jeering at cowardice, and incredulous of bluff. He finds he can win regard by deeds rather than words, by meeting demands for stunts, by never refusing a dare, by making good a boast. The cowardice of the sneak and the telltale meets with such open disapproval by the rest of the crowd that the earlier tendency to run to mamma with grief and grievances is soon checked. A boy learns that he must adjust differences within the group, without a weak leaning on outside authority. He learns, too, that he must stand up for his own rights or be despised as a weakling. **'Fraid Cats and Tattle Tales**

As free play is superseded by the game, the necessity of rules awakens a consciousness of what playing fair means. To prevent others from taking advantage, each child must watch the other player to prevent cheating. In turn, his own selfish desires are held in check by the knowledge that his playmates are just as watchful lest he transgress the rules. What an immense amount of argument and squabbling can be heard as children are learning this lesson of fair play. **Play Fair**

By ten or eleven a boy, at least, is learning lessons of group loyalty, how to stand by the others in trouble, how to share his good things with the rest, how to plan with them for added enjoyment. The girl, somehow, learns this less thoroughly, or shall we say, with greater difficulty and more slowly. Certain petty jealousies remain **Play the Team** as a divisive force, hindering the coöperation of the girls' group as a unit. Tendencies to snub the others, to retain ideas of caste and clique persist into adolescence, when girls find it so much more difficult than boys do to play the team game heartily. Where the play director succeeds in coaching a girl team it has been against heavy odds, and has required much continued stimulation. Even so, fewer girls than boys engage in team games; and when they do, the self conscious talk about the team is in marked contrast to the spontaneous enthusiasms of their brothers.

Good Work of the Others A moral lesson all may learn is that of admiration for honest effort as well as for brilliant results. Important lessons for the teen age are those of generosity to opponents in the hour of triumph over them, and of contest without bitterness of spirit.

How we could wish that these lessons, learnable in play, might be carried over into business, industrial and national relationships.

Summary Such motor control tests as exist and have been standardized are either of the laboratory "performance" kind, or gymnasium tests of strength and steadiness; they are not very suggestive in a concrete way as to what to expect from children in the way of ordinary tasks. A beginning has been made, with children under four, to specify what physical skills are normal. In general, motor control begins with the larger, older, fundamental muscles, so that fine coördinations cannot be made by young children.

Much awkwardness at different ages is due to the irregularities of growth. Increase in size is not uniform, it proceeds by alternate spurts and resting periods. All parts of the body follow this law; spurts in one part do not parallel spurts in another, so that children are constantly readjusting their habits of motor control.

Play life shows a hunger for physical activity suitable for the stage of growth reached. Children need space and

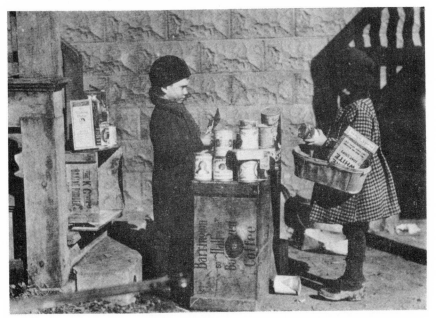

Playing store.

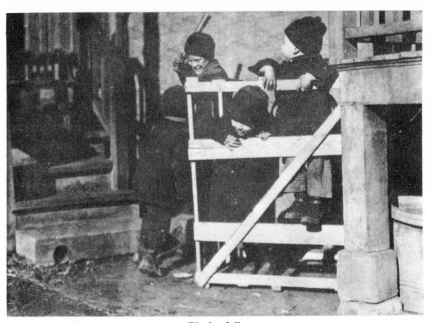

Playing jail.

time to play, as well as equipment over which they can exercise control. They also need play companions and opportune guidance to higher levels of development.

Boys are consistently more interested in mechanics and large constructive activities, in roaming and hunting, and, in the adolescent period, tend to specialize on a few violent team games and sports. Girls are more drawn to decorative constructive work, to dolls, to a greater variety of games, and are less violently active in the teens. Imaginative play shows marked age differences, as does the interest in languages. The most significant age change is in the progressive socialization from the individualistic play of the three-year-old to the team game of the sixteen-year-old. Educational values of getting information and exercising aesthetic judgment are involved in play, as well as the obvious values in hygiene and acquisition of physical skill. Moral values include the development of physical courage, but chiefly a recognition of the rights of others, as shown by taking turns, giving up, playing fair, appreciating others' efforts, being a good loser and a generous winner.

IV

The Development of the Intellect in Childhood and Youth

Some Limitations of the Earlier Studies of Intellectual Development

IN THE traditional descriptions of the development of the intellect, it has been usual to describe first the development of the senses, then the development of perception, of memory, of association, imitation, imagination, conception, judgment, and reasoning. In so describing these various aspects of mental development, the development of the mind as a whole has frequently not been clearly envisaged. In the simplest and earliest of childhood experiences and even in one and the same experience, all of these phases of mental activity may be involved. Further, such descriptions often gave the impression that we had to do with quite different processes in these various activities, whereas in perception and reasoning, for example, the same elementary processes occur; it is a difference of degree and complexity rather than of kind of process.

The Need for Information in Regard to the Development of the Mind as a Whole

Even in the current descriptions of the "perceptual", "ideational" and "rational" levels or stages of the development of the intellect, the continuity of these processes and the common elements involved are sometimes lost sight of. If a parent should wish to gauge the development of his child he might note that in various respects, as in sensory discrimination, as of colors and sounds, in his forming of concepts, in his acquirement of speech, and in the growth of his vocabulary, the child was the equal of, or was superior or inferior to the children described in the literature treating of the matter, but he might still remain in doubt as to whether *on the whole* (and that is what he usually would wish to know) the child's development should be considered normal (or average), retarded or accelerated. This unsatisfactory condition, from the standpoint of the parents' inquiry, may be attributed in part to the fact above emphasized that the literature had dealt with special *phases* of development rather than with *development as a whole*, and in part to another condition,— namely, that existing studies were seldom based on a sufficient number of children of different ages to make it possible to decide as to what was normal or what exceptional in a child of a given age.

Our knowledge in both of these respects has been greatly extended in recent years as a result of the initial contributions of the French psychologist, Alfred Binet, and of his collaborator, Th. Simon, and their many disciples, through the construction and application of tests of *general* intelligence. In order that this advance in our knowledge may be fairly appraised we shall need to review briefly the problems which confronted the psychologist in his earlier attempts at the measurement of intelligence.

It may be well to note, in the first place, that, in attempting to estimate or measure differences in intelligence, and to separate human beings into different groups, we meet in a new form, a very common difficulty. Clean-cut division between people has been the goal in many fields of testing. Dr. MacFie Campbell reminds us that "on one historical occasion a speech test was relied on as an infallible diagnostic criterion and that whoever could not pronounce the word 'shibboleth' satisfactorily was deemed an Ephraimite and was slain at the passage of the Jordan." And as Dr. Campbell adds: "The victorious men of Gilead probably worried little over the fact that diagnostic mistakes may have occurred; the test gave much satisfaction, because it was easy to apply, took up little time, and gave a clean-cut answer which did not require further thinking."

The Search for Tests of General Intelligence

73

Similar merits—easy to apply, take little time, and give a clean-cut answer—have been long sought for in mental tests. At one time it was thought that tests of the acuity of the senses would do, since all intellectual life must depend ultimately on some sensory experience. But it was soon found that individuals might have very defective sense organs, or, as in the case of Laura Bridgman and Helen Keller, be bereft of the chief avenues of sense and still give evidence of a very considerable development of intelligence.

Similarly since all thought and intellectual activity eventually results in action, it was and is still believed by many that tests of motor skill, of the precision and accuracy of movement, would give the desired differentiation. But some of the most intellectual of men are notoriously clumsy and awkward, if one confines attention to gross bodily movements or even to such fine adjustments as are involved, for example, in handwriting.

The next attempt was to devise tests of what seemed more distinctly intellectual processes,—the quickness of reactions, the speed, wealth and quality of associations, the extent and quality of memory, and the presence or absence or the degree of success in reasoning in concrete and so-called abstract situations. Here again it was found that an individual might have, for example, a very good memory, at least for some things, and in other respects be adjudged feeble-minded.

The Contributions of Binet and Simon In a word, in the long history of mental testing no single infallible test or "shibboleth" had been found. In the last two decades, however, a marked change has been made in the situation, due to the genius of the two Frenchmen named below. As not infrequently happens, the discoveries—for such they are—seem so simple that one wonders that they had not been thought of before, and their importance is at first minimized. Two important changes were introduced by Binet and Simon. The first and more obvious was that, since no single test was sufficient, a combination of a number of tests or problem situations might be used, the average of which would give a more representative value than any one test alone.

Up to the time of Binet, then, it is fair to say that the psychologist had followed the same method in his attempts at measuring intelligence as he had previously followed in his descriptions of intellectual development. Binet, however, recognized that the memory, for example, could not be tested apart from the senses, or association without involving attention and he gave up the attempt to separate the intellectual processes involved. He chose instead situations at first simple, then of increasing complexity and difficulty, but still within the possible range of the experience of the individual, in the meeting or solving of which his general mental development might be tested. This was Binet's general plan. Some of his tests, as, for example, the tests of rote memory differed, it is true, but little, if at all, from the earlier proposals for the testing of single capacities, and in other tests, as, for example, the arranging of five wooden cubes of the same size but differing in weight, in the order of their weight, a single capacity such as the sensory discrimination required, may seem to be the more important element involved. It was, therefore, not simply the sort of test which he applied, but his idea of combining or averaging the results of these single tests and problem situations as a measure of the growth of the individual which was the primary reason for the success of his method.

The usefulness of this method was greatly enhanced by a second and also very practical proposal: that comparison of individuals could be made in terms of the average development or attainment of children of various ages, the now familiar concept of mental age: that, for example, a boy of ten who can only pass mental tests which the general run of seven-year-old children can pass

The Concept of Mental Age

may be said to have a mental age of seven and give evidence of possibly three years of retardation in mental development.

In order to establish such mental age norms it was necessary to test large numbers of children of all ages. This has now been done in nearly all the civilized countries of the globe so that for the first time the psychologist is in a position to say what is normal and what is exceptional in the matters at least which the tests evaluate.

Even with this "battery" of tests which Binet and those who have revised and extended his series of tests have produced, some phases or specializations of mental development may be missed in the case of exceptional individuals. Before, however, speaking of such limitations which still exist in these attempts to determine intellectual development, we shall need to examine the tests of various age levels in order better to appraise the positive contributions which have resulted from their use.

What the Tests Test We must first have clearly in mind what the tests are designed to measure. They are not really tests of native intelligence as distinct from learning but are used to estimate the native intelligence by seeing how much has been acquired from the ordinary experiences of the individual as apart from special training. "Theoretically". to quote from a recently published statement of the writer, "it would follow that measurement of the actual progress of representative learning would furnish the best test of intelligence. For practical reasons most tests now in common use are not tests of the capacity to learn, but are tests of what has been learned. The assumption is made that if one samples the results of learning in matters where all the individuals tested have had an equal chance at learning, he may arrive at an estimate of the capacity to learn. But since it is difficult to find even simple experiences which are common to all individuals of a given age period, actually, again, one tries by sampling a large range of fairly common experiences to strike an 'average' which, despite the fact that a given individual may have missed this or that experience, will still be representative of the individual's learning."

With these considerations in mind a description of the tests at certain mental age levels will illustrate the means by which the intellectual development of the individual is gauged. Our examples will be taken from Kuhlmann's and Terman's Revisions and Extensions of the Binet-Simon tests.

Kuhlmann has standardized tests for the ages of three months, six months, twelve months, eighteen months, and two years. The following are the tests for the third month:—1. *Carrying hand or object to mouth.* A small block or other object is placed in the infant's hand. The question is: Has the infant sufficient motor coördination and control to carry the block (or his hand) to the mouth more or less at will and not merely through random or chance movements? 2. *Reaction to sudden sounds.* Does the infant "start" or wink when a telegraph snapper is sounded within a few inches of his ear, or when the examiner claps his hands behind the infant's head? 3. *Binocular coördination.* Can the infant follow with its eyes a bright light, such as an electric light, which is moved to and fro or up and down a few feet away from its eyes, and without showing especial incoördination even when the eyes are turned to extreme position? 4. *Turning eyes to object in marginal field of vision.* Will the child turn its eyes (or head) toward a bright light which is moved in the marginal field of vision? 5. *Winking at an object threatening the eyes.* Does the infant wink when a large object such as a hat, or the flat side of a book is "passed" suddenly toward his eyes?

The tests for the age of twelve months are as follows: 1. *Sitting and standing.* Can the infant sit unsupported for two or three minutes or stand unsupported for five

Tests of the Infant's Intelligence

Tests of the Development of the One-Year-Old Child

seconds or more? 2. *Speech.* Can the infant say, "ba," "dada", "nana", "mama", "papa", or other combinations of two or three syllables, or will it try to repeat such syllables or words when they are spoken to it. 3. *Imitation of movements.* If a rattle is shaken in front of the infant and then placed in its hand, or if its hand is shaken while holding the rattle, will the infant repeat the movement or are there any other movements such as nodding the head, pursing the lips which it can be brought to imitate? 4. *Marking with pencil.* Will the infant try to mark on paper if given a pencil and paper, especially after seeing the examiner mark on the paper? Or, if the examiner takes the infant's hand and makes some marks with the pencil, will the infant then try to make more marks? 5. *Recognition of objects.* If several objects, such as a ball, rattle, bell, or blocks are placed before the infant, will it reach for any one of them? On repeated trials does it show a preference for any one thing rather than another? The test is passed on satisfactory evidence that the infant discriminates objects, gives undoubtable signs of the recognition of persons or shows preferences in its choice of playthings.

Tests for Age Five The tests for age five are, according to Terman's revision, as follows: 1. *Comparison of weights.* Can the child tell which is the heavier of two weights of 3 and 15 grams respectively? 2. *Naming colors.* Can the child recognize and name the four primary colors, red, yellow, blue and green? 3. *Aesthetic Comparison.* Can the child tell which is the prettier of two pictures, one depicting an ugly and the other a pretty face? 4. *Definitions, in terms of use or better.* When asked what is a chair, what is a fork, what is a doll, is he able to define these words at least in terms of use, e.g., "a chair is to sit on", "a fork is to eat with", etc. 5. *The game of patience.* Prepare two rectangular cards and divide one of them into two triangles by cutting it along one of its diagonals. The test consists in seeing if the child can put the triangles together so as to match the rectangular card. 6. *Three commissions*. If the child is told to "put a key on the chair, to shut a door and bring a box to the examiner", is he able to execute these commissions?

The tests of the ninth year are as follows: 1. *Giving the date*—the week, month, day of month and year. 2. *Arranging five weights*, identical in appearance and size and weighing 3, 6, 9, 12, and 15 grams, in order from the lightest to heaviest. 3. *Making change.* For example, "if I were to buy 4 cents worth of candy and should give the store keeper 10 cents, how much money would I get back"? 4. *Repeating four digits backwards*—6-5-2-8. 5. *Using three words in a sentence*, e.g., make a sentence which has the words "boy", "ball" and "river" in it. 6. *Finding rhymes.* Three rhymes for each word (a) day, (b) mill, (c) spring.

Tests for the Ninth Year

The last two tests of year nine depend in good part on the individual's facility in the use of language. Similarly, among the tests of the higher ages are tests of the subject's vocabulary, of his knowledge of abstract words, of the fluency of his verbal associations, of his ability to read and report on what he has read, of his ability to understand fables. There is, thus, little question but that the linguistic abilities of the subject are given a little too much weight in the general estimate of the individual's development, especially in the upper ages of the revisions of the Binet tests. Children from homes where a foreign language is spoken, or from homes of certain social levels where there is little interest in reading or where even conversation is very limited in scope are at a disadvantage in these tests. The development of their intellectual abilities may, however, be considerable, only it has taken a quite different course. This is one of the limitations of this series of tests. For this reason, other tests (of skill in performance, of practical ingenuity,

Some Limitations of the Tests

etc.) are being proposed in which linguistic and, in general, scholastic training does not play so large a part. Even a child brought up in a cultivated home may sometimes show a surprising slowness in the development of some single ability, and it is always necessary before coming to conclusions about his mental development to take cognizance of other balancing factors. A perfectly normal child may occasionally be a year or more behind the average of his age in learning to speak. This sometimes happens in the case of an only child who is brought up with adults, and has had little acquaintance with other children. Such a retardation may be made up for by subsequent acceleration when the child finally essays speech. Before this occurs his development may be better gauged by his greater skill in using his hands, in his recognition of color and form, by his knowledge of direction and locality, in his appreciation of the niceties of dress, in his social behavior, etc., etc.

Such observations simply show the need of extending in practice the fundamental ideas of Binet which have been set forth. We may now turn to some of the findings and conclusions in regard to intellectual development which have resulted from the use of these and similar tests.

What Have the Tests Discovered in Regard to the Development of the Intellect? Although the tests themselves do not supply conclusive evidence in the matter it has been customary to assume that development is more rapid in the early years, say up to the age of five, and that the increments are decreasingly less up to the time of maturity when the influence of growth, as a factor more or less separate from training, ceases. The growth curve of the average individual may be pictured by the continuous line of Fig. 1, p. 81, although there is perhaps just as good reason for representing it by the straight dotted line. In either case the first really important finding of the tests is that the majority of individuals tend to follow the same general course of development as this average. This may be illustrated by the growth curves of a superior, a normal and an inferior individual Fig. 2 p. 82, So far as the tests can determine, the superior individual is superior to start with and the inferior individual inferior at the start. This is indicated on the chart by a small space

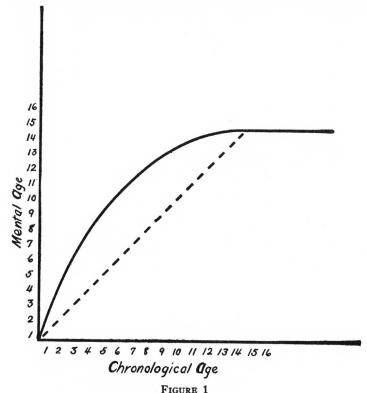

FIGURE 1

separating the beginning of the curves. The inferior individual develops at a slower rate and reaches the period of the cessation of growth at a somewhat earlier age than the average; the superior individual develops at a more rapid rate than the average and continues his development for a somewhat longer time. The characteristics and training of inferior and of superior children are discussed in detail in Chapters XIII and XIV.

**The Average
Adult
Mental Age**

It is a mooted question as to when intellectual development ceases on the average. By our present tests the increments are not measurable in the case of the average individual long after the age of fourteen or fifteen. This finding has led to much misunderstanding and controversy, and is indeed not easy to interpret. We have been

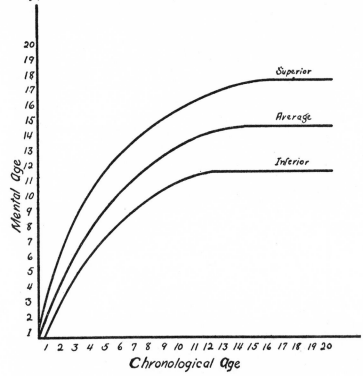

FIGURE 2

accustomed to think of the individual as developing until at least the infirmities of old age become apparent. And it is true that there may be a continuing increase in knowledge and in breadth of experience, but it appears that when the average adult is faced with numerous situations as new to him as to the fifteen-year-old, in which he has not had special training and experience, (and he cannot have had extended acquaintance in all the possible specializations of human knowledge and experience) the general level of his performance is no better than the fourteen or fifteen-year-old. However this may be, it is sufficient for the purposes of the present discussion to note that the feeble-minded do not reach the average of fourteen or fifteen years, while presumably the specially gifted or endowed may continue to develop intellectually much beyond the average period.

These differences in development are now commonly expressed in terms of the ratio of the chronological age to the mental age of the individual, the so-called "intelligence quotient," which is obtained by dividing the mental age by the chronological age of the individual, as explained further in Chapters XIII and XIV. A child of 10 with a mental age of 10 has an intelligence quotient (or IQ) of 100, a second child of the same chronological age but a mental age of 12 has an intelligence quotient of 120; a third child of age 10 and mental age 8 has an IQ of 80. Repeated tests of the same individuals have shown that the intelligence quotient tends to remain constant during the greater part of the period of growth. The special importance of this finding lies in the fact that one may predict the probable curve of development when the test is made in the early years of life. An IQ of 100 means that a child is likely to continue to grow at the average rate, one of 120 that his growth will be 20% more rapid, and an IQ of 80, 20% less rapid than the average.

The Intelligence Quotient and Its Significance

Similar facts have been discovered in regard to physical development. Repeated measurements of the same individuals have shown that the boy or girl who is taller than the average at five years of age is likely to remain taller, and the one who is shorter is likely to remain shorter than the average until at least the adolescent period. At the latter period in the case of growth in stature there may be a considerable shifting in these

Comparisons with Physical Development

relations. In how far this is true of mental development has not yet been determined. It must be noted that there are also individual exceptions to this general rule of the constancy of the intelligence quotient during the earlier years of growth. In these individuals the course of development is irregular and uneven. The reasons for these individual variations have not been sufficiently studied. Severe illness and social isolation may sometimes account for retarded development; a process of "hot housing" which is sometimes resorted to by over ambitious parents—may produce at least temporary acceleration in development. In others the cause appears to be inherent. As Cyril Burt has said in speaking of children whose growth has been retarded,— "Such children are creatures of deferred maturity. Their development is not arrested; it has been postponed. Although upon a lower plane, their mental growth runs parallel with that of many cleverer children, in whom the phenomenon is more familiar. There is many a sharp child whose cycle of growth is like that of the mulberry tree, presenting first a long delay, and then a sudden yield of flower and fruit together. Their existence is recognized in the double scholarship examination. In London at the age of thirteen a second examination has been instituted specifically for those who in the current phrase 'bloom late', and whose anticipated powers, therefore, do not ripen by the age of ten. In like fashion, among the classes for defectives, time and due season will here and there disclose a sporadic 'school autumnal'."

The Inter-relations of Mental and Physical Development In how far these peculiarities in mental development may depend on corresponding changes in the general physical or physiological development is a question, the answer to which must probably await a study of a sufficient number of individuals by means of both physical and mental tests repeated at regular intervals throughout the whole period of growth.

Such a comprehensive investigation was begun a year ago at Harvard University by the writer with the aid of a subvention of the Commonwealth Fund. Over 3000 first-grade children were examined with a series of mental, physical and scholastic tests with the intention of repeating these measurements annually on the same children or as many of them as remain in school over a period of ten or twelve years. The physical measures include height and weight and bodily proportions, dentition and ossification as shown by X-ray photographs of the carpal bones.

"Our present opinion", to quote from a recent statement of the present writer, "which may or may not be substantiated, but which is based on repeated observations on a relatively small number of individuals, is that we shall find . . . the following conditions: A child somewhat backward in mental development, whose yearly increments in mental age have been small and who on repeated examination proves to be correspondingly backward in general physiological development, may frequently make up for his slow start before he reaches maturity. The prognosis in his case would be better than in the case of a child of the same early mental level but who, at the same time, is found to be physiologically well along in the course of development. The fact that he has come on so well in general physical development in the early years without corresponding mental growth would make his prospects less hopeful. Similarly, some of our much heralded prodigies, who have rather petered out in later years, may prove to have maintained their relative superiority for a few years because of early maturing, supplemented by a kind of hot-housing."

The basis of the above expressed opinion may be illustrated by reviewing briefly the observations and test findings of two or three children whom the writer has recently described elsewhere.

Illustrative Cases

Among the cases observed in which slow or average development in the early years has been followed by rapid physical and mental development later on in the period of growth is that of a girl who at the age of 9 years and 11 months had a mental age, as determined by the intelligence tests, of 9 years and 10 months, and an intelligence quotient of 99. Three years later she attained in the tests a mental age of 17 years and 8 months and an intelligence quotient of 136,—a gain of 37 points. At the time of the first examination she was at about the 68th percentile in physical height of girls of her own age; at the end of the three years she was at the 87th percentile. The acceleration in mental development was thus accompanied by a somewhat corresponding acceleration in physical growth.

An Interesting Case. A girl who entered school at the age of six had, as a result of systematic instruction which her parents had begun when she was three years old, covered the regular work of the first four or five grades of school. She secured on examination with the general intelligence tests a mental age of between 11 and 12 years and an intelligence quotient well over 160. In a series of performance tests for which this previous coaching had not prepared her, she did but little better than children of her own age. Although physically weak, of slender build and frequently ill, there was some evidence of a certain physiological development in advance of her age which may have been in part the result of the intensive training and hot-housing to which she had been subjected. Her present superiority in the mental and scholastic tests would appear to be due in good part to these factors. If this is the case, the following are some of the possibilities in her subsequent development: (1) she "may continue her unbalanced development with a resulting freakish intellect or genius within very narrow limits; (2) the physiological changes of adolescence may be completely unsettling, with a nervous breakdown and the development of psychopathic traits; (3) the demands of general somatic development may become such that the initial acceleration in development proves purely temporary and the child settles back to the general level of mediocrity."

"A different result is indicated in the case of a boy first examined in 1918 at the age of five years and nine months. In four successive annual examinations his intelligence quotient has closely approximated 100. His parents are both of exceptional abilities, and, because of the child's general health and some suspicions of defective heart action, they have let nature take its course in the child's development. His present mental status is, it is believed, due chiefly to his native intelligence. Physical and physiological measurements and indices, including dentition and ossification, indicate slow development— a condition which may by the time of the pubertal acceleration lead to his passing well above the general average of his age. The prognosis is one which repeated measurements can alone, at present, test."

The above cases illustrate the possibilities in the current investigations of development. A further analysis of the relative influence of native endowment, physiological maturity, health and environment,—the last to include the effects of special training,—by means of repeated tests and observations of the same individuals, offers the promise of a better understanding than we now have of some of the persistent problems in the development of the intellect in childhood and youth.

The above account of the development of the intellect **Summary** in childhood and youth does not attempt to describe the many variations which may appear, nor to do justice to the complex of factors which affect the growth of the intellect. One individual may be characterized by an extraordinary plasticity or strength of memory, another be conspicuous for rare powers of imagination, and a third for an unimaginative but acutely logical mind. Further specialization of abilities may be found within these general divisions of the mind: one person's memory may be much better for some things than for others; another may reason well in mathematics and poorly in finance. These differences cannot be neglected in describing the intellectual development of any given individual; yet the fact remains that the most important recent advance in our knowledge of the growth of the intellect has come about through a method which obscures these differences by striking a balance or average of the individual's abilities to find a measure of his general intelligence. This chapter has dealt chiefly with the more significant findings as well as limitations of this method.

The chief advantage of the method is that it offers a means of viewing the intellectual development as a whole. The need of a correlative study of physical and physiological development has been pointed out above, and for many practical purposes, the study of the more strictly intellectual development must also be supplemented by and interpreted in terms of knowledge in regard to the emotional and volitional life of the individual, such as is given in other chapters of this book. It thus appears that although one's immediate concern be with the growth of the intellect, the subject is but a chapter in the study of the individual organism as a whole.

V

The Child's Moral Equipment and Development

Character Cannot be Isolated

IF OUR problem here were such a simple matter as the best diet for a normal child of given age, our study would hardly have to take account of much else. We could decide upon the proper food for the child without considering other facts about him. But the case is quite different when we are concerned with moral development. The moral nature is not something which can be understood apart from other life-problems. On the contrary, it is most intimately bound up with all that the child feels and does and thinks in every one of the many inter-related fields of his life.

In this respect, the child is no different from his elders. There was a time, for example, when scholars singled out for special study the tendency to imitate; and they told us that character was largely a matter of imitation. Yet why do we grown-ups imitate people who are unworthy of the compliment? Many answers can be given—we have never been taught any better, or we are indifferent, or we are the victims of our habits. All these reasons are bound up with others which have no distinctly moral significance. For instance, a weak will may be largely the result of poor health. But the same is true of the child. All sorts of conditions play their part in shaping his character.

Fortunately, these influences are more or less capable of control and wise direction. One such influence we may designate by the general term "knowledge". Sometimes children go wrong because the better way is un-

Knowledge, Feeling, Habit, Physical Condition, Each Plays a Part

known to them. Or even when they do know, they forget. But in recent years, the psychologists have had to remind us that it is also necessary to have the right disposition. Unless a child really wants to become the splendid type of man or woman we hope, all our holding up of heroes to admire will be of little avail. If the child does not genuinely care for the better things, it is because there are other wants which are stronger. Which desires, therefore, are more likely to be carried out? Plainly the right of way will be taken by those desires which the child is most in the habit of expressing. Hence neither feeling alone nor knowledge, but habit and practice have much to do with moral behavior. Habit alone, however, is insufficient; because bad habits must be broken; and in order to get the better ones started, there must be some sufficiently powerful incentive.

Nor must we leave out of sight the influence exercised by the condition of the child's health. Like their parents and teachers, children are less apt to be amiable and self-controlled when they are fatigued; and now the best schools and homes take every precaution to avoid unnecessary strain. Or sometimes we call a child lazy when his chief trouble may be that he is undernourished. It is a good thing that in our best juvenile courts to-day, there are psychiatrists who keep us from pronouncing the old final verdict of "bad" upon children who need neither a court nor punishment, but the attention of a physician and a nerve specialist. When we consider how difficulties in the way, for example, of a proper sex hygiene and sex morality, may be met by a careful study of the child's general health, his food, his clothing, his sleeping, his sports, the state of his nerves, we see how mistaken it is to look upon the moral nature as a single faculty sharply separated from the rest of life. There is no such thing as a distinct training in character apart from the rest of the child's development.

Our problem, therefore, is to be worked out in general along these three lines: (1) Any experiences at all which arouse distaste for what is vile and love for what is admirable, make it likely that the child will choose more wisely among the courses of conduct open to him. (2) Any knowledge which increases his understanding of human life offers a help to a sound choice. (3) Any training in persistent, resolute, efficient carrying out of sensible purposes increases the likelihood that the child's life as a whole will be effectively self-directed.

Use Every Resource

Before considering what resources his elders can bring to bear upon this development, let us look first at what the child brings on his own account. The old-fashioned training assumed that morality could be imposed from without. This was a mistake. We can force an external obedience; but a genuine character is always the outcome of what the child himself wishes at heart to do and to be. At a very early stage he already shows that he has likes, dislikes, impulses, propensities of his own. In recent years these have received close study; and thanks to the writings of such men as Hall, Barnes, Dewey, Thorndike, Freud and others, we know that, troublesome as these impulses are, they are also our best allies. Our cue is to try as far as we can not to antagonize them, but to turn them into fruitful directions. For example, many boys love to hunt squirrels or birds. A wise training will not stop with telling them that it is cruel to take life for sport but will direct the hunting tendency into a desire to get a good photograph of the wild creature, or to come close enough to make an accurate drawing, or to give a correct description at the meeting of the Scouts or the Wood-crafters. The mention of these groups suggests how another propensity, the gang spirit, instead of being combated, can be turned into the pride of membership in a club or other association where the groups work and play together in a wholesome way.

Use the Child's Natural Propensities

Here are some of the normal desires of the young which we can harness in the interests of moral growth:

Desire for Strength
1. Desire for strength: For example, a boy may not quit smoking for other reasons, but he may do so when convinced that the habit will interfere with his athletic achievements.

Desire to Earn a Living
2. Desire to earn a living: This is bound up with the self-respect and the pride in self-reliance to which many an appeal must be made.

Hero Worship
3. Hero worship: The child's first heroes are the people who perform the striking, dramatic, physical exploits. Their admiration for firemen, policemen, chauffeurs, baseball stars, can be used in the interests of courage, persistence, self-control. As they grow older, we must enrich their acquaintance with admirable types in worth-while biographies. At every stage, however, the strongest influence will be exerted by the living examples of friends, parents, teachers. It is well for parents to have frequently as their guests at home men and women of many different careers in order that the children may the better be able to choose their own careers and personalities.

Desire for Fellowship
4. Desire for fellowship: Jane Addams tells how a group of boys had infected one another with the drug habit. At the institution to which they were sent, it was at first proposed that the lads be segregated from one another; but a wiser counsel was followed, and the group spirit which had led them astray was enlisted to encourage them to work together for their cure. The love of fellowship is intertwined with many other desires. It shows itself, for example, in family pride, which may lead to the conceit of caste or, on the other hand, to a strong incentive to make good for the honor of the family name. School spirit is a familiar resource which every wise teacher employs. It should in time widen out into community spirit and into patriotism. The sacrifices

which people are willing to make for their country indicates how useful a contribution to moral nurture can be reaped from the social impulses.

5. Desire for distinction and independence: Along with the desire to be a member of a group like all other members, there is also the wish to stand out and to be one's own master. The athlete not only wants his school to excel, but he desires to be known as the one to make this possible. Individual praise is a familiar enough incentive. So is the wish to be master of one's own life. Our cue is to get the child to understand as early as possible that if we allow him freedom, it is with the expectation that he can be trusted to guide himself wisely. Teachers of history and civics have a splendid opportunity to bring home to young people the thought that freedom is good only to the extent that people use it to liberate in themselves what is most deserving of such freedom. The best kind of liberty for anyone of us is that which encourages and promotes the liberation of the highest life in our fellow-beings. *[Desire for Distinction and Independence]*

6. Desire for leadership: This is closely related to the preceding. It is good to gratify it by such methods as having the children take turns in leading games, occupying executive positions in the school-government or in otherwise directing their groups. The timid gain self-confidence; and the aggressive get the chance to work off their bullying tendencies constructively. *[Desire for Leadership]*

7. The will to power: Every game is at bottom a setting up of artificial obstacles for the sheer fun of getting the better of them, as we see in the working out of puzzles or in tennis. This propensity to make a game out of difficulties can be used to get children to do useful things that would otherwise be distasteful. It has long been used in the kindergarten. Experience there has shown that wisely directed play is the best beginning for *[The Will to Power]*

serious study. In recent years the principle has been extended into the grades.

We must beware, however, of misapplying this modern educational doctrine of Interest. It is good to have children make a game of the things they dislike to do. This does not mean, however, that they should do only the easy tasks or drop the harder ones the moment the latter become distasteful. Instead, we should use every possible means to have children go at the hard things with a hearty desire not to let the difficulty frighten them, but on the contrary, to let it serve as a challenge to the will to power. Otherwise, we shall run the danger of having them grow up morally flabby.

We have already seen how the will to power shows itself in the desire for leadership. Children can understand that to deserve to be leaders, they must train themselves.

The "combative instinct"—another expression of this tendency—should be directed into siding with causes which are just but which are as yet unpopular.

Desire for Justice 8. Desire for justice: Most people are willing to observe fair play when once they see clearly enough wherein it consists. Here, too, the earliest beginnings are laid in children's games. Normally, they appreciate readily enough what it means not to take an advantage denied to others. It is our part to cultivate still finer practices and finer understandings of just dealing. Pupil participation in the government of the school, for example, is an indispensable resource for civic training.

Benevolent Impulses 9. Benevolent impulses: Few people are born without desires to show kindness and mercy. It is good practice to get the children to begin young with the habit of considering the needs of those less fortunate than themselves. To make sure that their charities represent a genuine feeling, the objects must be people whom the children actually know to be in want. We must be on our guard against arousing these feelings too frequently without giving the children a chance to express them in acts of honest helpfulness. Otherwise we run the danger of encouraging sentimentalism.

10. Sex impulses: Capable of doing endless mischief, **Sex Impulses** these are also capable, when rightly trained and directed, of contributing much to the development of character. Chivalry is a single instance. The subject is dealt with elsewhere in this volume.[1]

11. Religious impulses: Where the religious beliefs **Religious Impulses** of the parents and the teachers are sincere, there can be no question of the stimulus they offer to worthy conduct. The same is true of the children. Search deeply enough, and at the roots of every strong character we find reverence. Whether, however, religious instruction should be given in public schools is another matter. Private institutions are free to do as they wish. But in our public schools it would seem wiser to avoid reviving the sectarian antagonisms which are likely to be aroused whenever questions of religion are broached. It is better to have all the best influences in school and community unite upon those moral teachings to which all our citizenship can subscribe with whole-hearted, unified effectiveness. The churches can make their offerings through the home, because there they are free to emphasize to the full whatever beliefs and practices they regard as most distinctive and precious. They can also reach the child through the inspiration they afford to the teachers and through their efforts, as power-houses of idealism, to encourage every spiritual influence at work in the community anywhere. The church can contribute largely in this way to worthy conduct.

All these impulses and tendencies are so intertwined that it is impossible to give a complete list which would satisfy everybody. Some educators would want us to

[1] See also Neumann, *Education for Moral Growth.*

include the parental instinct, the instinct of workmanship, self-respect, the "combative" instinct, etc. In one form or another, however, these propensities are mentioned in the list we have given. It is difficult to make a complete list.

Some Motives are of Higher Quality Than Others

Some tendencies, it is evident, represent a higher level than others. For example, it is better for a child to do things because he is convinced that they are right, than simply because he is praised by the teacher. There need, however, be no conflict here. Wise teachers will use the child's affection in order the better to cultivate his moral judgments. "Do it for my sake" is a useful appeal where the higher fails to evoke response. But it is unwise to keep the child long upon the level where this is the only incentive he accepts.

Respect the Child's Stage of Growth

In general we must beware of two extremes. One is not to direct our appeal too high above the children's heads. A child of seven cannot understand the injunction to return good for evil. To insist upon such a teaching at this stage, is to encourage him to become a hypocrite. We can be satisfied if we get the child, instead of doing injury, to drain off his impulses to anger in some harmless direction. Hyprocrisy and cant are by all means to be avoided.

Give the Higher Motives Every Chance

The other danger is that we may so frequently appeal to only the lower motives that the better ones get little chance to grow. It may be necessary for the teacher to say that the cheat will be punished if he is caught; but if the fear of punishment is the only influence upon which he calls, there is little likelihood that the child will ever grow into a being who can be trusted where punishment is not likely. We get men of honor when we treat boys as candidates for such trust. If we find that the higher appeal fails, then we must fall back for the time being on the lower. But we must never lose sight of the need to get the growth which comes only when the higher powers are given real chance for exercise. Trustworthiness grows by being trusted.

What resources from without can we bring to aid in the development of these inner tendencies?

Our leading help must be the providing of opportunities for practice. The chief influence in the forming of character is what the children themselves do. The way to learn perseverance, regularity, promptness, justice, kindness, team-spirit, initiative, responsibility, is to begin early to practice these essentials. The exercise must be secured in as large a variety of fields as possible. Promptness in attendance at school, for example, is no guarantee in itself that the child will be prompt in meeting all his engagements. Habits are in the main specific. Sometimes a habit of concentration in analyzing sentences may spread over into the work of arithmetic; but we can not always be sure that this will happen. Self-reliance in studying the textbook will not transform itself of its own accord into a habit of self-reliant willingness to side with an unpopular minority. Obviously we must try to get as much practice as possible in the latter case as well. In general, to instil needed habits, the familiar formula of William James will be found useful: (a) get a good start in a strong motive, (b) allow no lapses, (c) seize every favorable chance for practice, (d) do not rely on "don'ts" but offer a substitute for the habit to be displaced.

Character is Formed by Practice

In the cities, our schools and homes are now obliged to make provision for the forming of habits which the old-fashioned life was more likely to encourage without special thought upon the matter. In the old village days, boys and girls were expected to make things for themselves instead of buying them, to take part—and a quite responsible part—in the work about the fields,

Special Practices are Required in the Schools of To-day

the barn, the kitchen and the shop. Opportunities to start important things in this way and to gain the moral growth in holding themselves accountable for the outcome are far less open to children in cities to-day, and lamentably few for the dwellers in crowded tenements. It is for this reason that our schools, instead of confining themselves as of old to the teaching of the three R's, are more and more providing occasion through workshops, cooking classes, school-gardens, dramatic clubs, etc., for that real practice which alone can inculcate the habits needed for the building up of strong wills.

Industry, punctuality, obedience and temperance, however, are not the only kinds of habit required. Multitudes of people with these habits make the quite contented vassals of self-seeking politicians. Hence, as Professor Dewey has been telling us, the future citizens of our democracy must be trained in habits of intelligent initiative and of intelligent, free coöperation. Obedience, for example, is a virtue only when the child realizes that under certan conditions (e. g. a fire drill) instant, implicit response to orders is the best thing for himself and for his group. But a sturdy character requires that such obedience be intelligent in order that the child may not respond unthinkingly to any boss who happens to give him orders. Capacity for voluntary team-work is also needed.

Democracy Needs Training in Self-directed Group responsibility
For these reasons, it is quite fair to demand that the school make every effort to train its pupils in initiative and self-directed choice and responsibility. Children must have every wise opportunity to plan their own courses of action and to hold themselves to account for carrying these decisions out from the beginning to the end. Because they get such chances in their games, by organizing teams, for instance, accepting the responsibility for the success of their activities, deciding for themselves who is to play at this post or that, what challenges

to take or decline, they get a training in will which is not only as serviceable as that derived from obeying the school's rules to be punctual but is often more necessary. Teachers and parents will do well to study the modern "project" method for the occasions it affords for such exercise in self-direction.

Encourage Self-Reliance

Fathers and mothers know that one of the most promising moments in a child's life comes when he begs to be permitted to go on a far errand and pleads that he can be trusted. Parents find also that a steady allowance of spending money with the responsibility for its use vested in the boys and girls themselves is a better training in self-mastery than for father or mother to decide at every step whether they should buy things or not. It is easy to see why young folks reared in the strictest homes so often go wild when parental control is lifted. Untrained in the use of freedom, they abuse it when it comes later.

Provide Chance for Voluntary Coöperation

Along with the training in free self-direction, there must be practice in team-work. The best preparation for the character required for democratic citizenship is that which trains the child to take a free and real share in the responsibilities of the groups to which he belongs. This is why participation in the government of the school should be encouraged as far as possible. Even more valuable in some respects are the opportunities offered in collective enterprises whose success or failure depends entirely (as the running of the school does not) upon the children themselves. The best way to learn responsibility as a member of a group is to share in an enterprise which may go to pieces entirely unless all the members do their part. A school newspaper or a dramatic performance or any other such project, willed and put through by the children themselves, is an invaluable chance to learn how real is the responsibility of a group member to his group.

Practice Must be Enlightened

If character is to grow, the necessary practices must be guided by an understanding of their meaning. This requires an education in two directions—an increasing light upon the nature of one's choices, and a stock of ideals to inspire still better choices. We have already seen that hard tasks, otherwise disagreeable, are attacked the more cheerfully when the child appreciates what sense there is in doing them. Hence the value of an earnest, skilful, moral instruction designed to broaden and deepen the child's understanding of the excellence of right conduct.

The Best Suggestions are Concrete

Any suggestions we thus offer must be concrete. We never act out ideas of general "goodness" but always ideas of specific good deeds. "Be a good citizen at home" has a better chance of being carried into practice when the child knows that this can be translated specifically into "Go on errands for your mother cheerfully" or "Help your brother in his school-work."

The Best Suggestions are Always Constructive

Positive suggestions are better than negative. Better than "Don't giggle" is the advice "Grit your teeth". Instead of "Don't strike", recommend, "When you are angry, breathe deeply". The younger the children are, the more danger there is that holding up "horrible examples" may induce them to do the very things we are trying to prevent.

One of the chief obstacles to the child's accepting of moral instruction is his idea that morality is a life of "don'ts". The emphasis should therefore be put on the fact that the moral life is a way to reach those objects which at heart the child most deeply desires. Instead of emphasizing the harm, for example, in lying, it is better to put the chief stress on the fact that the truthful person is the one who is trusted and that he is also, in contrast with the liar, strong and brave. Moreover, emphasis upon things to avoid is likely to lead to the kind of character which does nothing more than conform to external regulation. The growing character which of its own accord does the sturdy, noble acts, is more likely to be developed by its loves than by its fears.

Suggestions come best from those who are admired or respected. The weak teacher who says that he expects his boys to behave like gentlemen is likely to be regarded as only coaxing them. A teacher who is respected will convey such a suggestion with much greater weight. The best moral teaching fails to impress unless the teacher is already held in high regard. **Those Who Offer Suggestions Must Be Admired**

The effectiveness of any moral teaching depends in a large degree upon the atmosphere at the time. Mothers, for example, find the quiet bed-time talks with their children an influence for good because at this moment there is less need for their words to struggle against the array of hostile ideas with which the mind is apt to bristle at other times. For similar reasons, the music and the address in the school assembly before the day's work begins, the church service, the atmosphere of ceremony on great occasions, all make it easier for moral teachings to be taken to heart. **Atmosphere Counts**

Modern psychologists tell us that indirect suggestions imparted in moments of mental quiet are often more influential than the most skilful direct exhortations. Say openly to a boy who is a confirmed smoker that he ought to reduce the number of his cigarettes, and it is quite probable that he will allow the counsel no admittance. Suppose, however, that he is in the workshop with his attention focussed upon the joint which he is framing. Now our chance of persuading him is better. A hint or two about the smoking while he is busy in this way may often be found to carry its point as if it had come from the lad himself instead of from outside. **Indirect Suggestions are Sometimes Better**

The many successes that are credited to the power of auto-suggestion in dealing with adults remind us that children too are more likely to work for their own better- **Trust is Essential** ment when they are encouraged to believe that such betterment is within their power to achieve. It is far better in the main to treat children with a loving trust in their better selves than to act as if we expected nothing from them but misbehavior. Trust in the better nature is absolutely essential to calling it out. Trust begets trustworthiness.

Value of Direct Moral Instruction

Should moral instruction receive a definite place in the school curriculum? The answer depends upon the teacher. Moral instruction is of the greatest usefulness where the teachers are in earnest, where they possess the necessary skill, where they see that moral instruction is only one item in the general program of moral education, and where all the moral forces in the school are called into play together. The advantages of scheduled moral instruction are: (a) the subject is given importance by having special time set aside for it; (b) it permits the teacher to bring together the results of the children's experiences and thinking in other fields; (c) it offers the chance to cultivate habits of moral thoughtfulness and to acquire standards of conduct of a higher kind than those which are merely customary.

Dangers

There are dangers which must be carefully guarded against. The subject must not be permitted to become tedious. If it is bad for children to think of science or literature with dislike because of poor teaching, it is worse for them to have such a feeling with respect to an ethical life. Wholesale introduction of courses in moral instruction everywhere is therefore not to be recommended. It is better to put the work into the hands of only those teachers who possess the necessary competence and enthusiasm. Much work is still to be done in our normal schools to train future teachers in this necessary field. In the meantime, great as the need is for moral instruction, it is better not to spoil things by poor handling.

Every subject when it is properly taught, offers something of moral value for the simple reason, mentioned at the beginning, that character is nothing isolated but the expression of all that we are. From this viewpoint, there is moral value, for example, in arithmetic in so far as sound character requires business-like methods. Let us glance here, however, at the specific contributions which each subject can offer to enlightening the moral judgments, elevating moral ideals and infusing them with power. Literature, history, civics, geography, science are especially fitted to give much.

There Are Moral Values in All of the Subjects Taught

Science is a tool by means of which the human race has attempted a better mastery over its physical surroundings. We should try to have our young people appreciate their debt to those who have made today's advantages possible. We should also want them to cultivate in their own lives the qualities of disinterested, persistent, truth-loving investigation by which the greatest scientists have been animated. Especially should we try to have them understand that science is only a tool (it may be misused and work deadly harm) and that its efforts must be constantly guided toward the elevation and the ennobling of human life.

Science-Teaching

History and civics and geography are full of moral values when they open the eyes of the children to important facts in the problem of how human beings should work out the task of living together upon this planet of ours. History is a record of certain successes in this direction and of many tragic failures. Both the triumphs and defeats should serve as inspiration to the better citizenship needed everywhere in the world to-day. It is obvious that this requires, among other things, such personal qualities as fairness, bravery, tolerance, respect for divergent excellence, coöperative spirit; and many opportunities to talk over these needs will present them-

The Social Studies

selves to the teacher who keeps in mind the best of the reasons for teaching the subjects at all.

Literature   Literature is invaluable because it deals with problems of human life in a highly interesting and beautiful manner. Sometimes characters in novels or plays are as real to young people as the actual persons whom they meet. To be as chivalrous as Gareth or Ivanhoe is often the unconscious wish of many a lad to whom the poem or the story appeals for its own sake as nothing more than an interesting tale. The cue for the teacher is to talk over these ideals in such a way that the pupils are stimulated to put their admiration into practices of their own. The old-fashioned methods made literature something to be studied, dissected, memorized. The new methods regard literature as something first of all to be loved. Otherwise any hope of spiritual value from it is quite futile.

Eliciting the moral values in the various subjects must not be understood here as a substitute for scheduled moral instruction, except in those schools where teachers are as yet unprepared for the latter work. To inform and elevate the children's ideals, every possible agency should be enlisted.

Biography   Much should be made of biographies. Nothing so quickens life as contact with life in the great souls of the race. Every subject in the curriculum has been made possible because human beings in the past have handed on these acquisitions of the human spirit. The lives of the greatest among these benefactors, in the sciences, in art, in the social and moral life of the race, should be known and reverenced. Respect for the past need not be a bar to progress. On the contrary, the truest moral progress will always be found to have its roots in a reverent appreciation of the gifts made possible by those who have gone before. We have already mentioned what the spirit of hero worship contributes to the forming of ideals.

The whole process of moral growth is shot through with feeling. Ideals are not matters of cold-blooded calculation. They are the suggestions which come out of the depths where knowledge and warm feeling are one. Hence the need for school and home and community to provide those experiences which touch the springs of feeling. Patriotic celebrations are outstanding instances of the way in which the heart is won over to the side of certain civic ideals. Other ideals can be stimulated in like manner.

Feelings
Must Be
Stirred

On this point we may quote the following from a pamphlet by Percival Chubb, issued by the Ethical Culture School of New York: "We plead for the incorporation of the festival in the regular activities of the school on the general ground that it is important to keep alive in the child those feelings of joy and gratitude, of admiration and awe, of which the festival has at all times been the expression. It is important that the child should have an imaginative sense of the great rhythms of life and the mighty presence and potencies of Earth the mother, Earth the sustainer of his life, Earth the august home of his labors. We should preserve in him, if we can, something of the child-man's responsive glow in the presence of the changes of nature—Christmas and New Year, with their returning light and length of day's; Candlemas, the old mid-winter feast; Easter, with its tribute to Flora; Thanksgiving and Harvest Home, with their grateful load of winter store. It is more important still that the child should recall continually on birthdays and death-days the great heroes and martyrs and sages to whom the race owes its priceless gifts of liberty and humanity; its inventors and voyagers and toilers, its singers and artists; as well as the great historical anniversaries and centennials which mark turning-points in man's advance along the centuries. It is by these commemorations as by nothing else that we can feed in the

Festivals
and Cere-
monials

young those emotions of admiration, reverence, and love which are the fundamental forces in education as in life. It is thus that we can develop—unconsciously, of course— that underlying consciousness of kind, of human solidarity, of coöperative unity, which may offset the crude and narrow individualism that everywhere menaces us."

Caution

In general the findings of modern study offer us both a caution and an encouragement. They warn us not to try to hurry matters by expecting of children a moral understanding beyond their years. Respect the child's stage of growth. Do not force matters. Ask instead whether the traits which we are tempted to root out immediately may not have something valuable to offer to the child's entire development and whether the worse expressions may not normally be outgrown with the years. A related caution is to beware of trusting the child's moral development to any one device or resource. Character, let it be repeated, cannot be separated from everything that the child feels, does, thinks.

Encouragement

The encouragement to be drawn from modern psychologic study is that the number of those who can be counted morally hopeless is relatively small. Even those impulses which so frequently lead to mischief offer instead a hope. They are currents of energy which we can allow to be harnessed either for good purposes or for bad. The child is neither an angel nor a demon but a being with all sorts of native propensities whose outcome is shaped by the direction in which we guide them. It is just as natural for a child's hand to shape a work of beauty or to extend a cup of blessing as to scratch and tear and maim. Everything depends upon the practice which the child receives in doing the better things, upon the inspirations he can be brought to accept, and upon the growing ethical understanding with which his mind can be enriched.

VI

THE SOCIAL TRAITS OF CHILDHOOD AND YOUTH

T HE term *Social* will be used in two senses in this chapter. It will be used to designate the primitive, crude beginnings of social consciousness and also the more fully developed trait which includes social consciousness of a high order involving altruism, morality, true citizenship and religion. The popular mind thinks of social generally in the more primitive sense. It is often assumed that when people are in groups or acting in organizations that there is always social coöperation. Nothing could be further from the truth. There may be large groups massed together as in the case of flocks of birds, herds of buffaloes, or tribes of savages, where there is mere aggregation but little of group coöperation. Such groups have doubtless assembled because of the primitive social instinct, gregariousness, but true social coöperation may be very remote. This primitive type of social trait—gregariousness—is manifested by all animal life. Children are no exception.

In this discussion a very broad definition of instinct is assumed. By instinct is meant the innate tendency of the individual to react in certain ways toward environment. Instincts are contrasted with behavior that is learned by the individual through his own experiences. Just where the one ends and the other begins is difficult to determine. Instinct as here used is almost synonymous with heredity. It consists of the fund of inborn potentialities or tendencies with which the individual starts life as a fund of capital. To be classed as instinctive, it is not necessary that actions manifest themselves at birth.

Meaning of Social

Relation of Instinct to Social Traits

Many of the most important instinctive tendencies like those of sex, morality, religion, etc., are deferred for a long time after birth. The child possesses at birth a fund of tendencies toward social reactions. These are manifested at varying times as the organism becomes mature.

Gregarious-ness Among Animals

There is a very striking tendency among animals to herd or band together. Note the familiar expressions which characterize the habits of many animals—herds of cattle, bands of sheep, herds of buffaloes, flocks of geese, swarms of bees, and nests of ants. When animals become separated from the accustomed group they give evidence of lonesomeness, even distress and grief. The way in which animals follow a leader is also well known. Among buffaloes some conqueror is always at the head of the herd, sheep follow the bell-wether, geese and ducks in their migrations are always piloted by the strongest gander, bees follow absolutely the queen bee, etc. Sir John Lubbock regards the action of ants, bees and wasps which are often combined to effect a definite result as examples of true social coöperation and involving some sort of means of communication.[1] Romanes cites instances among ants in which they carry coöperation to a high degree and says, "it is evident that they must have some means of communication. This is especially true of the Ecitons, which so strangely mimic the tactics of military organizations." He says they have officers, outposts, and scouts, besides the main armies and all act in unison. "In these mining operations the ants work with an extraordinary display of organized coöperation— the work seems to be performed by intelligent coöper- ation amongst a host of eager little creatures."[2] Romanes says that the lowest animals with definite social emotions and which recognize offspring are the hymenoptera,

[1]Lord Avebury, *Ants, Bees and Wasps.*
[2]*Mental Evolution in Man,* p. 91

including ants, bees, and wasps. He says there even is "evidence of parental affection in the care which spiders, earwigs, and sundry other insects take of their eggs and broods."[1] Jealousy, anger, and play are evident among fish. Sympathy seems to be displayed by the hymenoptera. Emulation, pride, resentment, love of ornament seem to occur among birds. Romanes believes that grief, hate, cruelty, and benevolence are displayed by cats. Revenge, resentment, and rage he ascribes to elephants and some of the monkeys. The highest social emotions manifested by animals below man are shame, remorse, deceit, and a sense of the ludicrous as displayed by dogs."[2]

Gregariousness rather than true social unity characterizes primitive groups of men. The tribe lives in communities largely unorganized. The laws and regulations are mainly monarch-made and do not represent the deliberations and contributions of the several individuals or of concerted group action. True, the group bands together for mutual protection and individual property scarcely exists. On the other hand, true communism is lacking because group effort is not exerted in property gaining and holding for the benefit of all. Naturally the mutual protection against enemies develops before organized community efforts to promote the welfare of all concerned.[3]

Similar traits are displayed by youthful gangs. Shielding and protecting are manifested before the promotion of welfare. Likewise in various labor organizations the idea of the protection of its members from predatory interests stands out prominently while the development of high standards of efficiency and service of its members and the organization as a whole is tardy in appearance. It is natural that these should be the first

Social Traits Among Primitive Peoples

---

[1]*Mental Evolution in Animals*, p. 344.
[2]*Mental Evolution in Animals*, p. 344-347.
[3]See Fiske, *Cosmic Philosophy*, Vol. II, Ch. 22.

stages. But they are only the beginning and it should be understood that they are the embryonic stages out of which the highest social traits may be unfolded.

Gregariousness in Early Childhood

Solitude is feared and shunned by all human beings. Miss Whitley has written.[1] "This desire for the presence of others shows itself in babies. Being left alone in the room will often call from the baby a cry of distress, and the adult human being seems to afford the greatest comfort to him. After babyhood, the instinct shows itself more particularly in desire for companions of the same age, though at adolescence there may be a desire for association with those older. It is true also that an adult, if left alone in a house, finds comfort in the presence of a child." With this tendency (gregariousness) as the foundation, together with the food-getting, hunting, and fighting instincts, it is easy to see how coöperation is developed; but without the gregarious instincts bringing individuals together, making their presence a satisfaction and their absence a discomfort, it is probable that the so-called social interests would have been very slow to develop.

Accentuation in Youth

The gregariousness of childhood is accentuated in youth. At this time they begin to seek their own crowd. They are eager for parties, dances, picnics, hikes, and they contrive all sorts of schemes for bringing about these occasions. Oftentimes the desire to pick their own crowds leads to clandestine meetings and they frequently run away from home to escape from the restraints that seem out of harmony with their ideals of good times and agreeable crowds. As Pringle has noted:[2] "It is a time when the adolescent feels that he and his group understand more fully and know better all that is essential to life and conduct than older people, who, as it seems to him, have lost step with the times; hence, there is a

---

[1]Norsworthy and Whitley, *The Psychology of Childhood*, p. 63.
[2]*Adolescense and High School Problems*, p. 91.

tendency for a time to be fundamentally impervious to adult influences. Fortunate is the adolescent who is surrounded by boys and girls of his age who are wholesome, enthusiastic, and right minded; when this is the case, he is quite safe, and his environment is his salvation."

Dr. Thomas Arkle Clark, Dean of Men at the University of Illinois, says:[1] "Men, young and old, are social animals. All of us like to join things. It is as difficult for me to refuse an invitation to become a member of a club or a fraternity or an organization as it is to resist the seductive talk of a book agent when he spreads his attractive wares before my eyes. I feel like a hero if I can summon the courage to turn him down. We joined church or Democratic party, I have no doubt, not so much from any strong religious or political convictions as from the fact that we were asked; we found it difficult to resist a chance to join, and we yielded. I am not arguing, however, that there is always profit in joining. Boys feel very much about joining things as men do. When they go into a high school fraternity, they are but imitating their fathers or their older brothers in college each of whom, no doubt, has his club or his fraternity." **Affiliation with Societies**

It was formerly taught by psychologists and is still believed by the popular mind that imitation is a mark of immaturity, a characteristic of children and the feeble-minded. We often hear the expression "mere imitation," describing a particularly unintelligent action. A newer view, however, regards imitation, as one of the most important modes of learning on the part of intelligent adults as well as of immature children. The one who can not imitate is uneducable; and the more imitative the more highly educable is doubtless a more correct psychological view. Childish imitation is apt to be uncritical while the trained adult's imitation is selective. The **Imitation and Social Consciousness**

---

[1]*The High School Boy*, p. 115.

important matter is to select things worthy of imitation. Some of us are apt to imitate ignoble things or things not worth while.

Beginnings of Imitation

The first apparent imitations of the babe are largely reflex movements and not conscious or purposive imitations. Tanner says,[1] "In the sixth or seventh month there are some clear cases of imitation, but even then they are relatively few, while from the ninth month on, the baby imitates all sorts of movements and sounds—combing his hair, shaving himself, sweeping, and other household tasks. By two-and-a-half years the child is into everything, imitating his elders and wanting to help in every way." Kirkpatrick says,[2] "Everything, from the crowing of the chickens to the whistle of a locomotive, from the wriggling of a snake to the preaching of a sermon, is imitated. Nothing in his environment, physical or social, escapes the child."

Adolescent Imitation

"To get an idea of imitation among adolescents, one needs only to observe any adolescent boys or girls with whom he may come in contact—their behavior in general, in school, their manner of reciting in the classroom, their actions on the street, in the home, at church, at a party, in any situation where groups are thrown together. I have frequently watched a group of high school pupils on their way to school, and have noted the same fashions in dress, in wearing the hair, and in slang expressions. If one wears an overcoat, it may be because the rest do, not because it is necessary; if one carries an umbrella, all must do so. Sometimes all ride in the street car; at other times every one walks and one would scorn to ride. Just now all carry their lunches in a crumpled paper sack folded in an approved fashion and carried in a certain way. One would stay out of school rather than carry a neat lunch box. The songs they sing, the phrases they use,

---

[1] *The Child, His Thinking, Feeling and Doing,* p. 295.
[2] *Fundamentals of Child Study,* p. 131.

the movies they attend, the shows they praise or taboo, the popular football heroes they acclaim, the things they approve or decry, all are largely the product of unstudied imitation which they have caught from the crowd.

It is usually believed that children imitate their elders, but a moment's consideration shows this to be a superficial observation. Whom do the high-schoolers imitate in their dress, their speech, their attitudes, and their prejudices? Whom do the college freshman copy? There is certainly a wide distance between the dress of the freshman and that of the professor. In the ideals espoused, the conduct followed, who are their patterns? One who knows a college campus or classroom is not misled into the wrong answer. The youth's everyday associates are the ones that slowly but surely determine his actions, his habits, his ideals."[1]

Language as a Social Development

Language has been developed solely because man is a social being. Necessity arose for communicating and understanding one another and language was invented under the stress of social necessity. No other index is so accurate of the child's social environment as his use of language. If entirely isolated from companionship, the child's language would be rudimentary and inarticulate, and many doubt whether it would develop at all. Under the stimulus of the group the child without set lessons, in an apparently haphazard, chaotic fashion acquires an astonishingly large vocabulary in a short space of time. Popular opinion greatly underrates children's vocabularies and even adults'. Even renowned scholars have made under-estimations of vocabularies, alike of children and of mature persons.

Extent of Vocabulary

We know, of course, that the business of communication of ordinary mortals is transacted with comparatively small coin. From all sides we hear a single adjective

---

[1]Bolton, *Everyday Psychology for Teachers*, p. 231.

describing every object and occurrence. A fad or craze often dictates the particular one. The words "nice," "lovely" or "beautiful" often do duty in the description of a book, a dress, a lecture or a sermon, a trip to the mountains, a picture, a character, or a piece of pie. Most people are not very discriminating in their use of modifiers. But even granting this to be true, their vocabularies are not so dwarfed as is often asserted. Their stock of substantives is frequently very much richer than we might suspect. But it is only because their stock of words is relatively small that they have been thought so insignificant. I was first led to question the current statements, relating to the extent of various persons' vocabularies, through a study of the language of children. I tabulated the vocabulary of a boy of three years and found that the number of words spontaneously used, and in a comparatively restricted environment, aggregated over twelve hundred.

This social desire for communication can be used advantageously not only in childhood but especially in adolescence when the desire to be impressive is so dominant.

Play The discussion of this important instinct as a means of utilizing other social instincts will not be developed here because of its treatment in Chapter II. Suffice it to say that it is one of the earliest manifested of the social traits and is by far the most important means of securing spontaneous expression and development of the other traits. It should be constantly in the mind of the parent and teacher in dealing with children from the kindergarten to the university.

Love of Approbation Very early in the child's life he is sensitive to the approval of those around him. Sometimes there is a bravado attitude but underneath it all approval brings intense satisfaction and disapproval stings and haunts, ofttimes even produces illness. How children hate to be blamed! And how radiant they become when commended! In early childhood it is the approval of the parent, the teacher, and other grown-ups whose praise is sought and whose blame is dreaded. Gradually, however, the sanctions of the group to which a boy or girl belongs come to be the powerful sources of motivation. "What mama and papa told me to do or not to do" is at first the inviolable law, but gradually even parents are questioned or disobeyed because of the mandates of the group. Take, for example, the code of children and youth with regard to informing on others in their group. Many a boy would sooner have his right hand cut off than be dubbed a "tattletale, tattletale!" The public opinion of the boy's or girl's world comes to be as binding as the laws of the Medes and Persians.

Miss Whitley has said,[1] "Man's attitude toward approval and scorn is part of his original equipment. By nature he is satisfied and made happy by approving looks, smiles, hand-touches of those about him felt to be equal or superior, or the admiring glances of inferiors, and he is made uncomfortable by scowls, frowns, derisive looks, and jeers. Love, respect, or admiration for those administering the approval or the disapproval, of course, intensifies its effects."

Arthur Brisbane writes in the morning paper that "Edith Schlenker, fourteen years old, tall for her age, was teased by smaller children in her school class. She stayed away from school, and her father, with good intentions, of course, scolded her severely. She jumped from the roof and killed herself. She was an only child. That short story reminds parents that it is difficult to realize the intense sensitiveness of young children."

Robinson Crusoe on a desert island had no motive for outdoing other people. His whole thought naturally

Spontaneous Rivalry

---

[1]*Psychology of Childhood* p. 66.

concerned himself. How to exist there temporarily and how to escape were his sole incentives. Man normally surrounded by his fellows, however, is stimulated to do things that others have accomplished and then to exult in outdoing them in a variety of ways. In childhood this impulse to rival and outdo others certainly is not from altruistic motives. It is sociable, but not social. Desire for praise, for satisfaction in others' discomfiture, dominate at first and may remain throughout life unless brought up to higher levels.

Rivalry is observable in children's games, in youthful contests such as baseball, shinny, skating, football, and various other sports. The same spirit may be utilized in "spelling down," in arithmetic games, learning geographical facts, and countless other schoolroom activities. Often youngsters will even overwork in their effort to outdo somebody else who may have been held up as a model.

Much exaggeration and even lying among children come from the desire to be superlative. Children feel that they must say that they can jump farther, run faster than their playmates, that their fathers are bigger, smarter, and richer than other children's. If necessary in order to be different and distinguished they can even have measles, or mortgages on their homes!

This desire to excel can be used to great educational advantage. A little judicious commendation, the arrangement of competitive games, plays, and forms of work will lend zest to their activities and yield fruitful accomplishment. Desire to excel may come to mean desire to be of most service, to carry the greatest happiness, to do the most good in the world. Self-feeling may disappear, except for the egoistic satisfaction of serving others.

Through imitation standards of conduct are developed

and spread in childhood and youth. William Dean Howells[1] has observed this with keen psychological insight and has related his observations in a highly entertaining manner. He says, "Everywhere and always the world of boys is outside of the laws that govern grown-up communities, and it has its unwritten usages, which are handed down from old to young, and perpetuated on the same level of years, and are lived into and lived out of, but are binding, through all personal vicissitudes, upon the great body of boys between six and twelve years old. No boy can violate them without losing his standing among the other boys . . . . and he cannot enter into their world without coming under them. He must do this, and must not do that; he obeys, but he does not know why, any more than the far-off savages from whom his customs seem mostly to have come. . . .

"There were some things so base that a boy could not do them; and what happened out of doors, and strictly within the boy's world, had to be kept sacredly secret among the boys. For instance, if you had been beguiled, as a little boy, into being the last in the game of snap-the-whip, and the snap sent you rolling head over heels on the hard ground, and skinned your nose and tore your trousers, you could cry from the pain without disgrace, and some of the fellows would come up and try to comfort you; but you were bound in honor not to appeal to the teacher, and you were expected to use every device to get the blood off you before you went in, and to hide the tear in your trousers. Of course, the tear and the blood could not be kept from the anxious eyes at home, but even there you were expected not to say just what boys did it."

Early in the teens boys congregate in groups. They may organize a game like marbles, baseball, football, or shinny, or may put off to the depot, or "the ol' swimmin' hole;" or they may go to the back alley or behind the

Public Opinion Among Children

Boys' Gangs

---
[1] *A Boy's Town*, Ch. 7.

barn to swap stories or to have their first smoke. Many
recent writers on the psychology of youth have paid their
respects to the boy's gang. Sheldon made a searching
study of boys' spontaneous organizations. He found that
1,139 boys had 934 societies. Similarly 911 organizations
were found among 1,145 girls. Forbush reported 862
societies among 1022 boys and Puffer who made a study
of the Lyman Industrial School for Boys found that 128
of the 146 studied belonged to gangs. The morning
paper chronicling some youthful depredation is most
certain to mention a gang or band to which an erring boy
belonged. Often the gang becomes a predatory society,
but even more often athletic clubs are organized. The
writer remembers a boxing club to which he belonged. It
met nightly in a back alley shanty during an entire winter.
It was organized because boxing had been forbidden at
school.

Swift says[1] "Gangs are the expression of primitive
tendencies. An environment incapable of draining off
these instincts into channels which make for social growth
perpetuates the racial impulses of early man. . . .
The acts in which gangs engage always have a social
content. A group may be large or small, but if the boys
have a common purpose which binds them together for
exploits and mutual protection they constitute a gang.
In the case of small boys, however, the bond of union often
breaks when they are caught. . . . The names of some
of the gangs among the inmates of the Lyman School are
suggestive of the aims and life of the lads. 'The Eggmen'
(because they robbed farmers), 'The Wharf Rats' (because
their meeting place was a wharf), 'Liners,' and 'Crooks'
are among those mentioned by Puffer." Sometimes the
name, however, is much more terrible than the activities
of the organization. The writer watched for many years
"The Dirty Dozen" which consisted of a dozen boys who

---

[1] *Youth and the Race*, pp. 246-249.

stuck together from the grammar school through high school; and now even in college and business life, about half of them still stick together. During the life of the organization the members did not smoke, swear, or commit any depredations. Every Sunday evening they went to the same church where they had fitted up a room, equipped it with cooking utensils and had their supper together, then went to the services, often appearing inattentive or irreverent, and waited for the girls at the steps. Every one later voluntarily shouldered a rifle or assumed some responsibility in the World War, two of them paying the supreme sacrifice while in the service of their country.

One of the social qualities much desired by youth and **Leadership** adults and admired by all, even by children, is that of leadership. It is possessed by different individuals in very different degrees. Even in childhood some possess natural qualities which mark them out as leaders—even in mischief. The great majority of human beings are really followers; which is a social trait and implies leaders and recognition of leadership. Doubtless most men might be leaders in something were the germs of leadership developed at the proper period.

Hero worship is very strong in children from ten to sixteen or eighteen, when they will do almost anything commended by leaders. Howells tells us[1] that the boys in "*A Boy's Town*" even looked up to not only the Whig politicians of the town, but also to some "dandies, whom their splendor in dress had given a public importance," to "certain genteel loafers, young men of good families, who hung about the principal hotel, and whom the boys believed to be fighters of singular prowess." They also even admired some professional drunkards "whom the boys regarded as the keystones, if not the cornerstones, of the social edifice."

---

[1]*A Boy's Town*, Ch. 20.

Swift has shown convincingly how it is possible to utilize the gang spirit of boys, and the same could be said of girls, in developing real leadership and the finest of loyalty to the leaders and mandates of the group. Puffer[1] has shown that leaders, even in the gang, excel in truthfulness, perseverance, bravery, reason, shrewdness, and independence. Mrs. Jacob A. Riis says she found that it was easy to convert the gang by first enlisting the fealty of the leader. Many a wise teacher had also discovered that disciplinary problems disappear when leaders in mischief are induced to array themselves on the side of the teacher.

Doll Play Undoubtedly one of the earliest manifestations of the parental instinct is in doll play. At an early age both girls and boys play constantly with dolls. Boys give up this play earlier than girls because of traditional attitudes of those around them toward doll play. Sully[2] writes that boys "not infrequently go through a stage of doll love also, and are hardly less devoted than girls." According to Miss Tanner[3] "The love of dolls appears to reach its height in the ninth year although strong from the third year to the twelfth. Many girls play with dolls until they go into long dresses and are ridiculed for their love of it; and not a few ladies confess to the existence of the passion." Dr. Hall believes that doll play is not wholly an evidence of the parental instinct but partly due to fetishism and religion. Sir John Lubbock also says[4] that the doll is "a hybrid between the baby and the fetish."

Hall has said[5] in his classic study of dolls: "The educational value of dolls is enormous. . . . It educates the heart and will, even more than the intellect, and to learn how to control and apply doll play will be to discover a new instrument in education of the very highest potency. Every parent and every teacher who can deal with individ-

[1]*The Boy and His Gang.*
[2]*Studies of Childhood*, p. 43.
[3]*The Child, His Thinking, Feeling and Doing*, p. 405.
[4]*Origin of Civilization*, p. 521.
[5]*Aspects of Child Life and Education*, p. 194.

uals at all should study the doll habits of each child, now discouraging and repressing, now stimulating by hint or suggestion."

Gradually the parental instinct develops and shows itself in the care for children, although in boys it appears to be almost entirely suppressed during the years when they are most influenced by the gang spirit. With the onset of adolescence the sex instinct matures with astonishing rapidity, becoming often an almost overmastering passion of the lower animal type. Sometimes gradually, sometimes almost in a flash the emotion of love for the other sex appears, and if there is fortunate choice in the object of affection the emotion becomes one of the tenderest and most altruistic in human life. King[1] in referring to this characteristic as a part of the adolescent "birth of a new self," has selected an apt quotation from Margaret Deland, which is here reproduced:

Appearance of Sex Attraction

"Elizabeth's long braids had been always attractive to the masculine eye; they had suggested jokes about pigtails, and much of that peculiar humor so pleasing to the young male; but the summer she 'put up her hair,' the puppies, so to speak, got their eyes open. When the boys saw those soft plaits, no longer hanging within easy reach of a rude and teasing hand, but folded around her head behind her little ears; when they saw the small curls breaking over and through the brown braids of spun silk, clustering in the nape of her neck; when David and Blair saw these things . . . something below the artless brutality of the boys' sense of humor was touched. They took abruptly their first perilous step out of boyhood. Of course they did not know it. . . . The significant moment came one afternoon when they all went out to the tollhouse for ice cream. . . . As they sat eating their cream together, Blair suddenly saw the sunshine sparkle in

[1]*The High School Age,* p. 98.

Elizabeth's hair and his spoon paused midway to his lips. 'Oh, say, isn't Elizabeth's hair nice?' he said. David turned and looked at it, 'I've seen lots of girls with hair like that,' he said; but he sighed and scratched his left ankle with his right foot. Blair, smiling to himself, put out a hesitating finger and touched a shimmering curl; upon which Elizabeth ducked and laughed, and dancing over to the old tin pan of a piano pounded out 'Shoo fly' with one finger. Blair, watching the lovely color in her cheek, said in honest delight, 'When your face gets red like that you are awfully good looking, Elizabeth.'

" 'Good looking,' that was a new idea to the four friends. Nannie gaped; Elizabeth giggled; David 'got red' on his own account and muttered under his breath. But into Blair's face had come, suddenly, a new expression; his eyes smiled vaguely; he came sidling over to Elizabeth and stood beside her, sighing deeply: 'Elizabeth, you are an awful nice girl.' Elizabeth shrieked with laughter, 'Listen to Blair, he's spoony!'

"Instantly Blair was angry; 'spooniness' vanished in a flash; he did not speak for fully five minutes." They presently started home, "but," says Mrs. Deland, with keen insight into the nature of youth, "childhood for all of them ended that afternoon."

Objectives in Sex Education   The great objective in sex education should be parenthood and family life in its highest and holiest relations. In general the higher the sex development, judged from the standpoint of true social or altruistic traits, the more the lower sex instincts have been brought under control and removed from consciousness. Irradiation of the lower into the higher channels of love, altruism, religion, etc., are the important objectives. The attention should be drawn away from direct sex emotions by activities, physical and mental, that shall develop what appear to be unrelated to sex, but in reality are intimately related to sex attraction and survival. The development of athletic prowess, bravery, chivalry, pride in dress, adornment, care of young, pride in family, skill in music and art, care for the weak or unfortunate, missionary zeal, religion, all are part of the psychic urge to develop and perpetuate one's own idealized life. They are all direct outgrowths of the parental instinct which in turn is directly related to sex.

John Fiske[1] has called attention to the fact the parental instinct is the basis of all morality. With the increased length of human infancy due to the helplessness of human young, parental care and solicitude became necessary. Even among the higher animals "the period of infancy is correlated with the feelings of parental affection, sometimes confined to the mother, but often shared by the father, as in the case of animals which mate. Where, as among the lower animals, there is no infancy, there is no parental affection. Where the infancy is very short, the parental feeling, though intense while it lasts, presently disappears and the offspring cease to be distinguished from strangers of the same species. . . . The prolonged helplessness of the offspring must keep the parents together for longer and longer periods in successive epochs; and when at last the association is so long kept up that the older children are growing mature while the younger ones need protection, the family relations begin to become permanent." Out of this germinal social consciousness there gradually develop sympathy, love, and altruism extending beyond the family to the tribe or clan, to the village, city, state, nation—all humanity.

Relation of Parental Instinct to Altruism and Religion

In addition to the belief in and reverence for a supreme being and wonder regarding origins and ends, religion is fundamentally social. It involves a love for one's fellows and a desire to be of service to them. Religious awakening is not characteristic of the little child. The child

[1] *Cosmic Philosophy*, Vol. II, p. 343.

is ego-centric. His love is more apparent than real. He may be affectionate for the purpose of receiving something in return. We know the traditional story of the little boy "so very good, just before Christmas!"

The Religious Instinct and Its Expression
But with the onset of adolescence the germs of true religious life evidence an awakening. Starbuck[1] has shown by a survey of thousands of cases that the great majority of religious conversions take place during the ages from fourteen to twenty. A few occur earlier and a few later but adolescence is the great birthday of religious emotions. These find expression not only in various forms of worship, including song, prayer, ceremony but also in the expression of love toward other persons, missionary zeal, and altruism toward all mankind. If not then exercised they are liable to become stunted and dwarfed. If properly encouraged in the normal individual there is the succession of "first the blade, then the ear, then the full corn in the ear." It is well to teach the young to "Remember thy Creator in the days of thy youth."

Educational Suggestions
To prepare for the responsibilities of adult citizenship the child and the youth must have opportunity to learn through actual participation in some of the activities of citizenship. These should not be make-believe activities nor exercises devised as practice courses. They should be natural activities arising out of every-day situations in connection with the youth's world. There are all sorts of real work that occur in connection with the home, the school, the church, and civic enterprises. The most important of these in which group action can be employed are obviously in the school.

Feeling of Joint Ownership
The most fundamental fact the child can be taught in the school—more important than arithmetic, Latin or book-keeping—is that he is a part owner of the school and that he is not only to share in its benefits and privileges, but more significant, in its responsibilities. He must be

[1] *Psychology of Religion.*

led to a feeling of responsibility through being given an opportunity to exercise his instinct for ownership through participation. The *machinery* of student government is unimportant, sometimes even a hindrance—the *spirit*, the *attitude* is everything. The opportunity for participation should include coöperation in the management of the school paper, the various forms of athletic organizations, the literary society, the school play, the debating club, school parties and picnics and numerous other forms of recreation and amusement. These are forms of coöperative organization into which the pupils easily enter and participate. They pertain directly to youthful interests and enterprises. But these should be only the beginning. Through these they may be enlisted in group participation in activities more directly related to the welfare of the school. Out of the development thus secured and the training in coöperation gained they will have acquired confidence and strength for wider enterprises. They need to be helped to understand their relations to an organization in which the personal benefits are not quite so readily understood. This is the next step toward understanding their relation to the city, State nation—the world.

Dewey has exemplified this in his exposition of the idea that "Education is life!" He deplores school activities arranged purely as school exercises. Every activity in the school should have real significance in the child's own life.[1]

While group activity should be encouraged a caution should be suggested. Many pupils become helpless because others stand ready to do all their thinking for them. Some become lazy because they find they can shift all their work to others who readily shoulder all responsibilities. It is just as in adult communities and organizations; the few who can and will do the work and

Coöperation Alone Not Necessarily Ethical

[1]See his *School and Society* and *Schools of To-Morrow*.

shoulder responsibility are allowed to do it. Still others use the group as a crutch to lean on. They become dependent and never tackle a thing independently and vigorously. To be able to work in solitude without props or crutches for the purpose of mastery and for the ultimate welfare of the group is just as important in adult society as is group participation. The good citizen must learn to do his part whether it be destroying weeds in his own fence corners or participation in a plumed parade where the multitudes will applaud. Is there not a serious lack in citizenship of this very quality of keeping one's own back yard clear of weeds? Neumann says,[1] "Coöperation in itself is not necessarily ethical. Everything depends upon its objectives. School life should be organized around the idea, not that each student is to do his utmost to get a better mark than his neighbor, but that all are expected to make a free offering of their best to the progress of the class and the school as a whole and, through these, of the larger community." Bearing this in mind, let us consider a few typical instances of the resources at our command.

Utilize the Gang Spirit Judge Lindsay has succeeded to a wonderful degree in utilizing the gang spirit in the development of better citizenship in the youth of the slums. He says,[2] "In a certain suburb of Denver, where the smelters are located and there are a great many cheap saloons selling bad liquor and tobacco to children, two celebrated gangs brought to the juvenile court for dangerous forms of rowdyism and lawlessness not only completely suppressed every serious objectionable feature among themselves, but also went after the men who were selling liquor and tobacco to boys. They prosecuted and sent several to jail, and did more to stop the use of tobacco and liquor among boys in that neighborhood than the police department or civil authorities had done in the history of the

---

[1]*Education for Moral Growth*, p. 204.
[2]*The Problem of the Children*, Report of the Juvenile Court of Denver, 1904, p. 107.

town." Swift adds:[1] "The members of the same gangs also prosecuted men for selling firearms to children, for purchasing stolen property, and for circulating obscene literature. Yet these were the lads who had been making the trouble in that neighborhood, who had been stealing the property which the junk dealers bought, and who were among the customers for the firearms and immoral literature.

If a gang can be made to suppress its own lawlessness and become the protectors of those upon whom it has been preying, what limit is there to the utilization of its enthusiasm and its spirit? This suppression of lawlessness, however, was not accomplished by violating the ethics of the gang, but rather by giving to these impulses a more universal social outlet. And this, after all, is what constitutes moral training. The gang is a close social corporation. The action of its members toward one another is often exemplary. Kindness, truthfulness, and helpfulness would leave little to be desired, if these virtues were not so narrowly restricted in their application. But outsiders are not included among the beneficiaries. Now, it is the extension of the point of view of the gang— the enlargement of its membership to include the greater social group which has been shut out and classed among its enemies—that is the first task of those engaged in training boys. When this is accomplished a large proportion of the school troubles disappear because they have originated in the traditional opposition of the school-master to the impulses which have all the sanction of racial passion."

In one public school in New York, the pupils contribute their help in the following ways:[2]

Illustrations From School Activities

"Do all kinds of clerical work: mimeographing, multigraphing, typing reports, act as secretaries to grade advisers and chairmen. Serve as messengers. Do

[1] *Youth and the Race*, pp. 272-274.
[2] See Annual Reports of the Superintendent of Schools, 1920-22, "High Schools," Board of Education, New York, p. 16.

printing for school. Assist weaker pupils in scholarship. Operate the telephone switchboard. Operate the school bank under the supervision of a teacher. Edit three school publications under the teachers' supervision. Build equipment for school (typewriter desks, fire-drill signs). Operate motion-picture machine. Aid in community activities: charity organizations, hospitals, city departments (block captains). Supervise lunch rooms. Supervise movements of pupils entering and leaving building, and passing through corridors. Patrol corridors during the day. Receive visitors. Make sanitary inspections of building. Take charge of classes when teachers are absent and substitutes cannot be obtained. Handle minor cases of discipline between pupils."

John A. Tildsley, District Superintendent for High Schools, New York City, writing on the question "Are Our Schools Successfully Preparing for Citizenship?"[1] says, "In our plan of training for citizenship, we enlist all school activities. We do not favor the school city nor any artificial self-government plan. We hold that the best form of student self-government is the government of each pupil by himself. To this end we are opposed to all rules for rules' sake. That is, we believe that no rule should ever be promulgated unless at the same time with the rule the reason therefor is also announced, the only valid reason being the possibility of better living conditions for the student himself. We favor the development of qualities of leadership, of the ability to govern others, of the creation of a coöperative spirit through the delegation to service squads and kindred organizations of actual tasks which need to be performed. With the task we delegate the authority needed for the performance of the task.

"Do we realize the aims we have set forth, such as the creation of a right attitude?—the government of each individual by himself?

---

[1] *School and Society*, Dec. 22, 1923.

"I have known a school in which on the first day of the term, with 3,800 pupils in the building, of whom 1,000 were there for the first time, every teacher has been at a faculty meeting from 9 to 10 A.M. and not a sign of disorder anywhere in the building! Is this successful training for citizenship?

"A civics teacher in Brooklyn noticed that the trees in the Bay Ridge section were in danger of destruction from bagworms. A crusade against these worms was instituted among her pupils. Over 50,000 worms were brought to the school to be burned and many trees were saved.

"As a practical application of our citizenship training, over 9,000 pupils are acting as block captains, coöperating with the street cleaning department in its anti-litter campaign.

"Two winters ago, during the Christmas vacation, at a time of heavy snowfall, several hundred of our high school boys, as a civic service, shovelled snow for several days and did far more work than the regular force—and so I might multiply examples.

"Seemingly we are realizing our aim, the creation of a state of mind. The question we can not answer yet is as to its abiding nature.

"A citizenship which shall save the State needs for most people what is almost a regeneration, a more enlightened self-interest, a habit of surveying problems, as something objective to one's self, of seeing with eyes undimmed by self-interest. The task is too great, too large to be accomplished in one generation. But in my judgment it is incumbent upon us school men to undertake the task, to carry on and leave the issue with the gods. The State is endangered. Only the schools can save it, and they by conscious, intelligent effort."

The term "social" is used in two senses (a) meaning Summary sociable or gregarious, and (b) meaning altruistic or concerned for the welfare of others. Even the lower animals and savages are gregarious in their habits. Children have instinctive tendencies toward the manifestation of social traits. These tendencies appear at first in the cruder form and only rather late in adolescence develop into the higher states. To join organizations, if only a gang, is perfectly natural and should be utilized as the starting point in the development of altruism.

Imitation, formerly thought to be a mark of immaturity, is one of the most important means of acquiring the ways of the group. The child should be helped to imitate the best in social groups and in literature, instead of that which lowers and degrades. The most important period of imitation is adolescence. Language is the common bond of the group, and would never have developed but for the social traits. Play is a fundamental instinct and furnishes the incentive to the acquisition of all that is deemed worth while by childhood. Through imitation and play the child comes to value the affection of his elders and those in his own group. Approbation and disapprobation are powerful factors in determining conduct. Howells in *A Boy's Town* has analyzed this social trait keenly and portrayed it strikingly. Rivalry is instinctive and should be used purposively in stimulating to desirable effort and achievement.

The gang, so naturally formed, may be made the nucleus of the finest kind of social coöperation. Leadership here, as everywhere, is admired and followed. The gang may be used to develop desirable leadership and also to secure coöperation in worthy enterprises. Gangs frequently excel in and praise loyalty, perseverance, courage, bravery, generosity, truthfulness, shrewdness, as well as some qualities less desirable. Enlist the leaders in worthy enterprises and the gang will follow.

The higher forms of altruism, love, care for the weak and unfortunate, morality, reverence, religion, all have sprung from the social instinct of parenthood. Fiske says, "Even civilization would have been impossible without the development of the family."

To secure the fullest fruition of the social traits, it is necessary to understand their instinctive beginnings, to recognize their periods of nascency, and then to develop them through actual participation in enterprises that are founded upon expression of the most worth-while instincts. Such opportunities are abundant in the home, the school, the church, and in real life.

VII

The Child's Mastery of the Arts of Expression—Language, Drawing, and Music

General Truths of Learning and Habit Formation

MAN is a changing organism. In a machine, if two wheels are connected by belt or cogs, when one turns, the other turns. In man, two nerve centers that are not connected in their action in any way, become connected, if they are active together or in immediate succession. A child may hear a gun many times, and at other times see it, without there being any connection between the two experiences, but if he sees a gun as it is fired, then ever afterward the sound of a gun will make him think of its looks, or the sight of it will make him recall the sound it makes. The visual cells concerned in seeing the gun are now excited by the auditory cells concerned in hearing it, as surely as one wheel moves another with which it is connected by a belt. All learning depends upon this fundamental truth—that brain processes that occur together tend to excite each other. From birth till old age such connections are being formed, and thus memory, learning, and acquired motor skill are possible. Infinite numbers of connections are formed in the first few years of life.

Laws of Association

Many of these connections are repeated countless times, and the more times any two sets of nerve cells are excited together or one excites the other, the more close and sure is the connection. This is the *law of frequency*. The first connection of the two processes has the greatest effect. This the *law of primacy*. If only a short time elapses between repetitions, the connection remains strong. This is the *law of recency*. If the processes are intense and concentrated, the effect of repetition is greater. This is the *law of intensity*.

If the results of the last of the two processes are pleasureable, this process will again readily be excited by the first, but if unsatisfactory it will be replaced by some other. A cat that jumps for some meat and gets it, repeats the act, but the one that does not get it and gets slapped, runs away. This is the *law of satisfaction and dissatisfaction*.

Upon these laws depend all the law and the prophets of learning and education. The certainty with which the sound of the word "dog" will call up the visual image of the written or printed word, "dog," depends upon the frequency with which the processes of hearing and seeing them have occurred together or in succession, the intensity of the processes, their recency, the accuracy of their first association (e. g. the sound "dog" unconfused with similar sounds such as "log," "bog," "fog,") and finally the satisfactoriness of the results in the way of feelings of success, approval, etc. Of all these laws the most fundamental is that of frequency or number of repetitions, hence the value and universality of drill exercises. Yet the best teacher is the one who economizes time and energy by substituting intensity of activity and satisfactoriness of results in a few repetitions, for the many repetitions of the unskilled teacher, utilizing only the law of repetition.

The connections between processes or ideas are formed in accordance with the previous laws but this is not the whole story. The processes being connected are themselves becoming different. Often they are at first indefinite and mingled with other processes, but gradually become more and more definite and precise. The sound of *o* is the more prominent when the child first hears the word "dog." Later the *g* and *d* sounds are distinguished and discriminated as different from other consonant

Changes During the Learning Process

sounds. In a similar way the visual word "dog," short in length and with the first part above and the last going below the middle, is more precisely seen as a word composed of three letters, each of a special form, different from any other letters. As the oral and visual words become more firmly associated, the processes of hearing and seeing them become more and more definite and clearly different from similar processes concerned with the other words. Learning is, therefore, not merely a connecting of processes in accordance with the laws previously stated, but it frequently involves very great changes in the processes that are being linked together by frequent repetitions so that they take place more quickly and accurately.

Three Stages in Process of Learning and Habit Formation There are three stages in the process of learning and habit formation. The first stage is that of learning, in the sense of getting the processes to become prominent enough to be recognized and to make repetitions possible. The second stage is that of making the processes more definite and getting them more closely linked with each other. The third stage is that of habit fixing in which there are no longer changes in the way in which the processes take place, but only an increasing certainty that when one takes place, the other will follow and that the activities will always be performed in the way in which they have been most practiced.

These stages are partly indicated in the curves of learning showing the results of experiments in learning by men and animals. The curves usually go up sharply at first, then more gradually and if the practice is continued long enough, improvement ceases, as indicated by the curve becoming horizontal.

The increase in speed is accounted for by (a) elimination of short pauses between; (b) omitting useless movement and finding better methods; (c) imaging less completely what is to be done; (d) overlapping of

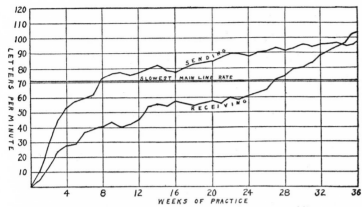

These curves show the improvement of one man while learning telegraphy.

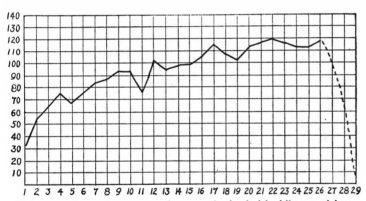

This curve shows the progress of a normal school girl while practicing five-one minute periods a day for five days.

processes, as in reading, when the eyes are several words ahead of the tongue; (e) some increase in speed of movements. The limit of speed at first is usually the rate at which one can think how to do the thing, while in the last stage it is the rate at which the motions can be executed.

When the rate and accuracy cease changing, the mode of doing varies but little and further practice fixes it and makes it so mechanical that it is difficult to change the way of doing and only by constant effort can greater speed and accuracy be secured, even temporarily. This fixing may take place long before the best methods and highest possible skill have been developed. The closer to the limit of possible improvement, the harder it is to fix the habit at that stage, for as soon as less conscious effort is made, there is a drop in performance. For practical purposes it is therefore often best not to try to push speed and accuracy to the highest limit, while for artistic purposes the effort to improve should never cease.

In practice, after the stage of learning how has been passed, there is always more than zero ability at the beginning. The one who has had the most practice of a similar kind or is most fortunate in hitting on a good method of procedure, will do better at first but may not end better, than one who starts with a poorer record. Children and beginners in any line generally improve faster than those who have had a moderate amount of practice, because they are in an earlier stage of learning.

Sometimes there are plateaus or even declines in the curves of learning—times when the individual seems to make no progress forward and may even go backward. This is often seen when a new and better method is tried, as when one advances in typewriting or telegraphy from writing by letters to writing by words, or from writing by words to writing by clauses or sentences, or a tennis player tries a new form of service. The change may be a good one, but efficiency may be less till better control is obtained.

Irregularity when one has nearly reached his limit is often due to variations in conscious effort and to the coming on of fatigue.

Speed Versus Accuracy In experiments in learning, several other truths have been discovered. If timing and records of amount done, lead all to try for speed, then all gain in speed, but many decline in accuracy. When told that only perfect work will be counted, all try for accuracy or perfection of form and improve in that respect, but for a time fall off in speed. This shows that the mental attitude while practicing determines the kind of an improvement made.

An experiment in learning to typewrite showed that when one division of a class practiced for speed at first and the other for accuracy, the first students gained rapidly in speed but soon reached their limit because of errors, while the others gained in accuracy first, then continued to gain speed till they were ahead of the other division in both respects. This gives the general rule that in all learning, speed should be sought, if at all, after the correct and accurate way of doing has been assured.

Some recent experiments have shown that if a class is divided into two sections, and section A is informed of the score made each time, while section B is not, the first section improves much more rapidly. If a change is made and pupils of section B are given their score while pupils of section A are kept ignorant of their score, then section B gains in speed while section A becomes slower. This is probably due in part to the fact that knowledge of improvement causes satisfaction and thus increases the effect of the repetitions. It is therefore very important that children should be given some means of seeing their own improvement in whatever they are learning. Praise or a teacher's marking is a partial but not complete substitute for one's own perception of success.

Knowledge of Results

This has been very clearly shown in a code experiment by asking a class when they had about finished the second stage of learning a set of number symbols, to use them in working a problem in multiplication instead of merely writing the symbols in order as they had been doing. It was found that very little improvement in using the code had come from writing it in order, since some who had practiced it only a few minutes in order could use it in the problem as well as those who had practiced it in order twenty-five minutes. From this it was learned that one improves in doing what he practices, chiefly in doing it in the same way and under the same conditions, and only

Results of Practice are Special rather than General

slightly, in doing the same or similar things in similar ways or under similar conditions.

It was decided that most practice should consist of doing what is practiced in the way in which one is going to use it and under the same conditions. If the thing being learned, however, is complex and difficult, then it will pay to practice it in the easiest way until it can be done properly. Much time is often wasted in school by practicing things for long periods of time in a different way from that in which they are to be used, e.g., practicing tables in addition and multiplication, instead of using the knowledge of combinations, as soon as a few are learned, in working problems.

Chance, Imitation and Ideas   When one tries to solve a puzzle, such as tracing a maze, or putting cut-out forms together, or tracing a star seen in the mirror, or reducing five squares to three in the following diagram by removing only three of the fifteen

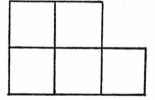

matches, he is likely to make a great many trial movements or images of movements before succeeding. The same is true in trying to learn the pronunciation of a new sounding word. If one can hear another pronounce the word he can learn with fewer trials. Directions as to how to do a new thing also help in shortening the time of learning, provided the right directions are given at the right time.

Extensive observation and experiment show that trial movements resulting sooner or later in success, and attempted repetition of the satisfactory movement is the most universal method of procedure in the first stage of the learning process.

A cat confined in a box from which he can escape by turning a button in the door, scratches and pushes in various places till the button is turned and he gets out. When put in again he is likely to do most of his scratching near the button and gets out with fewer motions. After a number of experiences he omits all the movements save those that turn the button and he gets out at once. In a similar way, a turtle, a pigeon, a rat, a dog, or a man learns to find his way through a maze in which there are many blind alleys. Most animals have no other way of learning new things. A cat is not at all helped by seeing another cat get out of a box. In other words it cannot learn how to get out by watching another animal turn the button. A child or man learns much more rapidly when he has such a chance to imitate.

It is also possible to give directions to persons as to how to get out or to find their way over a new route, and they can often learn by this *ideational* method without trial and error practice, but no animal can be taught anything new by the ideational method. In the case of man, movements involving new coördinations may be learned, in the sense of gaining an idea of how they should be made, by imitation and direction, but skill in execution is gained only by trial and increased approximation to accuracy. By hearing instructions as to how to stand, grasp the club, swing it, and so forth, and by watching others do it, one can begin the first stage of learning to play golf, but to complete that stage and pass well into the second stage of accuracy in driving, requires the use of the trial and success method. The same is true of skill in every accomplishment. Receiving directions and having opportunities to imitate, make fewer trials necessary but cannot bring success without some use of the more fundamental method of becoming accurate by a series of approximating trials. In the course of these trials one is guided usually by visual or auditory images but success is not reached until one gets the muscular feel of the correct movements.

Language and other forms of expression are learned by processes similar to those already described. In all of them, while being acquired, motor coördinations are important. Consciousness of how movements are being made is necessary but good training results in making purely mechanical the movements used in expressing ideas.

Since only the English language will here be considered, it may seem as if this title were wrong, but it is not. The child who learns English only, has four languages to acquire. (1) He has to learn to distinguish the sounds and to understand the meaning of oral words. (2) He has to learn to move his vocal organs so as to say oral words. (3) He learns in school to distinguish visual words and usually also to associate the visual forms with the oral forms and with the ideas for which they stand. (4) He has to learn to control his hand in producing visual words similar to, but not the same as, those he has learned in reading, and to use the conventional signs such as capitals, periods, question marks, commas, etc. These four languages are distinct, but are nearly always learned in pairs—one and two, and three and four being acquired at about the same time.

The first of each pair is concerned with understanding other people and the second of each pair involves motor acts producing words understood by others. All four languages become closely associated so that it is easy to translate one language into the other and often difficult not to do so; so that, when reading, many persons have a strong tendency to think and say the corresponding oral words.

This language is learned before the child goes to school. The discrimination of oral words develops first, followed and accompanied by learning the movements necessary in speaking them. Some children successfully perceive and learn to imitate them before they know their significance. Such children sometimes become as skilful as parrots in imitating words and phrases and with no more idea of their meaning. Other children learn the significance of words as soon as they distinguish them, but it may be a long time before they are able to control their vocal organs in uttering the words.

Various factors enter into this process of learning to control the organs of speech. The child starts life with (a) a few instinctively produced sounds; (b) he makes many others by more or less chance movements; (c) he repeats many of these sounds in a playful way (uses his vocal organs as playthings, sometimes as early as at the sixth month); (d) he imitates (at nine to fifteen months) various sounds including words, in a more or less playful way; (e) he voluntarily repeats words that he hears, at twelve to twenty months, usually with the purpose, then or later, of expressing his wants; (f) he learns to group these words more or less correctly into phrases, clauses, and sentences, usually omitting those that are to him unimportant.

At two years of age most children have acquired the art of vocal expression or, as is usually said, "have learned to talk." Some at this age use scarcely a score of words intelligently and intelligibly, while others control a vocabulary of ten or twelve hundred words. A vocabulary of from two to four hundred words is usual.

The pronunciation of these words remains more or less childish till three or four years of age. If there is little variation in the pronunciation of words which the child hears during the first ten years, his style of pronunciation becomes pretty well fixed and radical changes are not easily made later, although up until the age of twenty, some differences will result if a Westerner moves East, or a Southerner moves North and stays for a few years.

Even if he does not know it, his friends will notice a change when .he returns home. A foreign language learned after the age of twenty is practically always spoken with an accent. Children of foreign parentage often speak much better English if their parents do not speak English at all, than when they do. The child who hears good English in school and no English at home will speak much more correctly than one who hears poor English at home. No matter how well he may be taught the correct sounds, his habits will be influenced by the pronunciation that he hears most frequently.

Even in the homes of native Americans, a child sometimes acquires habits of incorrect speech because of hasty clipping of words and indistinctness of articulation by adults. The child is often worse than the parent, not only because, like the parent, he is hasty and careless, but because he has never learned to distinguish the correct sounds of words; e.g., a boy of twelve in a cultured home had not distinguished between the oral words "coal" and "cold" and used the latter to indicate what is burned in a furnace.

One who is interested in developing good pronunciation in a child must bear in mind the general principles of learning previously stated and carefully distinguish the stage of learning that the child has reached in pronouncing any word. In the first stage the child should learn what the exact sound of a word is, but he often practices the word before he knows just what its sounds are. During this period great care in pronouncing words in the presence of the child should be exercised that he may learn the right sounds. After he has the correct idea of the sounds, his early attempts to speak words will be more or less variable, as is always the case during the habit-forming stage. So long as the pronunciation varies and approximates the correct sound, there is no need for worry; but when the pronunciation begins to become uniform, the

142

habit-fixing stage is being entered, and if the sounds are not uttered correctly, pains should be taken to induce closer approximation to the right form. If, after this, the child hears a good deal of wrong pronunciation, care must be taken that the habit of correct pronunciation is kept fixed. This is less difficult if he hears words pronounced in various incorrect ways than if he hears one wrong pronunciation more frequently than any other.

The value of phonics consists in giving the child a clearer idea of the real sounds in words he is learning to use. The habits of pronouncing words are formed and fixed by speaking words as wholes and not by practicing the separate sounds, because the speaking of sounds in word combinations is an entirely different motor process from uttering them separately, e.g., "Three tall, slick, slim saplings" is difficult of utterance, not because the various phonetic elements are hard, but because this combination of them is difficult to pronounce.

Many changes in methods of teaching writing have taken place. A hundred years ago it was taught more as a fine art than as a means of visual expression, and artistic flourishes and shadings were much used. Later the idea of writing legibly and rapidly became more prominent. A half century ago the method of learning to write by special practice was carried to an extreme. The practice was also not so much to acquire a certain kind of movement as to secure the making of certain forms. In the Spencerian system there were only seven distinctly different elements,—straight line, right curve, left curve, loop, oval, reversed oval, and capital stem,—and there was much separate practice of each of these at a certain angle. So strongly was it believed that practice of these separate elements would make good writers that less than forty years ago a superintendent stated in an educational magazine that he would have a pupil practice one of these elements for a year, if that were necessary in order

Learning Visual Expression or Writing

to get him to make it perfectly. Few teachers were so extreme as this, but it took a good while for teachers to learn that the coördination of movements involved in making the elements separately is quite different from those involved in making them when combined into words. Most of the time spent in this separate practice was wasted. A few minutes of it helped in the first stage of getting a more perfect idea of letter forms, but further practice was of no value in learning to combine writing movements as required in writing words.

About this time it was discovered that the position of paper and body were important conditions favoring good writing, and vertical writing had considerable vogue. Later other systems were developed and the chief emphasis was placed upon the kind of movements made. Children were not allowed (during the writing lesson) to use whole arm or finger movements. This gaining of free, easy forearm movements is now given most attention in penmanship lessons. Great improvement has been made in the teaching of writing under the direction of special teachers, but the results are still unsatisfactory. Some of the reasons are as follows: (1) The forearm movement, although the best writing movement, is not as easy to acquire as the finger movement, especially if accuracy in writing is demanded at the same time. (2) It is difficult and often impossible to use it freely and successfully when the desk, chair, and position are not exactly right. (3) It is hard, after gaining freedom and skill in doing exercises with the forearm movement to keep the same movement and make small letters in various combinations, with sufficient accuracy. (4) Outside of the penmanship lessons, conditions are often very unfavorable for using the forearm movement, so that unless more care is taken by teachers than is usual, the majority of children will actually write in a different position and use a different movement, with the result that they get an entirely different sort of practice from that taught them in their lessons.

This is the reason why children often become poorer writers in the seventh and eighth grade than they were in the fourth or fifth. Many never acquire the mechanics of writing so as to be able to write a decent hand without giving special attention to the process. High school pupils often write what they have to say with no regard to penmanship, then copy what they have written, giving attention to penmanship.

There is no doubt that the forearm movement is the best for persons who write many hours a day under favorable conditions of seating and posture, but it is doubtful if it is wise to try to make all children acquire it when most of them will do but little writing and that under conditions unfavorable to the use of the forearm movement. Most teachers of writing, however, believe that the "muscular movement" should be taught because, even if not used later, it secures greater freedom of finger movements.

Whether this is a correct view or not, it is clear that much more care must be given to combination practice in the habit-learning and habit-fixing stage of learning penmanship. The freedom and accuracy of movement gained in the special practice in making "ovals", "m's", and so forth, must be developed in making all sorts of letter combinations where the comparatively easy rhythm is lacking, and then such movements must be used in all writing and not merely during the penmanship lesson. When pupils are to spell, take dictation, or do any writing they should be required to assume proper position and practice correct movements for a moment. During the writing, if many of them change to other positions and movements the teacher should again have them assume proper position and practice free correct movements for a minute or two. Only in this way can the special movement training be made to carry over into all writing and result in proper habit-forming and habit-fixing so that one can write whenever he wants to without thinking about how he is doing it.

Methods of Teaching

There are two fundamentally different methods of teaching writing and other forms of motor skill. These are (1) by separate practice exercises and (2) by combined practice and use. The first method is best adapted to class teaching and the second to individual teaching, and each needs to be combined to some extent with the other to secure the best results.

The most effective way of using the first method is briefly as follows: After a child has passed through the first stage of learning how letters look and the position and movements used in making them, he is ready to practice for accuracy and speed. His attention may then be directed toward better formed letters and when this aim has been approximated, part of the attention may be given to better size or spacing or slant, but with enough attention to form to prevent deterioration. When both these qualities are secured, a third purpose may be made prominent, but with some attention to the other two qualities. By this time the first quality is being produced in a fair degree as a habit that with a little further practice can be maintained without conscious attention. Thus, one purpose should be made prominent in all practice while other purposes are kept in mind only as much as is necessary to insure further practice of sufficient accuracy.

When all the qualities of good writing are secured in a fair degree and can be produced at a reasonable rate, the child should practice writing for expressing thought at the already attained standard of accuracy and speed.

If this policy is persistently followed, the style of writing will gradually become fixed and will be used under all circumstances with little or no attention to the writing process. The mind will be free to occupy itself with other things while writing legibly at a fair speed. This is a result far more desirable for most people than the ability to write well only by diverting part of the attention from the thought being expressed. The above outline of method is well adapted to class teaching where many are practicing under the direction of a teacher.

An individual child may learn to write successfully by doing the whole process as well as he can at once, under the usual writing conditions. Many children have begun writing words or sentences with only a very slight knowledge of script. This is quite possible if a child has before him copies of all the letters which he can look at when necessary. Not only may he copy print sentences in script but he may write sentences of his own, as in writing a letter to his absent father. In this case he will need some help in spelling. This method has the advantage of making the first practice more like the complex act that it must be in actual use.

If the child practices in this way he is sure to develop a habit of writing that will require no attention as to the mere mechanics of writing.

There is danger, however, that bad habits in one or several ways will be formed that will be difficult to overcome. If a child can have intelligent individual teaching he may be kept improving in all respects until a sufficient degree of perfection is reached. Even with a very intelligent teacher, however, it is hard to handle a large class by this method. No two children will need exactly the same directions and the teacher will not have time to see that each child practices in the way that will be most helpful to him.

The chief fault of both class and individual teaching is calling attention to errors. The teacher must see what is wrong in the results but must make the child think of the kind of movement which will give better results. Negative directions always do more harm than good.

The less the child attends to wrong forms and wrong movements the better. Only by attention to correct forms and correct movements while practicing can improvement be made.

A standard scale of handwriting with which children may compare their writing from time to time may be of great help. They thus gain better standards, learn to judge of their own work, and are stimulated to further effort by their success. After pupils can write an even, legible hand, tests of speed should be made occasionally to discover whether improvement in that respect can be made without decline in form. Rhythmical music while practicing penmanship is a great aid whichever method is used.

Drawing For many years *drawing* was regarded as a fine art, analogous to painting. The use of drawing in engineering industries, on the one hand, and the study of children on the other, have emphasized the usefulness of drawing as a means of expression in the field of form. Only a highly endowed and trained individual can use drawing successfully as a means of expressing ideas of beauty. However, everyone can acquire sufficient facility in drawing to make it a useful means of expressing ideas of objects and of their relations to each other. A training in the making of lines, sufficient to give facility in doing this, should be provided in the elementary schools, but no attempt should be made to secure artistic drawing from most children. Artistic expression should be provided for all, but this may be done much more satisfactorily in painting and by designing, using cut-out forms, or tracings, than by means of graceful, accurate lines in drawing.

Motor Skill Required to Portray Beauty This is true, not alone because only a high degree of skill can produce beauty by means of lines but because, in acquiring such skill, the child is inevitably retarded by the unsatisfactoriness of the results that he secures. His perceptions and ideas of beauty are always so much in advance of his motor ability that he continually has the dissatisfaction of failure. In writing, where accuracy only is required, this is not so inevitable.

In all these subjects but especially in drawing, teachers have usually taught in ways that increased critical perceptive judgment faster than motor skill. The effect has been most unfortunate in drawing, sometimes even when accuracy of representation rather than beauty was emphasized. This is evidenced by the fact that young children are generally willing to try to draw almost anything, while the older they get, the more shy they become in trying to draw any but the simplest objects. Nearly all kindergarten children, if requested, will try to draw the portrait of a man or a woman, while older children can scarcely be induced to make such an attempt.

Lines in drawing are used by a small child to stand for ideas in his mind, and it is not necessary that they should look just the same as the object represented. Crooked lines may indicate the stomach or other internal organs that the child has never seen, and be included in his drawing of a man as standing for what he regards as one essential of a human being. In drawing a house, a child makes lines or dots for whatever seems to him to be interesting and important, either the stove inside the house, or the wind that is making the windows rattle, regardless of what may be seen from any one point of view. So long as he is not impressed with the absolute necessity of showing things just as they look, he considers himself successful if his lines are so made or related to each other that he and others will know what he means. This is all that drawing as a means of expression demands, and this should be made the chief purpose in the teaching of the subject to most children. When this is done, drawing will always have meaning and will generally bring success, provided that care is taken in selecting the facts to be represented by means of drawing. Almost

How the Child Uses Drawing

any four-year-old child can draw a square or a circle so that everybody will know what is intended. He can draw a birch and an apple tree, so that one can tell which is the apple tree, or a potato and a turnip so that one can tell the potato. Such drawings, however crude, are successful and give the child the satisfactory stimulus of accomplishing his purpose. Improvement in motor skill will come naturally if the ideas to be expressed by the drawing are gradually made increasingly difficult. Only after considerable motor skill has been developed and some knowledge gained of the way perspective is represented, can a child draw a picture of a box so that one can tell where he was sitting when he drew it.

Teaching Drawing as a Means of Expression

If drawing is taught like language, as a means of expression, then the first essential is not beauty but understandability and every line drawn must be for the purpose of making the idea to be expressed more prominent. After success in this respect has been secured, it may be well to try to express the same idea with equal clearness and more beauty, but this purpose should be subordinate except for gifted and advanced pupils. If the purpose of making drawing a convenient means of expression to supplement or to be substituted for oral and written words were made the dominant one in teaching drawing, it would doubtless be one of the most popular subjects, and the pleasure and success of many adults would be greatly increased. When any other aim is made dominant, failure will be so frequent that little improvement will be made except by the few, and the typical child will leave school with less readiness to use drawing as a means of expression than when he entered.

Developing Accuracy, Speed, and Grace

On the purely motor side, the problems of developing accuracy, speed, and grace are very much the same as in other forms of motor training. The first guide is the visual image of what is to be made and that is compared with what is made; while a secondary guide is the motor feeling of free, correct movements of various kinds. Whether the special-practice method or the combined-practice-with-use method shall be made most prominent in training pupils to draw, is pretty much the same problem as in all motor training. In teaching a class, the first has advantages while the combined method may be used with little danger and many advantages as a rule in individual teaching.

In using the special-practice method, attention should be given to ways of using pencil, crayon, chalk, or pen and immediately after practicing special lines, there should be a drawing exercise in which, by means of such lines, some concrete fact is expressed.

In using the combined method, the teacher should look for the most prominent defect in the way in which pupils are trying to make the necessary lines and, without saying anything about the defect, should have the pupils watch her draw those lines by a better movement, then have them draw something requiring similar lines. She should not say anything about wrong ways of drawing and not so much about the right way as to divert the children from their main purpose of expressing something by means of the lines they are drawing and endeavoring to draw more easily, surely, and quickly. The best way of securing improvement, especially in the case of younger children, is by *showing*, rather than by telling.

Musical skill, whether in the use of vocal organs or of arm, hand, or fingers in playing an instrument, is acquired in ways similar to those used in other forms of learning. There is always a stage of learning *what* is to be done, and something of the *how* it is to be done, followed by a habit-forming stage in which there is a gradual approximation to accuracy, followed by a habit-fixing stage, as the same movements are repeated in a uniform manner.

Acquiring Musical Skill

Learning to sing differs from learning to talk chiefly in accuracy and in the number of muscles that must be

151

coördinated. The breathing muscles must be much more continuously and accurately correlated with those of the vocal organs, and the vocal cords must be more specifically and accurately controlled, while the tongue and lips mould the sounds. The ear reports the results of these combined movements and serves as the chief guide in perfecting and coördinating them, although visual imitation of another singer helps and motor sensations of muscular tension play a considerable part in the attainment of skill.

No matter how highly one may be endowed with a vocal apparatus he cannot under ordinary circumstances become a successful singer, unless he has also a "good ear" for music. His accuracy of muscular adjustment cannot become finer than his ear perceptions of the sounds he makes. Professor Seashore, of the State University of Iowa, has shown that the limit of improvement in perception of fine differences in pitch is reached after rather a small amount of practice. It follows from this that in judging the possibility of improvement in singing ability, not only must the vocal organs be considered but also the fineness of the organs for discriminating pitch. The construction of the vocal cords determines how high or how low notes may be sung, but the control of the sounds within those limits depends on the development of coördination of all the muscles concerned, under the guidance of pitch perception. Professor Seashore has invented a machine which makes it possible for a singer to see a vibrating marker that shows just how nearly he is producing the sound vibrations corresponding to each pure tone. In this way a visual perception and image are substituted for the oral impression in guiding the muscular action. Some singers can, by using this apparatus, improve more rapidly and reach a higher degree of accuracy of pitch, than when they depend upon their sound sensations and images to guide them. Qualities of voice other than accuracy of pitch must be guided by the ear.

The problem of getting the muscles of breathing and the vocal cords, tongue and lips coördinated under the guidance of the ear, is the same as when in writing, muscles are coördinated under the direction of the eye. In both cases the muscular "feel" of the right movements is also a guide as one attains skill.

In teaching singing as in teaching writing, either of two contrasted methods may be used,—(1) special practice for special ability in breathing, pitch, smoothness, etc., or, (2) practice in singing songs with only occasional attention to notes, scales, breathing, etc. A pupil with good vocal organs and a good ear can, by individual instruction succeed very well by the second method, but it is less surely successful than the first method in the case of class teaching of pupils of varying ability. Many teachers, however, using the special-practice method dwell too long on special exercises, instead of teaching songs with one excellency and then another made prominent.

Methods in Teaching Singing

In learning to play such an instrument as a violin, the process is much the same as in learning to sing, except that accuracy of tone is secured by movements of arm and fingers instead of those of the throat and chest. The ear is the primary guide to the accuracy of tone, supplemented by the muscular "feel" of the right movements. One who has not a good ear should never attempt to be a violinist. In the case of wind instruments the muscles involved are different but the ear remains the chief guide.

Learning to Play an Instrument

In playing a piano the situation is quite different, since accuracy of tone depends upon the structure and tuning of the instrument itself. Hence a person with little or no perception of pitch could learn to play a piano, being guided by the visual score as to what keys to strike. To secure other qualities than the orderly sounding of pure tones, a good ear for those qualities is needed as a guide. Images of how to move the hands may be gained from watching another pianist play, but the success of one's own efforts is judged primarily by the ear and secondarily by the "feel" of the hand and finger movements.

Some teachers of the piano use the first method, having a great deal of practice of separate exercises, while others approximate the second method of trying to do everything at once, but with special attention to improving now in one respect and now in another. When the pupil is intelligent and the teacher skilful, the latter method gives good results relatively quickly; but when these are lacking, the former method is surer. When there is difficulty in securing correct and free movements of fingers and wrists, it may be worth while to have a child practice the movements in a soundless way, while watching the hands of a good pianist, till he gains the "feel" of the right movements. Next, he may practice the movements alone, then try to keep the same "feel" as he practices a musical score which he has memorized, and finally to keep the same, as he practices a less familiar score at which he looks.

Summary   There is much similarity in all learning. New connections are formed between nerve centers and muscles concerned in native and acquired activities, in accordance with the laws of *repetition, recency, intensity, primacy,* and *satisfaction* and *dissatisfaction.*

The process is one of increasing adjustment and coördination of the parts concerned in speaking, writing, drawing, singing, playing, etc.

The first stage of learning is initiated and directed by conscious ideas stimulated by the performance of an act by another and descriptive of the essential elements of the act and the way in which they may best be combined.

The second stage is one of *practice* in *doing*, resulting in fixing ways of doing and increasing accuracy and speed, with decreasing conscious attention.

The third is the habit stage in which the acts are performed almost automatically, with nearly uniform speed and accuracy under the conditions prevailing during practice, except when fatigue brings decrease, or conscious effort increase, in one or the other.

Any change of ways of doing or conditions requires conscious effort and further practice before the act can be done speedily, accurately, and automatically.

In practice, accuracy should be sought before speed.

Some practice in doing things in easy ways or under special conditions may be justified where the acts are complex and likely to be performed in the wrong way, by many of those being taught; but such practice must not be long continued. The most efficient method consists in doing the act in the way that it should be done and under the conditions of its most frequent use, when such practice does not produce errors in ways of working that must be corrected by special practice.

The more completely the various arts of expression are made automatic processes that will function quickly and accurately wherever conditions and consciousness give them their cue, the better has been the training. Only then can the mind be freed from hampering details and the person become an efficient executive with subordinates in the form of habits to carry out with little or no supervision whatever he commands.

PART II

PRESENT STATUS OF OUR KNOWLEDGE
OF CHILD WELL-BEING

There is nothing in all the world
so important as children, nothing so
interesting. If ever you wish to go
in for philanthropy, if ever you wish
to be of real use in the world, do
something for children. If ever you
yearn to be wise, study children. If
the great army of philanthropists ever
exterminate sin and pestilence, ever
work out our race salvation, it will be
because a little child has led.

—*David Starr Jordan*

VIII

BRIDGING THE GAP BETWEEN OUR KNOWLEDGE OF CHILD WELL-BEING AND OUR CARE OF THE YOUNG

ALL the higher animals care for their young. Some animals, low in the scale of life, desert the offspring as soon as born. A few birds lay their eggs in other birds' nests and have no further care. But for the most part, all warm blooded animals care for their young. Even some fish prepare a nest and carefully guard the eggs until hatched. The common sunfish may be seen standing guard over its dish-like depression in the gravelly bottom, or chasing away any intruder. The human offspring has the longest period of infancy and immaturity of any in the animal series; consequently it has the longest period during which it must be cared for. Human life is motivated by two great fundamental instincts—that of self-preservation and the preservation of the species. Both these instincts focus upon the child, for on the one hand the child is a part of the parent self; on the other hand, he is the new member of the species —the hope of the future. Thus the end and aim of life is the care of the young. It is true that this aim is sometimes perverted, but it is important to note that when this is not the aim of life, it *is* a perversion.

It is of course true that many men and women have no children, but the majority of such people are nevertheless living and working for the children of others. The kind and quality of care given to the youth varies over a wide range: all the way from the simplest instinctive interest of the ignorant moron or imbecile, up to the intelligent care of the most highly developed individuals.

The Care of Offspring

While the former group is never disturbed by its ignorance of the problems involved, many of the latter group are perpetually conscious of their own ignorance of what is really best for the child. They are constantly seeking knowledge that shall enable them to give their children the kind of care that shall most completely fit them to best represent their parents and most efficiently serve and promote the welfare of the race itself. Between these two extremes there are all gradations, and the average is disturbingly low.

We Do Not Put in Practice All We Know About Children

While the most intellectual parents may be said to be using all the knowledge that the race has acquired in the care of its offspring, the masses are not beginning to use the information that is available. Thus it happens that in the group as a whole, the gap between our knowledge of child well-being and our actual care of the child, is enormous. That this gap must be bridged is evident on all sides. It is the purpose of this chapter to marshal the evidences of this need.

Are We Improving?

If the care of our youth were intelligent and efficient, we should expect to find each successive generation becoming more and more free from the problems, difficulties, and annoyances that previous generations had to contend with. Instead of this being the case, many of the most serious problems are increasing in magnitude and complexity. Crime, for instance, is decidedly on the increase if we are to judge from the increased number of inmates in our prisons and penitentiaries, the increase in cost of courts for the trial and conviction of the perpetrators of crime—and this in spite of the efforts of an army of workers who are trying to improve prison conditions and make the treatment of criminals more efficient. Some there are who claim that this increase is *because of* the work of these sentimentalists (as they are sometimes styled), but that this is not true is pretty clearly shown by the fact that our institutions for the care of juvenile delinquents, from whom most of the criminals come, are also on the increase.

In one State (Ohio) the need for accommodations for juvenile delinquents is so great that although the law states that a child committed to the Industrial School must remain until he is 21 years of age, unless earlier reformed, the officials have been obliged to establish a fiction whereby each child is reformed in *twelve months*. The two institutions, the one for the boys and the other for the girls, are thus regularly emptied every twelve months, in order to make room for the new cases that must be provided for.

The statistics show that *fifteen thousand* murders and homicides are committed each year, and the number is increasing in proportion faster than the increase of population. It costs the Government of the United States, *six hundred thousand dollars* annually to guard the mail sacks. There is *four thousand million* (4 billion) dollars worth of property stolen in the United States each year.

Nor is the situation any better if we consider the problem of the insane. In most states we are either building larger institutions or more of them, for the care of this class of persons. *One hundred and forty thousand* cases of dementia præcox alone, between the ages of ten and thirty, are admitted to the insane hospitals each year.

Finally, hoodlumism and sexual immorality are believed to be increasing enormously.

If it is true that "as the twig is bent the tree is inclined," we have a right to attribute most of this intellectual, social, and moral irregularity to our faulty care of the young. We have not succeeded in bridging the gap. Not only have we not bridged the gap, but we have not even located the difficulty or, I should say, the causes of the difficulty. The way in which we have attempted to solve these problems and produce a better

Juvenile Delinquency

Crime and Criminals

Insanity Increasing

The Cause

condition by changing situations which are mere incidents to the problem and in no way causal does not speak well for our boasted intelligence and progressive civilization.

One group of persons has laid all our troubles to alcohol. Another group lays it to the movies; and we spend large sums to censor the pictures. We pass laws prohibiting the exhibition of prize fight pictures, and the depicting of criminal acts. But with no effect upon the situation.

Another group attributes the trouble to the Sunday School, and points out the small proportion of children who are receiving moral instruction in the churches. Another group thinks the automobile is the most pernicious influence that has come into modern society. Still others declare the fault is with the schools, both public and private—that they teach too much literature, history, and science, and not enough morality.

Not a Rational Argument

All this is very childish and superficial. It is just as rational and intelligent as it would be to attribute an epidemic of typhoid fever to alcohol, automobiles, movies, Sunday School, public schools, or any other agency which was merely an accidental agent in spreading the infection, and in no way the cause of the trouble, which a few people might be intelligent enough to diagnose as due to an infected water or milk supply. But these intelligent people would be regarded as cranks by the masses, and no concerted action could be obtained to purify the water or stop the dairymen from distributing infected milk. Consequently the people would continue to die. This is a close analogy to the situation that we have been discussing.

New Knowledge

The analogy holds in another direction. Time was when we knew nothing about disease germs and their transmission through water or milk. We have been similarly ignorant until lately of the diversified natures of children and the consequent necessity for different kinds of care for different types of children. Even now these facts are known to relatively few, and the great problem of to-day is to get the general public to understand these facts, and to apply them in the care of the young. We will now examine the situation from this standpoint.

The first important fact to be considered, as bearing upon this problem, is the differences in intelligence. Until recently we have assumed and have acted upon the assumption, that all children had approximately equal capacity, and we explained the fact that they did not show equal accomplishment by the theory that they were either wicked or lazy; and the time that should have been spent in intelligent care of them was devoted to prodding and punishing them. Our views on this subject have been best summarized by Henry Fairfield Osborne, who says, "The true spirit of American democracy, that all men are born with equal rights and duties, has been confused with the political sophistry that all men are born with equal character and ability to govern themselves and others, and with the educational sophistry, that education and environment will offset the handicap of heredity." We now know not only that there are the widest differences in capacity, but we know approximately the proportion of children in any particular group that will have each grade of intelligence; and moreover we are able by our methods of examination to determine who they are. In other words, it is now possible to ascertain what is the capacity of each individual child. We know, for example, that approximately 5% of a group of children will develop the highest intelligence, and show marked ability; that 9% more will be almost as good; that 16% will be a little above average; that 25% will have what we have termed "average intelligence"; that 20% will fall a grade below this; that

Children
Differ in
Intelligence

15% more will never be able to do more than about fifth grade work, and finally, that 10% will have low intelligence, stopping at the fourth grade or lower. Now, any large school graded only on the yearly promotion plan, will divide up approximately according to those figures; and any class in such a school will tend also to show the same range of intelligence.

The Care of Children in the Public School We have a most excellent public school system. It has been evolved empirically by trial and error. We have found out, for example, what subjects can be mastered by third grade children, fourth grade children, fifth grade, and so on. And on that basis we have built our curricula. Now, it is evident that such an experimental procedure has taken account of the *average* child, but every teacher should know that in each room there are those who can do the work in half the time of the main group. There are others who can not do it at all. It is a liberal allowance to consider that the middle fifty per cent are well cared for by the existent course of study. We are not now speaking of the question of whether the subjects taught in each grade are the most valuable that could be taught, but only of the fact that such subjects as are taught are rightly placed and well adapted to fifty per cent of the class. It follows, then, that the other fifty per cent are not well cared for. Approximately half of these will find the work too hard, and the other half will find it too easy.

Dull Children Cared For The progressive, thinking educators of the country are satisfied that the dull group are better off in classes by themselves, than in the class with the average child. Therefore, they are advocating and are securing in many places special classes for the slow, backward, dull, and stupid children. Then the question arises,—What shall we do with these children after we have segregated them in special classes? The evolution of thought along this line is interesting. At the outset we thought it was only necessary to allow dull pupils a longer time in which to do the work, and so we prescribed the same studies as for the bright children, but allowed the dull ones longer time. Gradually, we realized that either they could not do the work at all, or they could not do enough of it ever to become sufficiently proficient to make practical use of what they learned. Then, taking our cue from the institutions for the feeble-minded, we decided to give them part time in manual training. This worked well, and gradually the time has been extended until, in those communities where the parents are intelligent enough to understand the situation, there is given to these children little else than manual and industrial training. In other words, we have learned to care for these children in a way that is *adapted to their natures.* But as yet no community has provided enough of these special classes and special curricula to care properly for all of the children, and many communities have taken no step at all in this direction.

At this point, it is easy to see why alcohol, movies, automobiles, etc., were thought to be the causes of delinquency and anti-social conduct. It is because children of low mentality, often coming as they do from homes where the parents have equally low mentality, can not adjust themselves properly to such situations as the movies give rise to, and as a consequence their deficiency becomes manifest. Thus the movies are found to be *not the cause* of the condition, but *the detector* of it. The same is true of alcohol; it is now generally accepted by thoughtful students that the person who abuses the use of alcoholic beverages, is a person of weak mind; or, as has been expressed, people are alcoholic because they are feeble-minded, rather than being feeble-minded because they are alcoholic. The *average* child in the public school is not injured by the movies. Up to three years ago, of the more than four hundred delinquent boys and girls

Are Movies the Cause of Delinquency?

examined at the Bureau of Juvenile Research of Ohio, not one ever claimed that his delinquency was the result of attending the movies, or that the misdemeanor he had committed had been suggested by the movies. Since that time, there has been so much discussion of the evil effect of the movies, that the children have discovered that it is a good alibi, and it is consequently given more frequently.

The evils of the old system of caring for these dull children in the same way that we have cared for the child of average intelligence were many. Space will not permit us to elaborate upon this topic; it will be considered at length in Chapter XIII. Suffice it to say here, that the attempt to make these children do the school work which they have not the capacity to do, has resulted in discouragement for them. And a discouraged person, whether man or child, is a dangerous person. He is ready for anything. Besides that, such procedure sent the child from school (when the time came to leave school) without his having been taught anything that he could use, either to earn a livelihood or to occupy his time. He was, therefore, an idle person, and the old proverb tells of the dangers of idleness.

A Concrete Illustration — Just as an example of what happens in such cases, the following instance may be cited: Of eighty delinquents examined in a clinic in St. Louis recently, of whom all but one were over thirteen years of age when they left school, four had been in the ungraded class; four were in the second grade when they left school (remember they were thirteen years or older and in the second grade); four left in the third grade; five in the fourth; eleven in the fifth; nineteen in the sixth; fourteen in the seventh (at thirteen all of them should have been in the seventh grade at least); of the rest, eighteen were in the eighth grade, and one was in the first year high school. Of another group of a hundred and forty-five delinquent

166

children in regular grades in the schools, two per cent were classified four grades above their actual mental ability. That is to say, they had been carried along, dragged from grade to grade in spite of the fact that they had no capacity for doing the work. Another four per cent were classified three grades above their ability; eight per cent were classified two grades above and twenty-two per cent one grade above their ability. These figures are typical of what is being found wherever such cases are being examined, and will be found to exist all over the country. In other words, we are not caring for these children as well as we know how to do. Surely it is necessary that the gap be bridged.

Let us turn now to the other end of the scale. We have noted that 25% of the children in any class in a public school are so much brighter than the majority of the class that they do their work in something like half the time that it takes most of the children to do it. What about these bright pupils? The public school is an institution for the care of children during certain hours of the day, and it is intended to promote their highest welfare by keeping them wisely occupied during all their time in school. If the work assigned for the class as a whole keeps a particular boy busy only half the time, then for the other half he is uncared for. In those circumstances, what happens? Experience tells us that one of two things happens: either the child uses his imagination and ingenuity to keep himself employed, in which case it is perhaps as likely to be useless or evil employment as good; or else, second, he falls into the habit of doing nothing, and thereby becomes lazy. In either case the school is not giving him the care that he needs. This is not the place for a long discussion of this problem; the answer is clear and definite: we need special classes for these bright children as well as for the dull.

How Are Bright Children Cared For?

Classes for Gifted Children

The treatment of gifted children will be discussed in detail in Chapter XIV, so that it will suffice to say here that the movement to give gifted children proper training has started and in a few places classes are in operation. The proof of the statement that there is a tendency for these children to grow lazy, is found in the fact that in more than one instance, such classes when formed are for the first two or three months almost impossible to handle because of the pupils' laziness which they learn back in the grades where they do not have to work. However, in due course, when they discover that there is really something worth-while to do, they wake up and from that time on their progress is rapid and their achievements surprising. Since we have begun to apply what we know about the mentality of school children, many a child has been saved and started on the path toward a higher usefulness by transferring him to a grade that was adapted to his intelligence.

A fourteen-year-old boy was recently examined. He had been expelled from one school and was in great danger of having the same experience at another. When examined it was found that his intelligence was three years ahead of his age; and during all his school life he had been in grades and had been given work that was far too easy for him, so that he had developed a contempt for the work assigned and incidentally for the teachers and school authorities who assigned it. This is likely to be the effect of failing to care for these children in accordance with their needs.

Result of Failure to Determine Mentality

Here we may note the facts about the rest of the one hundred and forty-five delinquent children referred to above. Only 27% were correctly classified; but 20% were in a class one grade below their ability, 7% were two years below, 4% were three years below, 2% were four years below; and one child was classified *five years below the grade where he should have been working.* No wonder that in our schools we develop laziness, indolence, idleness, contempt for authority, and other attributes out of which grow our misdemeanants and criminals. The gap must be bridged. We must apply what we know and train the young in accordance with their mental capacity.

When we referred before to the condition of the insane, undoubtedly some of our readers said to themselves, "What has the training of youth to do with insanity?" Formerly that might have been an unanswerable question. But to-day, we are in possession of information that makes the answer easy. It is doubtful if insanity is any more hereditary than tuberculosis; but as in the case of tuberculosis, so with insanity, the child may inherit a constitution upon which insanity easily grows. We now know that we have in our schools many children of a highly nervous temperament, and we also know that the wrong kind of care for these children may produce insanity, where the right kind of care would save them from it. Fortunately, the practice of disciplining the young through fear has largely passed out, and we should speed the day when the last trace of it is gone. *Do the Schools Cause Insanity?*

Appealing to the motive of fear, is one of the most dangerous procedures in the case of a nervous child. And there is no question that many of the patients in our hospitals to-day had the foundation for their insanity laid in school. Not only is that true, but it is also true that we can detect what might be called incipient insanity in many of the children in attendance at the public schools. We do not call it insanity, but psychopathy, instability, or mild mental disturbance. In this group, as in those already described, we are bridging the gap by recognizing these children and by giving them the kind of care that their mental condition requires. Such children are easily recognized in most cases by the well- *The Psychopathic Child* trained teacher. They have peculiarities that mark them off at once as not quite normal. They are not always known as particularly nervous children, but they show in other ways that in reality their nervous systems are not functioning properly.

The School and the Home

Such children are usually more or less solitary. They do not get along well with other children of the same mental level. They are apt to prefer adults to people of their own age. Their games may have a queer monotony which makes them seem peculiar, even in their own family. They have unusual and strong likes and dislikes in regard to food. They are frequently destructive, are apt to have violent tempers and their parents will frequently say that they have been recognized as peculiar from the time they were babies. They may be moody and they are rather easily depressed. Contrary to the feeble-minded who usually have a good memory and poor reasoning power, these children are poor in memory and better in reasoning. This results in their doing poor work in school in those subjects that require memory, such as spelling and geography and also it results in their being frequently very shrewd, cunning, and original in devising and planning pranks and other disturbances. They are the children upon whom the teacher can not rely, and concerning whose misbehaviors she is always worried, for they are different and the regular punishments do not fit them. No amount of punishment does any good. They promise well but fail to perform up to their promises. They are frequently cruel, sometimes kleptomaniacal, often guilty of lying, and sometimes of sex perversities. It is not necessary for any one unstable individual to show all of these symptoms, but any child manifesting several out of this group should receive a careful examination by an expert who understands the problem.

Some persons declare that it is the business of the

school to teach the subjects of study as they have been doing while it is the business of the home to attend to the morals of the young. This is a conservative attitude, and conservatism is frequently useful. But we are gradually breaking away from the old conservatism, and with satisfactory results. The appointment of school physicians was strenuously objected to originally on the ground that this was paternalism; critics said it was the parents' business to look after the health of their children. School lunches were even more strenuously objected to, but they have come to be quite general and are now recognized as of the greatest value. The story is told of a certain boy who needed a bath. The teacher sent him home at night with a note to his mother, asking that he be given a bath, saying that he did not smell clean. The mother replied, that she sent Johnny to school "to be teached not to be smelled". Nevertheless, she ultimately accepted the point of view, and a few days later sent him back with a note saying, "Smell Johnny now."

From a larger point of view, it may be asked, "What really should be the function of the school?" Someone has said, "It is the transmission of racial experience and the development of the individual psyche." The first impression is that this expresses it very well, but the more we analyze it, the more we see that it is inadequate. There are many of the experiences of the race that it is not necessary to transmit to the child. If they are worth keeping, they are in the records and can be referred to as needed. As to the development of the psyche, it may very well be questioned whether we have any power to *develop* the psyche, or whether our work is not rather to guide it in a somewhat more useful direction than it would naturally go. The hackneyed phrase of making a *good citizen* out of the child is much nearer the truth, if only we understand what is involved, and if we have at hand all the knowledge that has been attained of child

The Purpose of the School

welfare and if we do bridge the gap and put it into practice in our child training.

The Child's Natural Equipment It is clearly demonstrated now that the child is a bundle of impulses which have developed in the race, in order to enable him to cope with the environment in which he is placed. And if the environment of to-day and the requirements of the future were the same as those of the long past ages through which man has traveled, the problem of education would be fairly simple.

As a matter of fact, the environment has changed very radically, and with the result that many of the primitive inpulses which we have inherited lead to conduct which is intolerable in the present social group. This being the case, it should be our aim to develop in the young the power to *adjust themselves to new conditions*, and to acquire the *power of self-control*. For example, we now know that the instinct of self-preservation leads directly to the appropriation to one's own use of whatever he comes across that he conceives may be useful to him; and it leads also to the concealing of his own plans and purposes by deceiving others as much as possible. The instinct for the perpetuation of the race leads to uncontrolled sexual indulgence. In the times when men lived much apart and to themselves, all these were virtues. The hoarding instinct was basic in providing for the future; the deceiving instinct led to withholding from others information that might be used against the individual, and the sex impulse led to the production of many offspring to fight for the safety and welfare of the family.

In the modern world, we live close together and in a coöperative society. We have divided up the work of life, so that we are each dependent upon all the rest. Under these conditions, the instinct to hoard and accumulate becomes stealing. The instinct to deceive becomes lying, and unlimited sex activity becomes sex immorality.

Our problem, then, is so to care for the child that he shall come to modify his natural instincts thoroughly in the interest of the group as a whole. No one will deny that this is vastly more important than transmitting the history of the race or even the ability to speak and write correctly. It does not require, usually, that these latter arts must necessarily be given up, but it does require that whatever else is done, this transformation should be brought about. But in order to bring it about, each of the groups of children already described should have a different kind of care. The very dull child can not learn anything as a matter of abstract morality. His training must be concrete and definite. As already intimated, the bright child, if not properly cared for, may develop a contempt for the advice of his elders, and therefore not try to adapt himself to the rules of the group. And finally, the psychopathic child has a special difficulty in making the necessary transformation. Only the healthy child with sound nerves passes through this transformation without something of a shock. Therefore, the psychopath must be handled with the greatest care if his nerves are not to be more completely shattered, and he later to become an inmate of an asylum. *The Problem of Transformation*

There are many things yet to be learned about child welfare. There is much about the child's physical nature that we do not know; and also the details of his mental makeup and growth, and the effect of the many and diverse new influences in the environment. But we will gain knowledge of these in time. Meanwhile, the necessity for applying what we do know to giving the child the best possible care is paramount. It has been stated that four-fifths of crime and insanity could be prevented by proper care in childhood. It *Much Yet to Learn* is futile to graduate our children from school with high grades, if we are not at the same time doing much to prevent crime, insanity, and the whole long list of anti-social activities.

Summary   Man's greatest interest is in children. As usual it is hard to put in practice what we know.

However, something radical must be done because as a group we are losing ground. The anti-social element is increasing and the burden of the insane and feeble-minded is becoming heavier.

The explanation of all this is that we have mistaken symptoms for causes. The cause of crime, insanity, and delinquency is not anything so simple as the movies, alcohol or any of the other numerous supposed causes.

The cause is to be sought and found in man's inherited tendencies, which do not fit his present world, and we have not tried efficiently to modify them.

We now know better than ever before the nature of the child, the wide range of capacities in children and the necessity of adapting the training to the nature and ability of the individual child.

We have roughly *four* groups: the normal or *average* child for whom our methods and school curricula are pretty well adapted; the *subnormal* or *feeble-minded* child who can be made useful but only by special methods; the *super-normal* child who also is not well cared for in the regular school—he has gifts that should be cherished and cultivated. Lastly we have the *sick* child— the psychopath or unstable child. We are often making him worse and thereby filling our hospitals for the insane.

The schools must play the chief rôle in training the young because the home can not do so effectively. The school must not lose sight of the fact that the making of good citizens is accomplished more successfully by teaching children to control the natural tendency to steal and lie, than by teaching them to read and write.

We may continue to do the latter but we must not leave the former undone.

There is much yet to learn but we already know enough, if we put it into practice, to transform civilization within a generation or two.

IX

RELATION OF NUTRITION TO MENTAL DEVELOPMENT

I N CONSIDERING the relation of nutrition to mental development, let us first of all define what we mean by the term "nutrition" and also by the term "mind."

Nutrition and Mental Development Defined The use of the word "nutrition" to express two quite distinct meanings has given rise to much confusion. Instead of being merely equivalent to "nourishment" or "food," a better and broader definition is, "The process by which animals and plants take in and utilize food substances." This larger meaning includes not only the food itself, but also those factors which have to do with the assimilation of food and its utilization in promoting the growth and repair of the body. It is in this sense that we shall use the term in the discussion of its relation to mental development.

Still greater confusion exists in regard to the definition of what we call "mind." For many years, unfortunately, the mind has been considered as something quite apart from the body, but we are now coming to understand that it is a function of that part of the body called the nervous system, of which the brain is the chief organ. So then, considering mind in its relation to the entire body, and especially to that part called the nervous system, we study it in much the same way that we study other functions in their relation to the special parts of the body through which their behavior is observed.

Using the brain as a symbol for the physical basis of mental activity, we recognize that the better the body, the better the brain, and its power to function as mind is determined by the quality of its tissue, its blood supply, and other physical conditions. Therefore, the child needs a well developed and well nourished nervous system for mental efficiency, just as he needs well developed and well nourished organs in other parts of his body for physical efficiency.

When attention is thus turned to what the mind *does*, rather than to the more abstract problem of what it *is*, the whole subject of mental development becomes more clear. In a recent discussion Robinson[1] states the new trend of opinion as follows:

"Man is an integral part of the natural order; he and his environment are constantly interacting. Such well-tried old terms as the will, consciousness, selfishness, the instincts, etc., when reinspected in the light of our ancestral background and embryological beginnings, all look very different from what they once did. . . . .

"Mind and matter can no longer be divorced, but must be studied as different phases of a single vital and incredibly complicated situation. Mind is still in the making. An historical consideration of human intelligence, taking into account its animal and prehistoric foundations, its development in historic times, and the decisive childhood experiences through which each of us individually must pass—all these combine to reveal previously neglected elements in our minds, and untold possibilities in their future growth."

The relation between nutrition and mental development is shown in its simplest form in infancy. The well nourished baby crows and laughs; he eats, sleeps, and takes interest in the life about him, offering no difficulty in his relations with others beyond the effort to get what he wants. The poorly nourished infant is fretful, irritable, nervous; his sleep is disturbed, and

Nutrition in Infancy

[1]James Harvey Robinson, *The Humanizing of Knowledge*, p. 53.

everyone associated with him suffers because of his condition. Such an infant is rightly considered a sick child, and is treated accordingly. He needs mental treatment in the way of training and control, but this is futile without physical treatment to bring him into a normal state of nutrition.

Child's Negative Attitude Resulting from Malnutrition

Unless this malnutrition is promptly removed, further mental effects appear as the child grows older. Instead of a natural reaching out into the various forms of activity that are essential to his well-being, there appears an attitude of defence and a desire to be let alone which are fatal to normal social relationships. The child's interests are narrowed, and his whole attitude becomes negative. Unfortunate personality traits develop, such as self-centeredness, shyness, lack of confidence, selfishness, jealousy, fearfulness, depression, day-dreaming, and unusual attachments. As the sentiments and emotions develop, the situation grows more and more complex, and it is difficult to separate cause and effect and say how much the child's physical condition affects his mind, or to what degree his mental condition affects his body.

Brighter Children Are Heavier

The close parallel existing between physical and mental development was recognized by Bowditch as early as 1891, and the work of later investigators has served to emphasize his conclusions. In 1893, as a result of a study of St. Louis school children, Porter[1] reported that the brighter children were definitely heavier, and the dull children lighter, than the average child of the same age. A similar observation is made by Baldwin,[2] who has summarized with the results of his own researches data gathered by many other investigators both in this country and in Europe in a series of studies extending from 1836 to 1913.

[1]William T. Porter, M. D. "The Physical Basis of Precocity and Dullness," Academy of Science (St. Louis) Transactions, 1893, v. 6, pp. 263-80. "The Growth of St. Louis Children," American Statistical Association, 1894, v. 4 n. s., pp. 28-34.
[2]Bird T. Baldwin, "Physical Growth and School Progress," 1914, p. 96 ff.

178

The following statements from his report are significant as representing a practically unanimous opinion on this subject:[1]

"Dull children are shorter than precocious children of the same age, or average children." (p. 145.)

"Successful pupils are taller than unsuccessful, and the rate of growth is quicker than in the unsuccessful." (p. 145.)

"Dull children are lighter than precocious children." (p. 148.)

"The lung capacity was found to be much greater in children whose standing in school is high, and distinctly inferior in a school for laggards." (p. 148.)

"The tall, heavy boys and girls, with good lung capacity are older physiologically, and further along in their stages toward mental maturity, as evidenced by school progress, than are the short, light boys and girls." (p. 96.)

Underweight and Retardation in School Work

The same correlation between school progress and the nutrition of the child, as represented by the weight-height index, is shown in a more recent study made in Detroit covering 80,662 children, which reports a clear tendency toward an increase in percentage of underweight in proportion to the years of retardation in school work, while an equally consistent trend in the opposite direction accompanies each half-yearly step of acceleration in school work.[2]

Increase in Mental Power

It has been argued in this connection that these studies merely show that mental superiority accompanies physical superiority, without proving that the physically inferior child, if brought up to normal, would show a corresponding improvement in mental development. At the present time, it is true, we cannot say how much

---

[1]The relation between weight and height is generally accepted as the best single test of physical condition. As the child grows, every advance in inches calls for a corresponding advance in pounds.

[2]Packer and Moehlman, "A Preliminary Study of Standards of Growth in the Detroit Public Schools," Detroit Educational Bulletin, June, 1921, pp. 24-25.

improvement in the brain itself results from improvement in the general physical condition, but we do have conclusive evidence that the mental power of the child is actually increased. It is a change in power to function

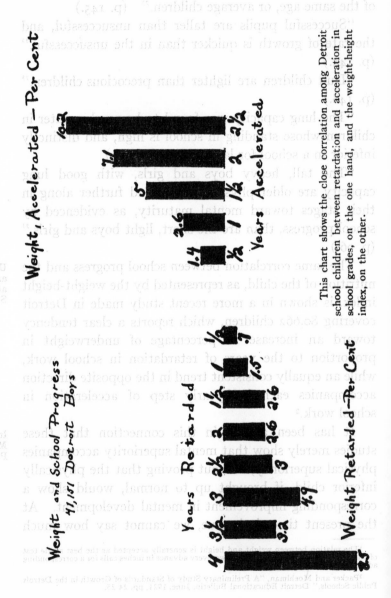

This chart shows the close correlation among Detroit school children between retardation and acceleration in school grades, on the one hand, and the weight-height index, on the other.

rather than an increase in native ability that we look for in bringing about improved nutrition.

Clinically, the physical changes that take place in the malnourished infant or older child as he returns to a normal physical condition are often remarkable, so great that the child can hardly be recognized. The mental transformation that accompanies physical recovery is frequently as great, so that it is a customary comment of parents and teachers,—"He is a different boy. His whole mental attitude has changed. You would not know him."

One of the common fallacies met with in discussions of the relation between mental and physical growth is due to the tenacity with which we hold to some exceptional case, as, for example, the weak or delicate child who despite physical handicaps has made striking progress in school. That this is not a typical experience, however, is shown by Whipple's[1] study of "gifted" children, in which he reports that of 128 students observed, 90 per cent were healthy themselves, and 83 per cent had healthy parents. *"Gifted" Children Healthy*

During the first year of life, the child's needs may appear to be met by attention to the physical essentials of health, namely, proper food, rest, air, and exercise; yet mental hygiene is also needed even in the first few weeks to ensure both mental and physical growth. *Essentials of Mental Health Necessary for Physical Health*

The first requisite is the teaching of *obedience*. The child's instinctive desires are expressed by crying if he does not immediately get what he wants, and if this method is successful, chaos soon reigns in the home, with the forming of habits that directly interfere with growth. Self-control through obedience is the foundation for all training.

A second need of the child is *mothering*, or *love*, which brings with it trust, happiness, and contentment. It is

[1]Guy M. Whipple, "Provision for the Education of Gifted Children in the United States," Mother and Child, September, 1923, Supplement.

common knowledge that it is undesirable to keep an infant too long in a hospital, however perfect the hygienic conditions may be. Mothering is necessary for growth.

A third factor is *regularity*, which has to do with habit formation, and gives the child a sense of order and security.

As he grows older, he needs to be taught responsibility, which gives him self-respect and self-confidence.

All these factors in mental training are best brought to bear on the child's development in the environment of a *good home*, where by the force of example as well as by training, the child develops proper habits of work and play, learns to have consideration for others, and finds out how to adjust himself to parents, servants, neighbors, and other children.

Standardized Program Ceases after Infancy Our greatest accomplishment in child welfare thus far has been in standardizing a program for infant care. This is one of the notable medical achievements of our era, and has resulted in a greatly reduced infant mortality. But when the period of infancy is passed, our record is not so creditable, and the pre-school years have come to be known as the most neglected period of life. In fact, most children pass through the whole growing period without the kind of examination that is needed to determine whether they are developing properly, mentally and physically.

Health Inspection in School Inadequate The opportunity afforded for the spread of infection by the massing of great numbers of children in our public schools has led to a certain degree of care with regard to contagious diseases, and we salve our consciences by a formal inspection of children in a hurrying line. But this sort of school examination, with children fully dressed, reveals little about their general nutrition, and anything like a thorough physical examination is almost unknown until the child becomes acutely ill. A beginning has been made in the wider adoption of the practice of weighing and measuring school children, but it should be followed by the incorporation of a broad nutrition program in the school system.

In a recent report of an orphan asylum, five pages were devoted to the subject of mental tests, while two lines were considered sufficient to sum up the results of the health inspection. Yet in this institution more than a third of the children were suffering from malnutrition. The mental examiners, it is true, call for a physical examination to rule out physical defect before they diagnose defects as mental, but there has been little attempt to see that the physical examination is adequate. Conduct and various mental qualities are graded and marked, but both in the school and in the home the physical condition of the growing child is treated with less intelligence than the farmer applies to his livestock, or the dog fancier to his puppies.

The result is that a third or more of all the children of this country are underweight, undernourished, malnourished; physically, and, therefore, mentally unfit. This neglected third is unrecognized in the home, the school, and the community, and we may well be startled by the significant fact that the major part of our discussions and conclusions concerning normal children is based upon observations of this group.

A clear distinction between the well and the sick would clear the way to a better understanding of individual differences and possibilities. A malnourished child who is toxic from focal infection, fatigue, bad air, imperfect digestion or assimilation, or any other cause, is a sick child, and his mental reactions are different from those of a child in normal health. Were this more generally understood, we should be the better able to cope with his difficulties.

The Malnourished Child is a Sick Child

These are the children who congest our clinics. They gain a place in open air schools, and remain there, with

Waste Caused by Malnutrition

183

little progress, until the age limit removes them. Teachers and principals spend profitless hours each year on a discussion of their promotion or demotion. More recently they have come to be a problem in industry when a working certificate is required. They appear in large numbers in the juvenile courts, and charity organizations know them through generation after generation.

In a prominent country day school it was found, after weighing and measuring all the children, that with one exception every problem of promotion and of discipline was in the underweight group.

"His Grand-father was Thin!"

Much time has been spent in discussing the respective influence of heredity and environment in both mental and physical development. We know little about heredity, for even when there seems to be tangible evidence as to the appearance of certain traits in successive generations, we are unable to state what might have been the development of the ancestor in question had he been placed in a more favorable environment. This is particularly true in the case of malnutrition. Time and again, when a certain child has seemed predestined to be thin because of his unmistakable resemblance to a thin forbear, we have seen him attain normal weight and maintain it, with a decided improvement in physical and mental condition. A practical attitude toward this important question is well stated by Kirkpatrick, as follows:

"From the individual standpoint, heredity should neither be ignored as of no importance, nor yielded to as inevitably fixing one's destiny. Instinctive and hereditary tendencies are the roots from which the physical, mental, and moral life develops. Some individuals develop more readily, and to a greater degree than others. All are of the same human characteristics, but each may make the most of his environment. Some cannot go as far as others in certain directions, nor as easily, but no one has exhausted his possibilities of development. The practical problem is to expend our efforts upon the useful characteristics which we possess in the greatest degree."

Whatever be the child's heredity, he needs the best possible environment to promote the mental, moral, and physical growth which his inheritance affords.

The question is often asked as to the extent of permanent damage done by malnutrition, and the degree of recovery and compensation possible after the causes have been removed. Animal experiments by Mendel and by Stuart and Jackson show that the organism has wonderful powers of recuperation, and remarkable ability to make adaptation in cases in which recovery is limited; yet if malnutrition continues throughout the normal period of growth there results an actual stunting, the vital organs remain undersized, and the length of the body lessened. In children who remain undernourished throughout the whole period of growth there is little evidence that they ever attain their own normal degree of development; while, on the other hand, undernourished children who are made "free to gain" and put on a good nutrition program respond promptly by an accelerated gain both in weight and in height.

Permanent Injury and Power to Recuperate

During the World War opportunity was afforded for the observation of malnutrition on a large scale, and Blanton[1] has reported a study made in Trier, Germany, with special consideration of its effect upon mental development. Some of his conclusions are:

1. At least forty per cent of the children in the Volkschulen are suffering from malnutrition to such a degree as to cause a loss of nervous energy.

2. While the percentage of stuttering, stammering, and other speech defects did not increase, there was

---

[1] Smiley Blanton, "Mental and Nervous Changes in the Children of Trier, Germany, Caused by Malnutrition," Mental Hygiene, July, 1919, v. 3, p. 343.

a marked increase in poor, lisping, slurring speech due to retardation or interference of the fine coördinations necessary for good speech.

3. Failure to pass grades increased from a pre-war average of 8 per cent to 15 per cent in 1917 and 1918. It is estimated that half of this retardation is due to malnutrition, and half to war conditions.

4. A similar lowering of the whole standard of school work, due in part to the same two causes, is noted. Half the children who in pre-war times did superior work now do average work, and the percentage of children who do inferior work has increased from 20 to more than 30 per cent.

5. Specific changes noted are: a lack of nervous and physical energy; inattention during school hours; poor and slow comprehension; poor memory; a general nervous restlessness while in school.

6. While children of good nervous stock, or superior intelligence, seem to withstand a serious degree of malnutrition extending over more than two years without greater impairment than a lack of nervous energy, children of poor nervous stock of inferior intelligence suffer a general, and sometimes a permanent, lowering of the whole intelligence level from even a moderate degree of malnutrition.

The problem of correcting malnutrition in children is in many instances a simple one, but in others it is one of the most difficult in all medicine.

Malnutrition can be Eliminated

Beginning work on this special problem in 1908, it was not until 1918 that I was able to demonstrate that every child in an entire group could be brought up to normal. Since then we have been able practically to eliminate malnutrition from ten orphan asylums and in the year 1923 nutrition work carried on according to our program in Rochester, N. Y., demonstrated that approximately 1000 of the most undernourished children of that city could be made to gain at the rate of 343%

in their own homes without seriously interfering with their school work. Similar results have been secured in other cities.

This was accomplished by ascertaining the causes of their malnutrition and removing them in nutrition classes by uniting the forces that control the child's health.[1]

It is of interest to note that the five chief causes of physical malnutrition, as observed in many thousands of cases, are also fundamental causes of mental unfitness. Taken in order of their importance, they are:

(1) *Physical defects*, or inflammatory processes, such as adenoids and diseased tonsils. This cause affects the mental condition by toxemias, clouding the mind, bringing about early fatigue, producing lack of concentration, poor memory, restlessness, and unstable nervous reactions.

Five Chief Causes of Malnutrition

(2) *Lack of home control.* While this cause is essentially mental, its physical results are so conspicuous that we list it second in the causes of malnutrition.

(3) *Overfatigue.* This cause is perhaps the one most generally overlooked, although its effects are both physical and mental. The constantly increasing activities and interests of present-day life have added to the burden of the growing child, and when he begins to fall behind in school, there is a tendency to increase the pressure by longer hours and home work.

(4) *Faulty food habits and improper food.* Aside from disturbed digestion and other functions, this

---

[1]The nutrition program adopted to secure these results has the following distinctive features:
1. Weighing and measuring as a means of identification.
2. Diagnosis based on complete physical growth, mental, and social examinations.
3. Removal of physical defects as a prerequisite for successful treatment.
4. Measured feeding (48-hour diet record).
5. Mid-morning and mid-afternoon lunches.
6. Mid-morning and mid-afternoon rest periods.
7. Regulation of physical, mental, and social activities to prevent overfatigue (48-hour list of activities).
8. Nutrition classes for the treatment of malnutrition.
9. Nutrition or diagnostic clinics for problem cases.

cause affects the nervous system at its source, and is reflected in every form of mental activity.

(5) *Faulty health habits* include all those factors commonly included under the term "personal hygiene," without which the child cannot thrive either physically or mentally.

Mental Unfitness

It will be seen, therefore, that most of the features of a program for dealing with mental unfitness are based upon removal of the causes which are associated with malnutrition. In fact, after working on the problem from the standpoint of physical unfitness, I found that the removal of these causes brought about mental changes in the child which corresponded with the aims of the mental hygiene workers. The parallel is sometimes less evident because abnormal conditions caused by sickness often persist after recovery from the original cause. These are the situations in which mental hygiene by itself is especially effective, but it is not effective when applied by itself as a cure for children suffering from such toxic conditions as listed above unless the basic cause is first removed. On the other hand, abnormal mental and social reactions, brought about by the child's physical condition, frequently disappear without special training when nutrition becomes normal.

(See illustrations on two pages following page 190.)

Another instance is that of a boy concerning whom it was not clear to either a psychiatrist or myself whether he was suffering from mental deficiency, retardation, or mental perversion due to abnormal physical and social conditions. It was evident that his mother was unable to grapple with the situation. He knew he could get his own way with her and did not hesitate to use both fists and feet in accomplishing his ends.

A good home school was chosen, where the boy for the first time in his life met with standards of living which did not bend to his whims and fancies. He soon recovered from the first shock and proved to be an example of the depth of inferior behavior to which an intelligent child can sink through indulgence and lack of training. Within a few weeks he had attained average weight, learned self-control and proved that he possessed normal intelligence. His teachers reported him to be a "perfect little gentleman."

Lack of Home Control

In any group of malnourished children we find lack of home control a factor in a surprisingly large proportion of cases, although its effect may be so conspicuously evident in improper food and health habits, chronic overfatigue, or the failure to have physical defects removed that the child's condition may seem to be due to one of these other causes. These are not only the children from homes which have become disorganized by tuberculosis, by the death or separation of the parents, or where the mother is the bread winner and cannot properly supervise the children's activities; but also in even greater numbers they are the "only child" or "spoiled child" types from well-to-do families or homes of wealth, where the children are over-indulged or left to the care of indifferent servants.

We can discover which of the causes of malnutrition are operating in any given case only by complete social, physical growth, and mental examinations. Each of the three is essential.

The social examination has been almost unknown in the past, yet it has to do with the child's interests, activities, and occupations, and is directly related to the factors of home control, overfatigue, and food and health habits. This record also includes the family history and the child's own health history, which may have valuable information bearing on his present condition.

Social Examination

The mental examination is given to determine mental defect, mental retardation or acceleration, and personality.

Mental Examination

The physical growth examination must be thorough,

not only to answer the question, "Has the child any physical evidence of disease?" but also the further question, "Is he growing properly?" The first step in this examination is weighing and measuring because we have as yet found no other single item of information that affords so much help in determining the child's nutrition. We are accustomed to follow the weight chart of an infant as an index of his condition, but the older child's weight line is an almost equally sensitive indicator of the effects of over fatigue, loss of sleep, slight indigestion, school tension, or any of the thousand incidents in his daily life.

Having through this series of examinations ascertained the causes of physical unfitness, the nutrition class brings together the home, the school, medical care, and the child's own interest, thus coördinating the various forces that safeguard health, namely, the home, the school, medical care, and the child's own interest. Weekly meetings are held, at which the attendance of the parents and the physician are essential. Home and school which have been "unhappily divorced," as Campbell puts it, are thus united, and the child's own interest is aroused through competition and coöperation. The class method gives the child a health objective. He has his individual weight chart which visualizes his physical condition, so that the mere mention of a habit that interferes with his gaining is often sufficient for its correction.

In scores of communities from Labrador to the Hawaiian Islands these classes are in operation; in the city of Rochester there are some fifteen hundred children enrolled at all times during the school year. As fast as one comes up to average weight and "graduates," another takes his place, and it is found that 70 per cent of the children maintain their new status after leaving the class.

Holt has characterized the class or group method as epochal in the treatment of children. It is a most

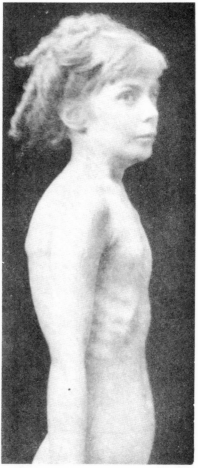 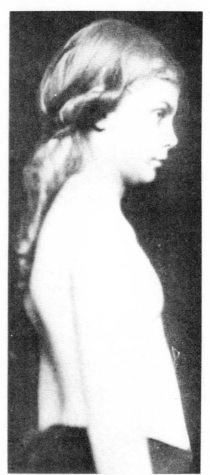

"BEFORE"   "AFTER"

The Case of Dorothea.

Dorothea, aged eleven, became tired on slight exertion, so tired that it took her nearly an hour to dress in the morning. She would sit and dream, rarely smiled, and her face looked distressed. She passed the school medical inspection, but was given a tonic by her family physician. The hospital diagnosis was "No Disease." The nutrition diagnosis was: underweight 21%; nasopharyngeal obstruction; cervical adenitis; carious teeth; spinal curvature; fatigue posture. Nutrition class treatment was begun with the resulting transformation in both mental and physical condition shown above.

These "before" and "after" pictures and the two following are those of a girl and a boy who illustrate very strikingly the physical and mental changes accompanying a return to normal condition from a state of serious underweight. These pictures are by the courtesy of The Woman's Home Companion and D. Appleton and Company. From "Nutrition and Growth in Children."

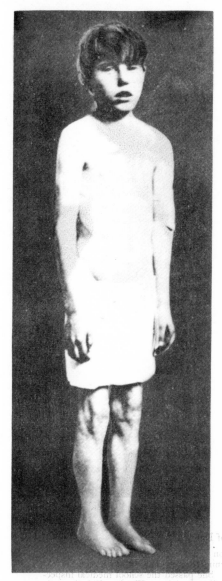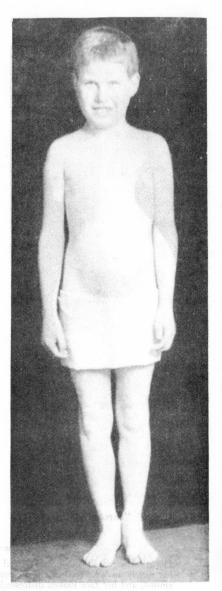

"BEFORE"   "AFTER"

Mental Retardation or Mental Deficiency.

Tom was 11% underweight, a mouth breather, with round shoulders, flat chest, spinal curvature, and flabby muscles. He was considered stupid, and kept after school in a vain attempt to hold him up to his grade. The right half of the picture shows him after his diseased adenoids and tonsils had been removed and he had followed directions as to diet and rest. The transformation in his condition can be seen to be mental as well as physical.

effective method of health education, and humanizes our child welfare work. It is based on the century-old maxim, *mens sana in sano corpore*, providing instruction as well as treatment, and appealing to the sympathies and affections as well as to the intellect. When a child has come up to the average weight line the improvement he has made is mental as well as physical. During the period in which he has faithfully followed the program of rest periods, diet, and general hygiene he has not only received a health education of the highest value but in the process there has been developed in him something called character.

Nutrition is not synonymous with nourishment or food but includes all the factors which have to do with the assimilation of food and its utilization in promoting the growth and repair of the body. The mind is a function of the body and our practical concern is with what it does rather than with what it is. Summary

Well nourished infants offer few problems. The infant that is ill nourished is fretful, irritable, nervous, and is rightly treated as a sick child. Continued malnutrition narrows a child's interests, develops in him unfortunate personality traits and induces a negative attitude toward life.

Bowditch, Porter, and Baldwin have shown that brighter children are taller and heavier and dull children shorter and lighter than the average child of the same age. A Detroit study shows close correlation between retardation in school and underweight for height.

Improved nutrition brings greater power of mind into operation. Malnutrition lowers the possibility of using mental processes. Whipple reports that "gifted" children are healthy themselves and come from healthy parents.

The physical essentials of health are proper food, rest, fresh air, and exercise, but mental hygiene is needed even in the first few weeks including training in obedience, mothering or love, and regularity. All these operate best in a good home.

Our present standardized program for infant care is one of the most notable medical achievements of all time but the remainder of the growing period is still neglected. So-called "medical" inspection in schools is a misnomer and is inadequate. The result of this neglect is that a third or more of the children in the pre-school and school periods are underweight, undernourished, and malnourished. These are sick children and should be treated as such. They congest clinics and open air schools, make up the greater part of the retarded and disciplinary groups in schools, and present a serious problem in industry. They compel undue attention and our standards of health and achievement are too largely determined by them.

Blanton reports that school children in Germany whom he studied showed the following results of malnutrition: a lack of nervous and physical energy; inattention during school hours; poor and slow comprehension; poor memory; a general nervous restlessness while in school.

The chief causes of malnutrition in the order of their importance are: physical defects, especially naso-pharyngeal obstructions; lack of home control or mental hygiene; over fatigue; faulty food habits and improper food; faulty health habits. Both physical and mental needs must be provided for in order to overcome this condition.

In order to determine the cause of any given case of malnutrition it is necessary to make a complete social, mental, and physical growth examination. The first gives a record of his history, interests, and activities. The second determines mental defect, mental retardation or acceleration, and personality. The third reveals physical evidence of disease and shows whether or not he is growing properly.

Any child who is habitually under average weight for his height is in need of a special nutrition program to bring him up to normal condition. His weight line is a sensitive indicator of the various factors in accomplishing or in retarding growth. The nutrition class, centering in the weight chart, coördinates the four forces which are essential in safeguarding physical and mental health: the home, the school, medical care, and the child's own interest.

X

Child
must be
Interpreted
To the
Adult

WHEN we talk of the mental hygiene of childhood we must of necessity address those who have the care and control, direction and education of the child in hand. We can hardly address ourselves to the child so we must speak to the adults who have his interests at heart. If, therefore, we are forced, by the necessity of the situation, to address the adults our first task must be to interpret the child to them. This might seem a strange statement at first but if we look back over the years and see with what cruelty children have been treated, murdered, sold into prostitution and slavery, deliberately deformed to use as beggars and mountebanks, abandoned, beaten and starved, we may realize to some extent the abyss which, in the past, has separated child and adult and we may safely assume, I think, that this abyss was created and maintained, partly at least, if not largely, as a result of

Ignorance
the Enemy
of Childhood

ignorance. In proof of this contention is the growing realization that children are the greatest asset of which any society can boast, for does not its further possibilities all depend upon the possibilities of their future? And therefore is not a nation's fate dependent upon what its children are and become?

Child thinks
Differently
from Adult

The main fact to bear in mind in order to bridge this abyss between the adult and the child and to come to some understanding of the child mind is to realize that the child thinks differently from the adult. Thinking is a highly complicated process and has developed in us

194

from the simplest beginnings. We have come a long way on the road of development from the child who reaches out its hand and thinks it can grasp the moon. Children are not just small adults. To be sure they are adults in the making but they are at a stage of development which so far removes them from adulthood that child and adult are, for the most part, strangers to one another. It is essential therefore that the adult should realize this and at least make an effort to understand the child by realizing the fundamental fact that the child's ways of thinking and feeling are just as understandable as ours if only we know on what they are based. The child who is afraid of all doctors because once he was hurt by a doctor has simply not yet learned to differentiate different persons and different sets of circumstances as we have and its fear is a perfectly natural outcome of this inability and confusion.

Children not just small Adults

Again the adult constantly makes the mistake of supposing that what the child cannot understand will not be attended to and so will create no impression. As a matter of fact the child is exquisitely alert to all that goes on about it and if it does not understand in the adult sense that does not prevent it from coming to its own conclusions as to what is meant, and that is just what it does.

Child Exceedingly Alert to all Impressions

Then again the child is not an isolated being. It is linked to the past by heredity; it is actively and constantly engaged in trying to relate itself in a satisfactory manner with the present in the form of its immediate surroundings and to that end is exceedingly alive to all aspects of its environment; and depending upon the nature of its inherited tendencies and upon its success with the present is its promise for the future. The child is not something that is formed and stationary; it is living, growing, developing and in the process it is plastic and there is considerable leeway as to the form and character it will ultimately assume.

Child not Isolated but Part of Surroundings

Childhood the Golden Period for Mental Hygiene

It is because the child is plastic, capable within limits of being moulded by circumstances, that childhood is the most important period of life and the golden period for mental hygiene. It depends upon how the developmental period of the first few years is negotiated what the future has to offer. Success or failure at this time means health and the possibility of happiness or illness and suffering.

Hereditary Possibilities Cloud Chapter at Birth

What the child brings with it into the world in the way of hereditary characteristics is the material which cannot be changed and is the stuff with which we and the child must work in the future. We may profitably think of the child as starting with a certain equipment, and life, in the processes of education and development, as presenting the possibilities and opportunities to this raw material for its unfoldment. This is a very different conception from that, now only beginning to be extensively given up, namely, that the child should be pressed, beaten if necessary, into the form that its elders think it should assume. It is a concept which concedes much more to the individual while not forgetting, however, the claims of society for a reasonable degree of conformity.

Education and Development are Unfolding Process

The whole developmental period of childhood has these two aims, the maximum unfoldment of the individual possibilities consistent with the necessary degree of conformity to social standards.

Authority and Reality

Into this two-way stream is projected the child who must learn to adapt itself on the one hand to the world of reality about it, consisting of the persons and things in its environment, particularly the parents and those who stand in similar relation to it, and the background of authority represented by these elders. These are what Miller[1] aptly refers to as the barrier of reality and the barrier of authority at which life demands a certain practical adjustment as the means of progress. I shall suggest briefly certain difficulties which ensue when these barriers can not be surmounted.

[1] The New Psychology and the Teacher.

Many parents act as if they owned their children instead of being, as is implied in what has already been said, the trustees of their childhood for future generations. They but hold their children's lives in trust for the future and more and more the parent is being held accountable for how that life turns out. It is being appreciated as fundamental that juvenile delinquency in a very large number of instances is traceable to home influences, more particularly those of the parents. The past abuses of children, already referred to, were based upon the theory of parental ownership. If a parent needed money he sold or bound out his child to service in order to obtain it. The theory of ownership was obvious. *Parent does not Own the Child*

The barrier of reality may be impregnable. Juvenile delinquents come from situations where reality is overwhelming, where circumstances are destructive and unconquerable, and so the child tries every means to escape, including the anti-social. *Reality may be Overwhelming*

If authority is too powerful and arbitrary it may crush out all initiative and capacity for individual development in the child. On the other hand, if the child cannot be so easily subdued, it may make of him a rebel, an iconoclast, a sceptic, incapable of conforming to any authority. The object of education as regards this aspect of authority is well put by Miller[1]: "It must be our aim, therefore, to bring up children so that they respect all racial experience, and at the same time learn, in due course, to challenge all authority. Authority must not be regarded as ultimately binding, nor must it be disregarded without respectful consideration." *When Authority is Too Strong*

Now, on the other hand if reality is overwhelming, the short cut is by the pathway of phantasy, day-dreaming, creating an imaginary world in which wishes come true to replace the real world in which they do not. *Reality Overwhelming*

If on the other hand authority is too weak, if the parent, the representation of the racial traditions and of

[1]Op. cit.

When Authority is too Weak and Reality made Easy

conformity, is too weak then the instinctive forces of the child are not sufficiently restrained; they run wild and lead to serious results. More of this later. If reality is made too easy, by inherited wealth for example, or by wealthy and indulgent parents, the same results may follow. The instinctive tendencies are not brought gradually under control and direction in the course of growth and development. Strength of character, just like muscular strength, is developed by overcoming difficulties, not by following the path of least resistance.

Relation of Parent to Child

All of these considerations spell certain conclusions as to what should be the relation of the parent to the child. The parent, as the responsible trustee of the child's possibilities, needs to set the stage, so far as in him the power lies, in such a way as will insure the maximum opportunities for the unfoldment of the child's personality along the necessary lines of social conformity. Two things are necessary. The first, and least important, is the ordering of the environment in such manner as will insure a reasonable amount of success to the child's efforts and thus provide stimuli for further endeavor. Nothing discourages more or is better calculated to destroy all initiative than an impossible task. Secondly, the parent needs to be a good example, a good model for the child to copy and try to emulate. This is, of course, especially true of the parent of the same sex as the child. The relation of the parent to the child is such that quite instinctively the child desires to be like the parent. The parent is the first model and it is very important that it should not fail. When neither parent is a worthy model and the two parents are at war with one another the child has nothing to hitch to and often becomes hopelessly confused, helpless, and impotent when he undertakes life as an adult. He has never had any training in one direction. He has lacked a model and cannot develop one on the instant.

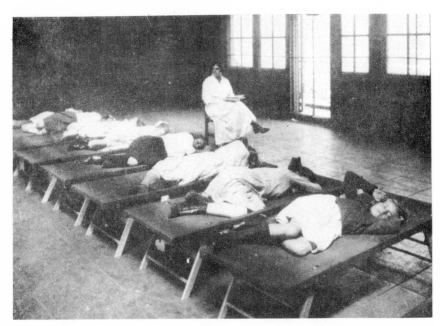

Complete relaxation; modern city life is apt to make children too tense.

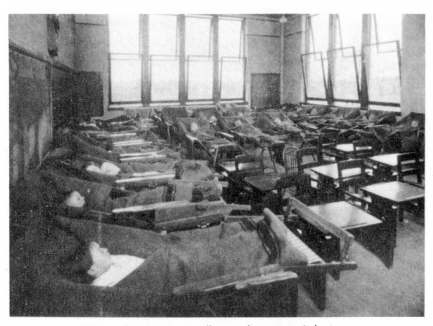

Children should study as well as rest in sunny and airy rooms.

In this matter of the influence of the parent upon the child, what the parents *are* is much more significant for the child than what they *do*. The child reads truly the deeper meanings that lie behind their conduct and the effect of their treatment upon him depends more upon their real feeling for him than upon what particularly they may do. If, for example, the parent is unable to see with the eyes of his child and is really patronizing and lacking in respect for his efforts, then no matter what words he may utter, his underlying attitude will get through and the effort will be to make for a feeling of inferiority in the child and for a lack of affection for the parent, which will remove him from the position of a desirable model.

What Parents are More Important than What They do

So much for the present—for the child's environment, personal, parental and material. The persons and objects of the environment either hinder or facilitate the child on his developmental pathway. What are the forces within him that drive him forward? These are the instinctive drives of self-preservation and race-preservation. They are fundamental, primitive, asocial and amoral, and it is only as a result of the refining forces of education that they can function in a socially acceptable way. The crude instincts are never permitted open expression after the early period of infancy. They must find progressively more and more refined ways of expression as the child becomes older and begins to take a place in the social group.

Nature of Child's Instinctive Tendencies

The crude, undirected instincts come out in open expression in infancy and if they are not adequately directed by education, example, and precept they may continue to do so. If they are too severely repressed by a system of bringing up that stresses the repressive feature by a continuous and uncompromising system of "don'ts" they may be snowed under, so to speak, only to short circuit in undesirable ways. The concept

Repression Alone Not Enough

of unfolding of the personality in the pathway of control and direction is an essential concept to guide all educational procedures.

Tendency of Parents and Teachers The tendency of parents and teachers is to attempt to mold the personality of the child in the form that *they* think is the right one. This tendency is almost sure to be a wrong one because the personality make-up, that is, the components that go into the making of a personality and their relation, is altogether a too complex affair to warrant anyone in attempting the application of any hard and fast rules. The impetus and initiative must come from within the child and it should be the function of parent and teacher alike to attempt to find out what it is that is seeking expression and help the child in the unfolding and development of these tendencies. Ernest Jones[1] has well compared this situation to the similar situation in the case of the poet. The

Inspiration inspiration of the true artist must come from within and any suggestions from outside are of no avail unless, perchance, they happen to coincide with what he feels as a spontaneous impulse of his own.

Nervousness and Mental Illness The various forms of nervousness and mental illness have as one of their most important components the failure, on the part of the individual, to develop in that orderly manner which presupposes the gaining of control of the instincts and their practical guidance in forms of activity that are both personally acceptable and socially useful and at the same time offer adequate forms of expression.

This process, or what is generally termed *sublimation*, begins very early in life, and failures that become manifest in adulthood are dependent upon disturbances in the orderly sequence of events during childhood; so that the period of childhood is of the first importance for mental hygiene, that is, for all those efforts that are calculated to prevent the subsequent development of

[1] Papers on Psycho-Analysis, Chapter xxxvi. The Child's Unconscious.

nervous and mental illnesses. Education does not concern childhood alone, nor even the school and college period; but is a process that goes on throughout life, for when it stops we but mark time until the end. Therefore, the earlier that wholesome efforts at helpfulness and guidance can be initiated the better, and the longer wrong ways of thinking and feeling hold sway the more serious the results and the greater the difficulty of undoing what has been done before new ways can be initiated.

If the unfolding of the individual does not go on smoothly; if, because of native equipment or of uneven emphasis during the early years an unbalanced type of personality comes to adulthood, there are many, in fact innumerable signs that make it manifest and indicate the nature of the difficulties from which the individual is suffering and which must be overcome in order to make a reasonably adequate adjustment and success of his life. These disturbances may occur in either of two directions, corresponding to the two great fundamental instincts, namely the self-preservative or ego-instinct, and the race-preservative, or sex instinct. In other words, the disturbance may manifest itself in the love life or in the nature of and working out of the ego-ideal. In many instances the disturbance is widespread enough to involve both realms. *Indication of Early Unbalance*

Every exaggerated character trait is evidence of an unbalanced personality make-up and is evidence also of the existence of the opposite trait. Between these two extremes the individual is forced to vibrate without ever the possibility of coming to rest. For example: the vain, proud, strutting personality is obviously out of balance and, too, he is distraught because he must everlastingly vibrate between this feeling of vanity and a realization of its emptiness and his real lack of qualities that justify it. He is never able to gain a true estimate of his worth *Path of Opposites* and regulate his life in accordance with his real assets and liabilities, but must always proceed upon a false evaluation and so he frequently fails.

Feeling of Inferiority   The feeling of inferiority is perhaps the best illustration of an unbalanced personality for our purposes. This feeling of inferiority may have many roots. The child who is persistently undervalued, whose opinions, remarks, and queries are always laughed at, whose efforts are invariably criticized for their shortcomings rather than praised for what they accomplish—all these serve to rob the child of any basis for self-confidence, of any feeling of self-respect. They deprive him of the sense of the joy of accomplishment and of success, and they imprison him behind a wall of relatives who repel his love. All of these results become exaggerated in the case of the "unwanted child," the fundamental antagonisms of its environment are so deeply grounded. A sense of inferiority may be fed also by the circumstances that result from physical deformity or lack of comeliness. The cripples and the "ugly ducklings" have a hard road to travel. The other children are cruel and teasing and in every direction they are forced to a recognition of their inadequacy to meet the more favored individuals on common ground.

The number and character of neurotic symptoms and traits of character is legion, but perhaps none is more common than the feeling of inferiority. Almost every neurotic has this feeling, a deep sense of inadequacy, which is developed beyond the warrant of the facts and leads to a self-depreciation which is in reality an undervaluation which may be sufficient to paralyze all effort; and in any case it is the basis of much unhappiness and dissatisfaction and too, much failure, because the individual is conquered by the difficulties of a task often before he undertakes it.

Dependence   This feeling of inferiority is a part of that dependence upon the parents which is the lot of all children at first but which should gradually grow less and less as age and strength and knowledge prepare the child for independence.

These feelings of inferiority and dependence are fostered and fixed by faulty attitudes of the parents and other adult members of the household and by wrong traditions in the family, which not infrequently have been handed down from the previous generation so that the parents repeat the mistakes of the grandparents.

Just as the feeling of inferiority is fed by failing to realize the necessity of providing opportunities for success and by treating the child's efforts with that lack of respect and consideration which implies that they are considered of no moment, so the state of dependency is prolonged beyond the safety point by over-anxious parents who will not let their child take any risks whatever, unmindful of the fact that life itself is a great adventure, in its very nature full of risks, and that strength of character can never be developed by removing difficulties but only by overcoming them.

To guide the infant and child through the formative period of life is a most delicate task. The idea that anyone is equipped to do it by instinct just because she happens to be of the female sex is absurd. This period of life is charged with the greatest possibilities and fraught with the most imminent dangers; and the most consummate skill is needed to develop the former best and to avoid the latter successfully. **Importance of Childhood**

There is probably good warrant for the belief that civilization would be impossible without altruism, and that the maternal instinct is the basis of altruism. But it must not be forgotten that altruism and the maternal instinct did not come into the world ready-made and in full flower, but that they have had a long and painful history. In their beginnings they were but feeble **Altruism**

Infanticide

sparks and there still seems to be danger that they may be snuffed out. If one doubts this he needs only to read the history of infanticide to have all his doubts vanquished. For example, Frazer says of the Polynesians[1] that they "seem regularly to have killed two-thirds of their children. In some parts of East Africa the proportion of infants massacred at birth is said to be the same. Only children born in certain presentations are allowed to live. The Jagas, a conquering tribe in Angola, are reported to have put to death all their children, without exception, in order that the women might not be encumbered with babies on the march. . . . Among the Mbaya Indians of South America, the women used to murder all their children except the last, ..." China has been the country where infanticide has proverbially been practiced on a large scale. Numerous edicts have been published against it from the seventeenth century on until the reign of Koang Siu which began in 1875, and during which there were many proclamations and warnings to the people to take their children to the orphan asylums rather than throw them in the river.[2] An instinct that is as liable to go so far astray as this is surely not to be blindly trusted.

Instinct must be Guided by Intelligence

The nicety of adjustment that has to be effected cannot be left to instinct but must be guided by intelligence. If the child's life is made too easy it will not develop sufficient robustness with which to meet life adequately when it grows up: if its life is made too hard it will lack the stimulus of success and fail to develop initiative and a sufficient optimism and self-confidence. If either too much or too little emphasis is placed on any tendency there is the danger of an unbalanced personality. If the parents lack desirable traits or possess undesirable ones they are to that extent bad models for the child. Besides all these, social conditions altogether outside the

[1] The Golden Bough.
[2] Payne, G. H.: The Child in Human Progress.

204

family may be controlling as regards certain factors, such as the prevalent scale of wages, the ability to get food in sufficient quantity, local conditions of sanitation, etc.

The most important single factor for the child is the quality of the love of his parents. Parents need to have that rare quality of love which is single-minded in its desire for the welfare of the beloved. If it has a selfish component such as a sense of ownership, or the desire to have the child take up a certain career as a matter of parental pride, or later to make a certain type of match that will further the social ambitions of the parent, then the love has certain qualifying characteristics which may make for an unbalanced type of personality on the part of the child. Without going to further length in the setting forth of principles I will present briefly a few examples of distortions and corrections to give some idea of how personality distortions actually occur.[1] Take, for example, a girl cited by Miss Jessie Taft[2] whose physical ugliness was the basis of a crippling sense of inferiority. The case runs as follows, in her words:

"I have in mind a girl whose physical make-up was fairly adequate but as a very little child she was clumsy, pigeon-toed, and inclined to be afraid to use her body. Her parents laughed at her attempts to walk and run and her frequent falls. This exaggerated her timidity and encouraged her not to try any unusual physical feats. There was no gymnasium work in the schools she attended. She grew very rapidly and at twelve was far too large and heavy for her age. Children called her "Fatty." Her mother said that great big girls should not run about like tomboys, but sit still and be ladylike. Her consciousness of her physical ineptitude increased to a painful extent. She took part in no sports or games that would betray her weakness. She was in deadly fear of walks, because there might be fences to climb. She

Sense of Inferiority

[1] Unless otherwise specified these examples were furnished by Miss S. T. Schroeder, Psychiatric Social Worker to the Out Patient Department of St. Elizabeth's Hospital.
[2] The Neurotic Child. Int. Proc. Conference of Women Physicians. Vol. iii.

dreaded the simple feat of climbing in and out of wagons. This lack of confidence extended to every part of her life. She was sure no man could ever care about her. She compensated in an over-development of intellectual interests but even here she had not the confidence that her ability warranted. Middle age finds this girl just beginning, through analysis of her own behavior, to get a legitimate self-confidence, intellectually and socially, as well as the free use of her body." Such a case needs little comment. To her natural handicaps the parents added ridicule which prevented her from making those efforts which might have, in part at least, overcome them. The radiation of her lack of confidence in her bodily adjustments to her intellectual sphere is very illuminating as is also the effort at compensating for a physical defect by mental development. The case also shows the characteristic neurotic under-valuation. She really possessed much greater ability than she felt she did.

Another case showing how a sense of inferiority may produce serious symptoms is that of an intelligent boy of thirteen, who having lost his parents, was living with his sister and her husband. In this home he not only missed the affection of his parents, but he was scolded and punished by his brother-in-law for doing things, or not doing them, quite natural to a boy of his age. By nature he was not aggressive, was easily discouraged and rather shy and reserved. With this make-up and his particular home situation to deal with, his reactions threatened to become abnormal. He began to steal, for two reasons: in order to obtain money with which to buy candy, etc., and also to cover up a growing feeling of inferiority. He thought it smart to be able to steal. By far the worst effect was on his disposition. He became sullen and insolent, resented any criticism, and cried very easily. Placed in a different environment, this boy responded quickly to encouragement and praise, though he was also taught to receive adverse criticism. He lost all his sullenness, became contented, a willing worker, and eager to please. This case shows how an anti-social act like stealing may be resorted to to overcome a sense of inferiority. It also illustrates the possibilities for curative treatment which possibilities are relatively very great in the early years.

Physical handicaps and a resulting sense of inferiority **Phantasy** may be compensated for by an over-development of the tendency to day-dream, to phantasy as is shown by a boy eleven years of age, born with physical disabilities and having had several severe illnesses during his life. He had no roof to his mouth, had a cleft palate and marked speech defect. To compensate for these drawbacks he turned his energies inward, until he became highly imaginative even to the point of having hallucinations. He imagined himself doing things which he wanted to, but could not. He also developed other traits. He became cunning and crafty, dishonest, and untruthful. Here we see the child dreaming of the things he wants to such an extent that he is beginning to lose touch with reality and is no longer able to tell the difference between the real world and his phantasies (hallucinations). This method of compensating for misfortune is very common and in fact is perpetuated in many of the well-known fairy tales. Quite frequently the hero of the fairy story is the poor, often simple-minded, son of a woodman or the unhappy, disappointed younger sister (Cinderella).

The following case is self explanatory. It illustrates **Incorrigi-** how, what seems to be incorrigibility may sometimes **bility** yield to simple common sense efforts if real attention is paid to the child for the purpose of finding out the meaning of his conduct. This is the case of a boy nearly fifteen years of age, but rating in the intelligence scale four years below that. It was thought, however, that his emotional difficulties did much to cause his retardation. This boy had a flashily-dressed mother, who worked away from the home all day and took no interest in making a real home for her children, in consequence of which they had to be placed out. This boy was put in one home after another and he became difficult to control. He paid no attention to work or school. He was said to be untruthful and unreliable, dishonest, and an habitual runaway. He also assaulted a little girl. As to his emotional life, he was idealizing his mother, having been separated from her for some time, building phantasies of her. Once the reason for his running away was to seek relatives in the vain search for a home of his own. He had dreams of death. If he shut his eyes he hallucinated easily. When thirteen he joined a church, prayed night and morning and always after stealing—to ask for forgiveness.

Finally, having been placed in an institution, where his conduct remained the same, it was decided to use, as a motive for good behavior, his greatest desire, to live at home with his mother (which could then be arranged). A marked improvement began almost at once. He did better in all his studies, had no more bad dreams or hallucinations, was smiling, and said he felt much happier.

Early Experiences The following case shows well how an experience in early life may condition late conduct in a thoroughly incomprehensible way unless the early experience can be disclosed in explanation.

A boy thirteen years of age, measuring eighteen years in the intelligence scale, was said to be giving trouble by stealing right and left, irrespective of any object's value or use to himself. Many things he afterwards gave away. By analysis, an episode was unearthed which occurred when he was four years of age. At that time he knew a little girl, and the two became mutually curious on sex matters. In order to get excuses to see her he would take anything at hand in the house to show her. In later years, when his adolescent sex feelings were developing, he found he could get a feeling of relief by simply stealing something. He had no interest in girls and in fact had a positive dislike for them. When he was gotten to see the connection between the episode when he was four years old and his present habit of stealing he entirely lost his desire to steal and did so no more. This boy had quite a talent for inventing things and later patented an invention for some automobile appliance from the royalties of which he supported his family. His interest in the opposite sex was awakened through a *transference*[1] to a *young woman worker*.

The next case shows well how easy it may be to acquire **Bad Habits** a bad habit that would seriously handicap the whole of the later life, and, too, how easy it may be to prevent this untoward result by the use of common sense.

A little girl four years of age, rather sensitive and impressionable, and of the type who early began to show talent in the artistic line.—For some time her mother had noticed that one of her boy playmates had the trick of obtaining what he wanted from his parents by screaming spells. As she had been expecting, her little daughter flew into the house one day screaming in much the same manner as the boy, and demanding some trivial thing. She was told to stop at once, that her mother knew exactly what she was up to. The child stopped instantly and looked at her mother in amazement. She was told that if she tried to do it again her mother would punish her. Two days later she repeated her trick and she received the promised punishment, which put an end to the child's experiment. By wrong treatment this might easily have developed into a bad habit formation.

---

[1] An affection based upon an earlier parental ideal which, in this instance, the young woman in some way aroused again to activity.

Child
Delinquency
often due to
parents

The closing admonition of this chapter, and perhaps the most important thing that can be said to parents, is, that whenever there is a neurotic or delinquent child in a family the most likely place to find the explanation is in the parents. Parents should take to themselves this lesson and when their child shows signs of nervousness not look exclusively for the explanation in the child and try to correct it by changing the diet, the school, etc., etc., but look first to themselves. Examine honestly their attitude and feeling for the child and see if therein may not lie the cause. Quite usually the parents have not the slighest idea of what is really the matter but the psychiatric social worker and the psychiatrist have learned where to look for the trouble and now it is time that parents should realize, at least, that the trouble may be with them.

Childhood
has Rights
as such

And finally, that the child should not be considered solely as an adult in preparation, that his right to consideration are not based solely upon the fact that he is an adult in the making but that he has rights of his own as a child and the best way to insure that he will become a healthy adult is to respect those rights.

Summary

The purpose of this chapter has been to set forth certain fundamentals which must be taken into consideration if the problem of the child in its various ramifications is to be adequately dealt with, and like all such fundamentals the results will be measurable largely in terms of the degree in which they are made conscious and subjected to conscious critical intellectual control and direction. Briefly these fundamentals are as follows:

I. The child is not just a small adult, but in his processes of thinking he is distinctly different from the adult, so that he is as little easy to understand by the adult as is the adult by the child. This necessitates that the child should be interpreted to the adult. Figuratively speaking, the child's language has to be translated into the language of the adult, before it can be understood. It is this basic fact that constitutes the most potent factor in the ignorance which has hitherto surrounded the subject of childhood. It is the factor to which the term ignorance is ordinarily applied when ignorance of children is referred to and is therefore basic in any intelligent program.

II. The child stands at the parting of the ways between the past and the future. It comes into the world with certain tendencies represented in its hereditary make-up that are unmodifiable. It presents other factors during its early years that are dependent largely upon environmental influences and which are capable of large modification. All children are not alike. Each differs from the other in the nature of these inherited tendencies and the quality of these acquired tendencies. It is therefore obvious that the same rule will not necessarily apply to any two children.

III. The function of education in the broad sense of the influence of the environment, including the home, the school and social institutions, is to deal in the first place with the inherited group of assets and liabilities with which the child comes into the world and to so influence it as to bring about by an unfoldment the maximum development of the assets and to minimize, as far as possible, the handicaps and the liabilities. This means more intelligent parenthood, more intelligent educational systems with greater stress upon the individual problem and as free as possible access to all the possibilities of the social environment as opportunities.

IV. The various forms of nervous and mental illness displayed by children are an expression of a lack of balance in this complicated process of adjustment referred to above. Here, as elsewhere, in the field of medicine, the best treatment is prevention, and prevention can only be exercised on the basis of a reasonable survey of the individual child and a reasonable capacity for favorably controlling the factors that influence him.

If man is ever going to learn to manipulate his human environment with anything like the success with which he manipulates the rest of his environment, and it would seem that the destiny of civilization may easily be involved in this condition, then are the questions that center around the child, the incarnation of the future of the race, fundamental.

XI

The Prevalence and Treatment of Sense Defects

THE human body has been aptly and properly described as a "living machine". Like the lifeless machines in our factories it is made up of a great many parts which work together for a common end. Like them it takes a constant supply of power or energy to keep it running—in the case of the lifeless machine, electrical or mechanical power—in the case of the body, the energy derived from food. Both kinds of machines are subject to the same broad and fundamental laws of chemistry and physics. If they are well built and carefully operated and protected from injury they work smoothly and well; and when the human body works in this way we are accustomed to say that it is in good health.

The human machine is of course far more complex in its construction than the roaring looms in a cotton mill or the delicate machines which take a bit of shapeless metal and turn it out in the form of a screw or a knife-blade or a gun barrel. At every step we make, scores of muscles must contract and scores of nerves must send out their messages to keep the movements in perfect mutual harmony. Day and night, the heart and the blood vessels must drive the blood to all parts of the body and regulate exactly the amount delivered to each tissue. Hour by hour the breathing mechanism must operate; and behind all these obvious activities the marvellous chemical processes of digestion and assimilation keep up the supply of necessary energy and make good the constant wastage of living tissue which constitutes the very essence of the whole life process.

The Living Machine and its Imperfections

213

Our first impulse as we consider the workings of this living machine is to wonder at its complexity and effectiveness; and such a feeling of wonder is fully justified. The human body is indeed a marvelous mechanism, but it is by no means a perfect one. If it were, it would be a miracle and not a manifestation of the laws of nature. No man ever lived whose body was at all times and in all its organs in perfect health; and the majority of us fall very far short of that ideal of health expressed by William James when he said, "Simply to live, move and breathe, should be a delight."

When our young men were examined for military service in 1917 and 1918, there was brought home to us all a very forcible realization of our shortcomings as a nation from the standpoint of physical effectiveness. More than forty per cent of the drafted men, presumably at the age of maximum vigor, showed physical shortcomings of a more or less considerable nature and above six per cent were so seriously defective as to be wholly incapable of military service. This was no peculiar or unique condition. Our Civil War examinations revealed the same general situation and so did the military records of all the countries which took part in the World War. It is merely an illustration of the fundamental truth that the human body is generally a somewhat imperfect machine and sometimes a highly defective one.

Physical Defects of School Children
Ill health is due to many and various causes—to inherited weaknesses, to bad hygienic habits which overtax even the powers of a normal constitution, and to accidental violence or the attacks of microbic enemies. We are not concerned here with the results of accident or with acute attacks of germ disease. These conditions are serious enough in themselves and they often leave behind them as after effects more or less permanent physical impairments. Accidents and acute illness are, however, obvious conditions which force themselves

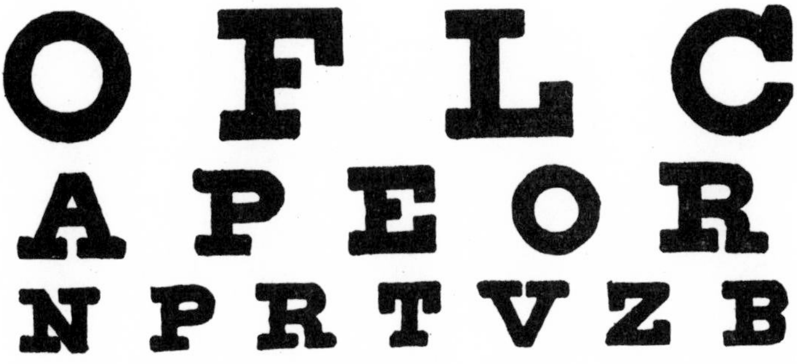

O F L C
A P E O R
N P R T V Z B

FIGURE I.

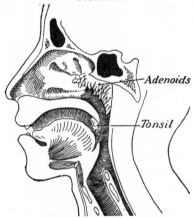

FIGURE 2

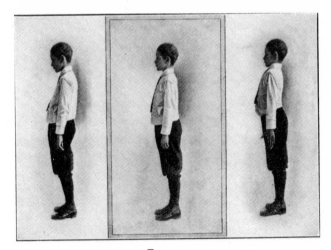

FIGURE 3.

From "Healthy Living," Book 2, by C. E. A. Winslow.   Used by permission of the
Charles E. Merrill Company.

upon our notice. It is the physical handicaps of those who are "up and about" and apparently well, with which we must deal in the present discussion. It is such defects that are likely to be overlooked; and when unnoticed and uncorrected they lay upon the child of the present and the adult of the future a burden of lowered vitality and inefficiency which it would be difficult to overestimate.

The regular and systematic examinations of school children by school physicians and school nurses, which have been made with increasing frequency and care since the plan was first introduced in the United States in 1894, have given us a clear idea of the prevalence of physical defects among children of school age and have shown us exactly what types of defects should be looked for by parents and teachers. There are differences between the results reported from various states and cities, as might be expected. Absolute perfection in any organ of the body, as has been pointed out, is rare; and the extent of deviation from the normal which shall be classed as a definite defect must depend to some extent upon the judgment of the physician. In some cities the school doctors set a high standard and class as defective a child who might in another school system be regarded as normal. By striking a mean between the high and the low figures recorded for a number of cities which have a good school medical organization, it is easy to obtain figures which give us a fair average for the actual incidence of more or less serious physical impairments.

The commonest defects of school children are those which appear in the form of decayed teeth. If we set a really high standard, competent dentists tell us that 85 per cent of American school children have dental defects; but even if we include, as most school physicians do, only the most serious dental defects we shall still find 20 to 40 per cent of our children with teeth in urgent need of dental care. Defects of vision come next, affecting from 15 to 30 per cent of all school children to a serious degree. Abnormal tonsils and adenoids will appear in 10 to 20 per cent of any average group of school children. Malnutrition is much harder to define than the local defects mentioned above, and here, there is a particularly wide difference between the results reported from various cities. The figures for the proportion of undernourished children vary from 2 to 20 per cent according to the standards set. Defective hearing is found in 1 to 2 per cent of our school children; grave orthopedic defects in more than 1 per cent, and heart disease in a slightly smaller proportion. These are the principal problems which we must consider in seeking to remove the handicaps of physical insufficiency from the growing generation.[1]

Remediable Nature of Physical Defects Before proceeding to consider these various types of physical defect in greater detail, it is important to emphasize the fact that our purpose in calling them to the attention of the parents of the nation is a very practical and constructive one. By taking thought, a man cannot add a cubit to his stature; but he can add pounds to his child's weight, and he can secure the removal of the greater part of the burden imposed by uncorrected physical defects. In nearly all the sorts of handicap which have been catalogued, prompt medical care and the observance of the rules of personal hygiene will restore an affected organ to normal condition or so supplement it that further damage is prevented and comfort and efficiency secured. Physical defects are indeed common; but they are also correctible.

In the city of Providence, for example, where the medical examination of school children is carried out under one of the most efficient health officials this country has produced, Dr. Charles V. Chapin, it was possible to obtain the following results during the school year 1921-

---

[1]The figures given are much lower than the estimates of Cornell and other authorities; but the author has preferred to err on the side of conservatism.

1922: Of cases of carious and decayed teeth found by the school inspectors, 88 per cent were adequately treated; of cases of defective vision, 80 per cent were corrected by the prescription of proper glasses; of cases of enlarged adenoids and tonsils, 56 per cent were relieved by surgical treatment; of cases of malnutrition, 80 per cent were remedied by proper diet and hygienic care.

An excellent illustration of what may be accomplished by a systematic attempt to relieve the physical defects of school children is furnished by the records of the Department of Schools of the city of Boston. Statistics for examination of eyes and ears go back to 1907 and show that in that year 31.5 per cent of the children had defects of vision, and 8.1 per cent defects of hearing. By 1916 these figures had been reduced to 12.9 per cent and 2.8 per cent, respectively; and the continued progress made in reducing these and other abnormalities during the following five years is indicated in tabular form below:

Percentage of Children Showing Specified Defects
Boston City Schools.

Year ending June	Defective vision	Defective hearing	Defective nasal breathing	Hypertrophied tonsils	Cervical glands	Skin disease	Defective teeth
1916	12.9	2.8	7.3	18.5	18.9	3.1	....
1917	11.6	1.8	6.3	14.1	7.4	2.8	....
1918	11.6	1.0	5.8	13.4	6.9	2.2	48.2
1919	11.5	1.8	6.1	12.7	4.7	1.9	44.3
1920	11.4	1.7	6.4	13.3	3.2	1.6	43.3
1921	11.1	1.5	4.7	12.3	2.1	1.6	40.6

The striking results which can be attained by the correction of the physical defects of school children is nowhere better illustrated than in relation to the problem of defective eyesight.

The eye is one of the most complex and beautiful mechanisms in the human body. Its main essential

Defects of Vision

parts are three—the lens in front which forms upon the retina behind a picture of objects at which one looks; the retina itself, a sensitive surface in which the light rays set up chemical changes corresponding to the parts of the picture formed by the lens; and the nerve connections which in a still mysterious way transmute these chemical changes into sensations of vision. In addition to these fundamentals, however, there are most complex arrangements for regulating the amount of light admitted to the eye by enlarging and contracting the pupil and for changing the shape of the lens (which is not rigid like the glass lens in a camera) so as to focus on objects far off or near at hand.

In only rare cases is this delicate machinery perfectly adjusted to the various uses to which the eyes are put in the course of civilized life—uses far more taxing than those to which the eyes of primitive man were ever subjected. If the lens is curved too little or is too close to the retina there is difficulty in seeing objects near at hand. If the lens is curved too much or is too far from the retina we get the opposite condition—near-sightedness. If the lens or the transparent cornea in front of it is irregular in shape the light rays will be bent so that they will not come to a clear focus thus producing the defect known as astigmatism.

Physical and Mental Effects of Defective Vision

Defects of vision are insignificant among very young children; but they increase steadily during the period of school life under the strain of the demands which our educational system must necessarily make upon eyesight. The results of such defects upon the health, happiness, and school standing of a child are serious and far-reaching. Aching and smarting in the eyes themselves, headache, abnormal fatigue, train sickness, and other types of nausea are among the more direct results of the attempt to read and study with uncorrected defects of vision. If eyestrain continues, the eyes may often become inflamed and laden with crusts. The stooping and strained position adopted by the sufferer in the effort to see clearly produces definite abnormalities of posture in many cases. Stress produced upon the nervous system leads to nervousness and irritability and in some cases to definite and severe affections of the central nervous system.

The influence of defective vision upon success in school and in the general social life of the child is sufficiently obvious. Medical inspectors and teachers are very familiar with cases in which the correction of visual defects has resulted in a complete revolution in the relation of a child to its work and its play; and the pathetic thing is that the child with poor eyesight has frequently no conception of its deprivation, but struggles to see the blackboard or pores over the dancing pages of a book in the belief that the world has the same blurred appearance to all his fellows. The same sort of handicap prevents participation in many sports and games, and robs the child of the normal pleasures of country life, the recognition of birds and flowers, and their subtle and appealing differences.

The detection of certain of the commoner defects of eyesight is exceedingly simple. Thus difficulty in distant vision may be tested by the standard letters in Figure 1 opposite page 214 and lack of clear vision of near objects by noting the ease with which fine print can be read. Other defects of vision are more subtle; and every child who has habitually "sore eyes," inflamed eyes or eyelids, who squints or blinks, whose eyes are painful in strong light, who suffers from headaches, who cannot read writing on the blackboard easily, who must hold a book less than one foot or more than fifteen inches from the face, or who must hold the head in an abnormal position when reading should be promptly examined by a competent oculist (not an optician). The prescription of properly adjusted eyeglasses is such a simple remedy

The Correction of Defects of Vision

for the complex evils which flow from eyestrain that it is quite inexcusable not to apply it.

Whether glasses are worn or not, it is important to observe certain simple rules of hygiene in regard to the use of the eyes—to avoid reading or sewing or other fine work with insufficient light or with glare directly in the eyes, with flickering or unsteady light (as in moving trains) or when one is in a reclining position.

Defects of Hearing   Defects of hearing are less common than defects of vision but are obviously of peculiar importance in relation to school work and demand immediate and serious consideration on account of the acute nature of the trouble which is frequently involved.

The symptoms of abnormal conditions of the organs of hearing are, on the one hand, earache or discharges from the ear, and on the other hand, defective hearing. The simplest test for the latter condition is made by the watch test. The eyes should be closed and one ear stopped with a finger and under such conditions the tick of the average watch should be clearly audible at a distance of two feet. The existence of defective hearing is often suggested to teacher or parent by habitual inattention, an expressionless voice, or imperfect articulation.

The cause of defective hearing may sometimes be an extremely simple one, such as the presence of hardened ear wax in the outer ear, which should be removed by a physician. The more serious types of defective hearing, with earaches and discharging ears, are generally due to conditions of inflammation in "the middle ear," a chamber behind the ear drum which is connected to the back of the throat by a passage known as "the Eustachian tube." Inflammation of the middle ear is usually due to infection with bacteria which have passed up through the Eustachian tube from the nose and throat and is therefore closely connected with respiratory diseases and with abnormal conditions of the tonsils and adenoids. Such infections are dangerous in the highest degree and may even prove fatal. Severe earache or any earache which persists for more than twelve hours should be referred to a physician for treatment.

The problems of tonsil and adenoid development offer an excellent illustration of what has been said in an earlier section in regard to the imperfections of the living machine. The tonsils are roundish organs which lie on each side of the throat in the general position indicated in Figure 2 opposite page 214. The adenoids (shown in the same figure) are finger-like, spongy growths which develop in the back of the throat where the passages from the nose open into it. There must probably have been some reason why these organs were developed in the course of evolution but they are evidently not of essential importance now, since their removal is often so highly beneficial; and they are peculiarly liable to abnormal development and to disease. When the adenoids become too large they obstruct the passage of air from the nose to the throat and children thus affected become "mouth breathers" and are apt to develop a narrow jaw and a peculiar strained expression. They sleep badly, frequently wake up crying, and are likely to be irritable and cross and backward in their studies. Adenoid growths greatly increase susceptibility to colds and infections of the middle ear.

Normal tonsils are not visible at all as projections at the side of the throat when one looks into the mouth, but in many children they have become so swollen as to be obvious even to the layman as swollen obstructions extending far out behind the back of the tongue. The character of the tissue of the tonsils is quite as important as their size. A small tonsil with irregular or "ragged" surface, providing a favorable breeding ground for bacteria, may be more dangerous than a larger one. The

(margin note) Enlarged Tonsils and Adenoids

particular reason why enlarged or unhealthy tonsils are so dangerous is that they furnish a gateway for the entry of disease bacteria. A marked susceptibility to local infection (tonsillitis) is the direct result, and repeated attacks of tonsillitis offer a reasonably certain indication that the tonsils require medical care. Unfortunately, however, the danger does not stop with the tonsils themselves. The germs which enter at this point may find their way to other organs of the body. Gland infections and ear infections are commonly associated with tonsillar disease; and heart disease in children is very frequently, perhaps most frequently, due to this cause. There are few more serious menaces to the general health of a child than seriously diseased tonsils.

The remedy for enlarged or diseased tonsils and adenoids is a simple surgical operation; and when a condition of this sort is suspected on account of any of the symptoms described above, the opinion of a competent specialist on nose and throat diseases should be obtained as to whether such an operation is or is not desirable. In young children it is often best to wait and see if adenoid growths will not disappear of their own accord. The judgment of the physician must decide in any given case.

Dental Defects Of all the organs of the body, none are perhaps more liable to disease than the teeth. If bitter experience had not taught us otherwise, we should probably have supposed these hard, shining, ivory-like structures to be among the most resistant portions of our anatomy; yet they yield with peculiar readiness to the decaying influence of microbic life. When a cavity is formed in the enamel, or hard protective outer coating of the teeth, the softer dentine underneath is rapidly attacked and ultimately an abscess may be formed at the root. The final result of such a decay (known as "dental caries") may be exceedingly serious since the bacteria from a tooth abscess are likely to pass on to the general circulation and cause rheumatism, heart disease, and other grave conditions. Abscesses of this kind are not always painful and may exist and work marked damage to the general health without a suspicion on the part of the victim as to the real cause of the trouble. Similar effects may be produced by inflammation of the membrane which surrounds the roots of the teeth beneath the gums (pyorrhea).

Nutrition experts and dentists are agreed that the prevalence of dental decay is very largely due to faulty diet. Among certain peoples who live under primitive agricultural conditions dental decay is practically unknown in spite of the fact that toothbrushes and dentists are also absent; while it is said that the teeth of such peoples rapidly break down under the artificial conditions of American city life. Attention to the principles of nutrition, to be discussed in a later paragraph, will, therefore, go far to reduce the danger of dental decay.

The next step in the care of the teeth is of course the maintenance of the greatest possible cleanliness in the mouth by the use of the tooth brush, at least twice daily, supplemented by dental floss when necessary. The brush should be used with a rotary or an up-and-down motion, and not horizontally, so as to detach food particles from the spaces between the teeth where decay generally starts. *Prevention of Dental Decay*

Most important of all, however, is the systematic examination of the teeth by a competent dentist, and their thorough cleansing by the dentist himself or by his assistant, the dental hygienist. In no field of hygiene is the superiority of prevention to cure more manifest than in the care of the teeth. Every child should have his teeth thus examined and cleansed every six months. If this be systematically done, cavities can be filled on their first appearance, there will be no pain, and no danger of serious decay; and the total expense will be only a fraction of what it is sure to be if the teeth are neglected until toothache indicates that the destruction of dentine has gone so far as to reach a nerve. The first set of temporary teeth should be safeguarded with the same care as the permanent teeth. Above all, the first permanent molar, which appears at the age of six years, is of very special importance since its size, position and early appearance help to guide the other permanent teeth into proper position.

This question of the general development of the teeth as a whole suggests the fact that regular dental examinations are of great value for other purposes than the treatment of dental decay and pyorrhea. For various reasons, the teeth often develop so that they are crowded together in an irregular manner which interferes with their efficient action in chewing and makes it hard to keep the spaces between them clean and free from decay. Sometimes (often as a result of adenoid growths) the palate becomes narrow and arched. These abnormal developments of the teeth and palate may often be corrected by special methods of dental treatment with marked improvement in appearance and benefit to health.

Problems of Posture Among the important points which we consider in estimating the physical condition of a child is posture, or the way in which the bony framework of the body is held in position. In standing, the head, body and legs should be poised one above the other so that a line dropped from the front of the ear falls within the forward half of the foot. The shoulder blades should be flat across the back and the feet should be directed straight forward. In sitting, the body should be bent only at knees and hips and the head, neck and trunk should be kept in one straight line. The healthy normal foot should have a well-marked arch under the instep and its toes should be freely developed, not cramped together, and free from corns. Examples of posture, Figure 3, opposite page 214.

The commonest defects of posture are (a) stoop shoulders and flat chest, (b) lateral curvature of the spine

(c) bowlegs and knock-knees (d) lameness and (e) flat foot (or broken arches). These conditions may often be present in only slight degree and may seem to be of little moment from the standpoint of general health. We must constantly remind ourselves of the complex inter-relationships which exist between the different parts of the living machine in order to realize how far-reaching the effects of faulty posture may prove to be. A flat chest limits the functioning of the lungs and favors the development of tuberculosis. Lateral curvature if unchecked may lead to grave deformity. The tilting of the foot in a slightly abnormal fashion may produce stresses on the nerves of the back of a most painful character and recurrent lumbago is often cured by the addition of a sixteenth of an inch to one side of the heel of a shoe.

The causes of such defects as those cited are as a rule to be found either in defective nutrition, microbic infection, or bad postural habits. Bowlegs and knock-knees, for example, are commonly symptoms of lack of certain elements in the diet of the infant. Most cases of hip disease, hunchback, and paralysis are due to bacterial invasion. On the other hand, round shoulders, and lateral curvatures are very largely the result of bad habits,—habits, however, which may have been fostered and developed by badly arranged seats and desks. The fact that poor vision frequently leads to a stoop-shouldered habit is an interesting example of the way in which one physical defect may be the cause of another.

It is of vital importance that the shoes of a child should be of a hygienic kind, everywhere as broad as the sole of the foot and wide enough in front to permit the toes to move freely. The inner edge of the shoe should be straight, so that a line drawn back from the middle of the great toe will touch the heel and the heel of the shoe itself should be low and broad. If a child is given proper shoes and a proper seat and desk he should not develop new postural defects; and those which already exist can, in large measure, be corrected by the use of special exercises prescribed by a specialist in orthopedic surgery.

Other Special Defects   In addition to the common defects of school children which have been discussed before, mention must be made of such prevalent conditions as swollen or sensitive glands in the neck, speech defects, various forms of nervous instability, and heart disease. Enlarged or swollen glands may be of no serious significance or they may indicate the development of tuberculosis. They should be promptly referred to a physician for examination. Defects of speech are generally associated with deafness, adenoid growths, or mental conditions. Such defects are largely remediable, particularly in the case of stammering.

Among the common signs of mental instability are restlessness, purposeless motions, difficulty in controlling the muscles, quick, involuntary, spasmodic movements, nervous exhaustion, and undue emotional excitability. Medical supervision and above all the enforcement of a correct hygienic régime as to diet, sleep, fresh air, and the evacuation of the bowels will often bring about a radical change in the psychology of the child.

Finally, a special word should be said in regard to heart disease, fortunately rarer among children than most of the conditions heretofore mentioned but of unique importance on account of its grave significance in after life. Exactly the same general principle which has been emphasized in connection with other physical defects holds in regard to heart disease,—the principle embodied in our homely phrase, "a stitch in time saves nine." Heart disease in children is generally the result either of a previous attack of acute communicable disease or of infection from decayed teeth or diseased tonsils. When the primary cause has been removed, the heart, like any other organ of the body, will to a large extent repair itself under hygienic treatment. Where such a condition is found there is, therefore, no reason for undue apprehension. Under the systematic supervision of a cardiac clinic, such as have been organized in most of our large cities, the child with incipient heart disease should show material improvement and frequently complete recovery.

The problem of nutrition is, when all is said and done, the most fundamental of all problems in the upbringing of a child. The chief business of a child is to grow,—to grow in mind and in character, but above all to grow in strength of body, since intellect and behavior are both closely knit up with physical well-being. This subject must naturally therefore be discussed in other chapters of this book especially in Chapter IX; but some reference must be made to it in even the briefest survey of the physical defects of children.

The Problem of Malnutrition

In the organized efforts made during the past five years for the improvement of child health, much stress has been laid upon malnutrition and particularly upon underweight as an index of undernourishment. Plans have been worked out in many schools for the systematic weighing and measuring of children and the comparison of the results with a standard scale indicating the normal weight for a child of a given age and height. This movement has been a most useful one in bringing home to the individual child and the individual parent the importance of good hygienic habits. It has been made clear, however, in recent years that underweight is only a very rough test of undernourishment. Different races have quite different normal weights for the same age and height; and the rate of growth is different at different seasons of the year. A substantial proportion of children who are considerably underweight are really in a perfectly normal condition as regards nutrition; while on the other hand children who are really undernourished may have a normal weight for height and age. The physician's examination must be the final test.

Of the frequency and the seriousness of real malnutrition there can, however, be no doubt. Rickets, for example, which is a very common disease of young children is the direct result of the lack of certain specific elements in the diet. It is believed on good grounds that defective teeth are largely due to deficient diet. The part played by undernourishment in lowering resistance to tuberculosis is among the most familiar phenomena in medical science. Yet in spite of these facts, undernourished children are by no means confined to famine-stricken Russia or the suffering nations of Central Europe. A recent study of the actual diets of several thousand children in Gary, Ind., a typical American industrial community, showed that only ten per cent of these children were receiving completely adequate nourishment.

Requirements for Proper Nutrition The diet of the child must not only supply the total energy for the life and growth of the body but also the particular kinds of substances necessary for the constant rebuilding of living tissue,—proteins, salts and vitamines. If a single one of these substances be insufficient in amount disaster will follow. The foods which are of particular importance in supplying the common deficiencies of a child's diet are fruits, leafy vegetables (such as lettuce, spinach, beet greens, and the like) and, above all, milk. A growing child should have a quart of milk a day.

If a child is undernourished it is obviously either because the right kinds of food are not set before him or because he has formed bad habits of eating and refuses certain necessary foods. The first condition can be controlled by intelligent planning of the dietary with the advice of a physician, a public health nurse or expert in nutrition. In order to obtain a well-balanced diet at a minimum cost, it has been estimated that, of the total amount of money spent in a given week for food of all kinds, one quarter should be spent for milk, one quarter for vegetables and fruits, about fifteen per cent for bread, cereals and other grain products, about ten per cent for meat, fish and poultry, ten per cent for butter and other fats, five per cent for eggs and the remaining ten per cent for sugar, cheese, and other miscellaneous foodstuffs. If such a diet as this be set before a child and if the child be taught to drink milk and to eat green vegetables and fruits, there will be little chance of malnutrition.

The responsibility of the school for the health of the child is a threefold one. In the first place it should provide as a regular part of the curriculum for systematic instruction in the basic principles of physiology and hygiene so that the child may understand something of the wonders of the body-machine for which he is responsible, of the dangers which threaten him and of the ways in which he can be kept in a condition of maximum health and vigor. In the second place, the school should supply opportunities for the actual practice of health habits and particularly for supervised physical exercise and play. Finally, it should provide for the systematic medical examination of all school children so that diseases and physical defects of all kinds may be promptly detected and, so far as possible, cured. _School Health Services_

The teacher, the school nurse and the school physician all play a part in the performance of this latter task. The teacher should be constantly on the lookout for the symptoms of communicable disease (coughing, running nose, inflamed eyes, rashes, and the like) and for such signs of physical defect as have been discussed in the preceding pages. The school nurse should see daily all such children as may be referred to her by the teacher and should pass on to the physician those who are in need of his attention. In addition to such emergency examinations the school physician, with such aid as he may desire from school nurse and teacher, should make a complete and exhaustive examination of every child, at least three times during his school life for the detection of physical defects and deficiencies. It is the duty of the school nurse to follow into the home each case needing attention, to give advice in regard to the hygiene of childhood, and to persuade the parents to have any physical defects which have been found promptly and completely remedied; and there should be school clinics maintained at public expense for the correction of such defects as will not otherwise receive attention. It is the poorest sort of economy to spend money on the education of a child so handicapped by physical ill health that he cannot profit by the opportunities which are placed before him.

Summary Finally, what is the message of medical science to the parent, in regard to the responsibility which rests upon him for the physical well-being of his child? It can be summarized in a very few words.

The human body is a marvellous machine but by no means a perfect one. It is subject to manifold diseases and defects and many children are seriously handicapped and endangered by such diseases and defects,—often without the knowledge of themselves or their parents that anything is wrong. If the conditions in question are promptly discovered they can generally be remedied by appropriate medical treatment or change in hygienic habits, or both, often with astonishing improvement in the health, happiness and mental and moral progress of the child.

If you who are reading these lines live in a city where there is a good system of school health sypervision, it will only be necessary for you to follow the counsel of the school doctor and the school nurse in order to insure the best results which medical knowledge can produce. If there is no such system in your schools, or if your child is below school age, the responsibility must rest with you; and it is important to remember that a large proportion of the serious physical and mental handicaps of childhood have their origin in the pre-school period.

The wise automobile owner does not wait till his car runs into a ditch before he calls in the repair man. He has his car overhauled and "tuned up" once in so often as a regular precaution; or, at the very least, he takes it to the service station when he hears the first "knock" or unusual sound which indicates that something is going wrong. Physical defects do not generally "knock" so obviously that the layman can hear them; so the only safe rule is to undergo regular medical examination. Your child should be examined by a physician, well or ill as he may seem to you to be, once a week during the first weeks of life, once a month during the first year, once a year up to school age, if you want him to have the fullest development, the strongest body, the most abounding vitality of which he is capable. This is the essential message of modern medicine,—that the doctor should be used as an agent of prevention and not merely for the disheartening task of repairing damage already done. It is on such a use of the resources of medical science that we can base the hope of a stronger and finer race of Americans in the days to come.

XII

THE TREATMENT AND PREVENTION OF DELINQUENCY

Question:
Treat Child
or Environ-
ment

THE first nice discrimination to be made in the treatment of delinquency in childhood, if we are to act intelligently, is whether and how much the child is to be treated and whether and how much environmental conditions are to be treated. It is curious and interesting to observe how opinions range, in the family circle or in the juvenile court room, all the way from doing everything *for* the child to doing everything, by way of discipline, *to* him. To strike the balance that fair-mindedness and effective action call for requires more earnest consideration than most people give the matter.

How poorly founded are off-hand opinions about the treatment of delinquency is seen both in the fact of the wide divergence of views concerning it and in the poor results so frequently obtained. It seems to be much the same as the treatment of ill health before the days of modern medicine.

The
Punishment
Attitude

The way to treat bad behavior in children say, in substance, some men and an occasional woman, is to knock it out of them. Even a clergyman argues, "The rod is good. I'm thankful to the old-fashioned school teacher who used it on me. Boys have too much deviltry in their make-up to be successfully treated in any other way." Or perhaps some judge proclaims that the law of the adult courts calculated to make the individual feel the consequences of his acts is to a very considerable extent what is needed in the treatment of juveniles. These are typical utterances and attitudes.

On the other hand, one hears from some mothers, **The**
fathers, yes and I have heard it, too, from employers who **Excusing Attitude**
have lost considerable sums through some child's stealing,
that the circumstances were such, the temptations so
great, or the suggestions of companions so strong that
really the delinquent should be excused. Their idea is
that, above all things, one must be charitable in the face
of such a situation. "I don't think he will do it again,"
or "You can't expect young people to have much sense
about such things" are what these people say.

Now the answer to both is the fact of the large number **Both Atti-**
of failures resulting from each method. Anybody who **tudes may be Wrong**
has had considerable experience knows of instances where
children have been beaten and beaten for misbehavior,
without any essential change in conduct; the main results
often being development of sneakiness, of self-defense
lying, a hardening of character, a hatred of those in
authority. Autobiographies of some habitual criminals
give much evidence of a bitter reaction to early punishment. And we definitely discover children who are not
self-conscious or self-analytical enough to attribute the
source of their tendencies to it, nevertheless developing
their most undesirable traits simultaneously with severe
punishment inflicted.

But then, the predictions of success for the opposite
let-alone form of treatment often do not come true. The
child may persist in going out with bad companions or in
pilfering at home. The employer perhaps finds to his
chagrin that the excused young employee accepts new
chances to take goods or money. Many such instances
are to be found in our recorded cases.

Of course, there is a measure of success in each method.
The clergyman may have been right about his own case,
and about success with some others. The forgiving
employer is, on occasion, rewarded by seeing reformation
follow his kindness. Undoubtedly there are good out-

comes subsequent to other off-hand kinds of treatment or non-treatment. No one can deny this any more than he can deny the fact that some patients get well of fevers in spite of anything that is done or not done. But we cannot logically attribute so much to either their moral or medical treatments as proponents of various set theories would have us attribute.

Moral Self-Healing

A better statement of fact would be that some young people have it in them to recover moral health rapidly. Perhaps there is less inner urge toward delinquency, perhaps there is better characterial fibre than in some others, perhaps there is less stress from the outside. Anyhow, some children do right themselves quickly without being steered by others morally and proceed in conduct ways on a steady keel. If it were not so this would be a sorry world; many offenses are committed and not repeated, many of us have been secretly delinquent and have recovered. For the sake of all—and sometimes mothers and fathers have to be told this by way of encouragement —it is well to think of the power of recovery in the moral world as one thinks of the healing power of nature in the world of physical health and disease.

Better Methods of Treating Delinquency

The foregoing is by way of introduction. After all, the aim in this chapter is to consider ways of effectually treating delinquency which is not so slight and self-curable that it needs no treatment. And of course these ways must be better directed than are the off-hand undertakings of those who have only one narrow point of view. We must turn to what there is of a science of treatment of delinquency and build from the materials we find there.

We can carry the analogy of the development of medical science still further. The handling of cases of disease in earlier times was according to ill-founded theory, or by following tradition or old wives' sayings. And then there came the new era of studying the causes of disease, and following soon upon the heels of this came new methods of therapy which our generation has seen one by one develop to conquer age-old ills. With regard to delinquency we are just now opening the era of the study of causation, with already most encouraging results from therapeutic endeavors based on better knowledge of the particular and immediate origin of the tendency to misbehavior.

And exactly as modern medicine has shown from a scientific basis that in many instances of ill-health both the individual and the environment have to be treated in order to restore good physical condition, so even more frequently one finds that these two phases of the situation have to be met in handling a case of delinquency upon the basis of what is fundamentally wrong. But the analogy stops here with generalities. One has rarely in medical practice, for instance, to deal with other persons as causes of a continuing trouble. But in studying delinquents we frequently find that the attitudes of others than the delinquent himself make strongly for or against his delinquency; other people form a part of his world that requires treatment.

So we have (a) the child himself, sometimes in body but always on the mental side, if we count the character aspects of his mental life; (b) the physical features of his environment, as when he lives under or frequents conditions that are inimical to his moral health; (c) the people about him, the company he keeps, and unfortunately sometimes his own family. Any or all of these may be factors in the production of the delinquency; and we can deal wisely with any factor, even with the child himself, only after we have come to some well-founded conclusion regarding his part in the problem of misconduct. This makes necessary a careful inquiry into the whole situation if well-calculated curative work is to be done, and I would warn against starting this inquiry from preconceived

Three Factors Always to be Considered

notions concerning the sources of trouble that may be unearthed.

First, the Physical Foundations of the Delinquent's Personality

We may very naturally and very practically begin by considering the young delinquent himself. First, perhaps, is there anything peculiar about him from the physical standpoint that stands in the way of his doing better,— anything important to be noted about the physical foundations of his personality? Pertinent are the following as some of the main points for inquiry:

Is the child weak physically or easily fatigued, so that the exigencies of life as met in school or at work, on the play-field or in home duties, bear too hard? (Of course mere smallness of size or of musculature means nothing; plenty of small people have really very superior physical qualities.) The point for us is whether there is any sort of bodily weakness that causes an "easier way" to be sought in sneakiness, unfairness, dishonesty, withdrawal from moral realities. Are the standards of accomplishment set so high anywhere for this given physical organism that the reaction against them is in the direction of getting desired ends by less arduous and by perhaps illegitimate means?

Localized ailments and defects may also be thought of as possibly reacting upon the whole organism, body and mind, so that there results a condition favorable to the development of delinquency. Thus, pathological growth of adenoids and tonsils, chronic infection of ears or teeth, serious obstruction in the air passages, to name some of the commoner ailments of children, can very readily bring about states of general ill-health which form a poor background for the development of good character traits, or of even normal powers of resistance to external suggestions and temptations.

Of course, none of these defective bodily states directly produce delinquency. Many, many children have these troubles and do not become delinquent. Perhaps the growth of a tendency towards misconduct proceeds by a path as roundabout as that we have observed in a number of instances of delinquent children with heart disease where excuses have been made by nurses, parents, and the child himself for not conforming to school and other discipline. One school physician forbade a boy to come to school because he would have to climb a lot of stairs. But this very boy, through knocking about the streets in his authorized idleness, became the leading spirit in an active gang of young burglars; he himself, in spite of the school doctor, doing the climbing over the transoms and other places.

It is very important to note the open avenues to delinquency for a child whose time is not well occupied in school or in other ways. We have known whole careers of misconduct to date from even temporary exclusion from school for sickness or for other reasons, provision for occupying the children's time not being made by either school or family. Perhaps the best source of help in prevention of delinquency here will be developing the new profession of "school visitor." *Open Avenues to Delinquency*

There is another type of physical trouble which affords a foundation for the growth of misbehavior trends,— the sort of ailment which produces irritability in the child. Perhaps the trouble cannot be made clear by the child himself—we find many young people very vague about even such a matter as headaches; perhaps the irritability is not recognized as such; perhaps they are only partly conscious of the difficulty. Relief from the headaches and discomforts of eyestrain makes a great change in feelings, as also from chronic ear troubles or from variously localized abnormality of structure or function. *Factors Which Produce Irritability*

However indirect defective physical conditions may be as causes of delinquency, when they are found in the person of the delinquent there should be no cavilling over the point that the child's chance for overcoming his

237

undesirable tendencies is enhanced by his being in good physical condition. And it is in recognition of this, rather than through belief in the direct physical cause of delinquency that has mainly led juvenile courts to be anxious about the health of the delinquents who come before them. The newspaper quip about Johnny's coming before the judge for throwing stones at windows and being sentenced to have his tonsils removed alludes to that modern consideration for the offender himself which has its rationale in the effort to obtain a sound physical basis for reformation.

The Problem of the Ductless Glands

Some day we may know much more than is at present known about the glands of internal secretion, the thyroid, pituitary, thymus, suprarenal, and other glands, which unquestionably condition many features of our physical, intellectual, and emotional life. At present the best authorities insist that much of what is stated popularly concerning the relationship of the activity of these glands to conduct trends is either very weakly founded or has no basis at all in known fact. Commercial interest has led to exploitation of the subject. We shall have to wait for much more scientific research before we can be well on the way in this method of control of human behavior tendencies.

Nervous Troubles the Chief Cause of Instability

Of all physical ailments, nervous troubles stand in the most direct relationship to delinquency when they involve instability of personality so that the individual is more liable to be beset by impulsions or obsessions and is more prone to be unduly suggestible. Notably, chorea is likely to leave in its train a tendency toward irregular behavior; so also some other organic diseases of the central nervous system. Sometimes an accident involving even slight concussion of the brain or where fright is one of the main effects may bring about abnormal lack of inhibitions, even in the sphere of social behavior.

Lately we have been studying the case of a boy who, previously normal morally, began a downhill path of

238

misbehavior almost immediately following an accident with internal injuries and severe fright. He has become a truant because the confines and tasks of the school room are too irksome; he has given way to impulses toward mischief and rebellion; he has readily fallen in with suggestions toward delinquency. His father confesses he endeavors to correct the boy by the only treatment he knows anything about, the rod, and the school people have apparently made no careful study whatever of the situation. The treatment that is necessary in this case—quiet life, perhaps in the country, removal from companions, a school régime with frequent change of occupation, recreations away from the excitement of city streets and night life—really belongs to the realm of mental hygiene. Indeed, the boy himself tells us soberly, "There's something come over me. I'm different. I don't want to get in wrong, but I can't endure sitting there in the school room so long. I ought to go away somewhere where it's quiet. I want to get my mind right again."

While this is an unusual case, the fact that boys and girls are able to size up the situation with regard to themselves very well has been observed by us many times. The atmosphere of a sympathetic inquiry is very apt to permeate a young delinquent's own mind and quicken his own powers of analysis, with the result that not a little light is thrown upon the possibilities of rational treatment. Indeed, the treatment itself often begins with such an inquiry.

But in considering possible physical bases for misconduct we must not make the mistake of believing that they are all on the side of physical weakness. Superabundant energy, general physical over-development, premature general and sex development are all recognizable in some instances as very specific foundations for misbehavior. The irritable restlessness of strength at the flood tide of adolescence when "A boy's will is the wind's will," the

Physical Exuberance May be a Cause of Delinquency

stress and urge of the chemistry of the blood of youth, the invitations of the world extended to the prematurely ripened young person, so often grown in body before there is corresponding growth of will or of world experience,—all of these are very real phenomena to be intelligently recognized and appropriately met by curative adjustments.

There should be Positive Treatment of Delinquency

With all of these points in mind as explanatory, the guardian of a young person who shows tendencies to delinquency should never sink into easy satisfaction with mere explanation. That is an attitude only too prone to be taken by those who are attracted to somewhat fatalistic biological or social theories concerning the basis of delinquency. There is much to be done about the individual case, not only from the standpoint of whatever physical treatment is possible and whatever social adjustment seems advisable, but also through aiding and insisting on self-discipline and self-mastery. The adviser will do well to aim at this by getting the child to see himself in his relationships to the world, by straight-forward presentation of facts and socratic drawing forth of reasonable conclusions from him. That there is a physical handicap may well be a challenge to manly achievement. The respect and reward of the world for the handicapped winner, paid to a Steinmetz, victorious over a half-sized, mis-shapen body, is a point well worth thorough presentation to all of that class of young delinquents we are now considering. That to run from a bad start and still win in the race of life is profitable and glorious, is an idea and argument which most will listen to. And, after all, the delinquent must be helped to see the pleasurable returns of self-discipline and right doing.

Nor does the existence of any sort of physical basis for delinquency necessarily deny the wisdom and value of discipline from without. But such discipline must be in accord with the needs of the given child and adapted to his temperamental traits.

Coming now to the mind of the child, we may say at once that several aspects of mental life are vastly more important to be understood in relation to delinquency than are physical conditions. This is because conduct of all sorts and at all times is the direct expression of mental life. Our acts are immediately the results of mental activity. There is no one fact that I would counsel every one interested in delinquency to keep so well before him as this inescapable relationship between mental life and conduct.

The Mental Life of the Delinquent of Chief Importance

Are illustrations necessary? If a boy pilfers, he does so because he has in his mind the idea of taking things. If a girl not previously intending to steal suddenly appropriates something in a shop, she does so with such an idea in mind as, "It's pretty, I'd like it." Or, when mischief is afoot with a crowd, the idea of pleasurable excitement is there, the fun of the chase, or satisfying some grudge; or perhaps the thought of the stigma of being called "yellow," if suggestion of misdeeds comes from companions. The reader would do well to consider other situations involving delinquency within his experience and carefully study the factor that mental life, immediate or remote, is in the production of delinquency. It is all the more important to know well this fundamental fact for the explanation of conduct, because accurate knowledge of the specific part played by mental life in the given case offers by far the best chance for direct curative attack upon the cause of the trouble.

Much has been made in recent years, as everybody knows, of the discovery by intelligence tests that among delinquents in juvenile courts or in correctional institutions there is a very much greater proportion of the feeble-minded than in the general population. But here again it is not the bare fact of feeble-mindedness which causes the delinquency—there are many mentally defective persons with good character traits. The army intelligence

Are Delinquents Feeble-Minded as a Rule?

tests showed clearly that plenty of people with intellectual capacity far enough below the average to be denominated mentally defective can be thoroughly good citizens. Case studies by any of us who have had large experience prove the same point.

Even in the mentally defective it is some specific idea or picture in the mind that leads to the misconduct. We might instance, perhaps, the remembrance of pleasure to be derived from the possession of money or other things as inciting the feeble-minded boy or girl to steal. Without such thoughts developed there is no stealing. Or truancy, or running away from home, or indulgence in bad sex practices—typical delinquencies of the feeble-minded—what are these but response to some mental picture or idea of pleasurable returns?

That the feeble-minded, especially the morons, those who belong to the highest group of defectives, are found with relative frequency among delinquents is simply due to their poor inhibitory powers, specifically, their lack of capacity for checking undesirable ideas, just such as spring up in the minds of many other children who do check them—this and their being prone to form simple habits easily, mental and physical, good or bad. With their less active ideational world it is no wonder that they easily accept into their mental life suggestions from without and fail to check undesirable inner mental associations by better thoughts. "When I go by the market, it always makes me think of taking stuff there and then I go and do it," said one defective boy to me.

The Treatment of Mentally Defective Delinquents The problem of the treatment of the mentally defective delinquents is often more simple than the treatment of the bright delinquent. The feeble-minded are satisfied with simpler pleasurable returns, with less complicated recreations and occupations. There is no doubt that a large share of defectives who are regarded as delinquents could be placed safely in country homes or colonized, some of them first needing proper institutional training. The good results of work in this direction are nowadays being published. The more difficult can be made largely self-sustaining in institutions. And some of them are controllable in their own families if the environment is suitable. But all such hopeful treatment must be undertaken before there is long-standing formation of the habit of delinquency. Our experience in tracing the development of criminal careers leads us to give the deepest warning to parents and public authorities in this matter. Allowing the mentally defective child to crystallize his own character in a bad mold through habitual delinquent ideation and delinquent reaction to his environment represents social and moral neglect that often brings dire results to the individual and to society. No inconsiderable number of chronic thieves, vagrants, and even more desperate criminals were defective children whose amenability at an earlier age should have been utilized to their own and to society's advantage.

While discussing delinquent children who are not quite normal mentally, we must include an important group other than the defectives. Not that we would exaggerate the size of this second group; in numbers it is relatively small. Nor do we want, either, to over-emphasize the relationship of delinquency to mental abnormality as a whole—in studying misconduct problems in children one finds those who are normal outweighing heavily in number the abnormal.

This second principal group consists of those who show evidences of poorly balanced mental processes. The trouble is not due to original mental defect, but to erratic mental functioning which may develop rapidly or be a matter of slow growth. To name the principal conditions which are to be noted, there is inability to control ideas, association processes, impulses; there is liability to form false judgments, to have false memories; there is the

Erratic Mental Processes may Cause Delinquency

tendency in all cases for the individual, on account of malfunctioning of his mental life, to be out of line with the world about him.

We cannot say that all children are mentally diseased who show any such manifestations; as a matter of technical classification, these erratic aspects of mental life range all the way from definite mental disease (psychosis) to aberration that is quite minor and temporary, such as may occur with chorea, head injuries, brain diseases, and disorders of some glands of internal secretion. During adolescence some children show exhibitions of peculiar mental behavior that is nothing short of aberrational although it may be merely a passing phase of their lives.

And then there is a sub-group composed of individuals, who show just a moderate lack of good mental balance beginning in childhood and lasting perhaps all their lives, with particular difficulties arising during periods of physiological and other stress. These persons we cannot denominate psychopathic personalities simply because their mental processes show in miniature or on occasion some of the phenomena which are characteristic of mental disease. Such individuals are frequently very far from being defective; indeed they may be brilliant from a purely intellectual standpoint. Their trouble, as in all cases in this group, has to do with maintaining good mental balance; there is weakness in control or in coördination of various departments of mental life. It is quite obvious that conduct difficulties may arise through the confusions and erroneous judgments and lack of control over impulses and ideas which characterize these faulty mental functionings.

The treatment of delinquency in any members of this group should be based on competent diagnosis, determining whether or not the child belongs properly in this category of those with poor mental balance, and secondarily, whether or not there is anything much that can be done in the way of medical therapy. In only a few such cases, we regret to acknowledge, will our present medical knowledge help us to effect a cure. But the healing power of nature itself will in some instances lead to self-therapy, as in cases of adolescent mental disturbance which we have witnessed recover without medical assistance.

The classification of the somewhat erratic individuals into types of personalities, such as is the fashion to-day in many psychiatric clinics, without study of their background in experiences, upbringing, and other features of environment, is a very inadequate procedure from the standpoint of treatment. The particular features of a given individual's environment that lead him into misconduct is perhaps the main point to be known. If we study him with common-sense thoroughness we frequently find that certain members of the family, certain companions or neighborhood allurements, certain school classes or special teachers, arouse a tendency to bad behavior which is not at all shown under other conditions. I could give hundreds of illustrations of this. For the treatment, if we decide, as in most cases we have to decide, that the individual's own personality is not immediately alterable, we must try to place him under environmental conditions where his undesirable behavior trends will be least likely to be brought out. *Environmental Conditions are always Important*

Here again I do not want to be misunderstood as believing that there is little value in discipline. On the contrary, I think discipline that is educative, that includes self-discipline, is of more value in most of these cases than anything else. With some psychopathic personalities the steady regime of a really good juvenile correctional institution over a prolonged period offers the best chance for beneficial treatment.

In our work we have seen many children who in one set of circumstances, with nagging parents, with an excitable family, with a teasing or otherwise irritating relative, or living under poor conditions for sleeping, and so on, have shown markedly psychopathic personality traits and yet who under quieter and better conditions have seemed entirely different individuals. One boy's eccentric behavior was largely in response to his brother's nasty talk, some of it in undertones at the meal table when it actually turned him against his food. The real instigator was accounted the good boy and the victim was regarded as delinquent because he ran away and stole either to get away or to get amusements outside his home. The proof of the value of analysis of the case is in the fact that our boy showed no delinquencies when placed in another family. After a time he grew more stable and was quite able to do well at home, the brother in the meantime having been persuaded to change his mode of thought and conversation.

A Good Environment may Counteract Erratic Tendencies

So it may be confidently asserted that the person with moderately erratic tendencies, who is guided into good habits of mind and body, perhaps if necessary placed in another home environment, is often able to get along well. Thus, the social aspects of a case are by no means the least or last consideration either for discovering the causes of trouble or for curing the trouble. One finds, unfortunately, however, that meeting the family upon a common-sense level of reconstructive effort is in many cases not so easy, not even when one is dealing with intelligent parents. A very good mother of a very unstable and badly behaved (and, because of her neurotic condition), utterly spoiled child, said, "Then you tell me that I who have done so much for my child am not the proper person to bring her up. That's too hard to believe."

Nor do we always get coöperation from teachers and principals who either have preconceived notions of what a child needs, particularly in the way of dsicipline, or who feel that the school system cannot be disrupted to give special privileges to a child who is not physically crippled. In fact it sometimes is much worse than that, for the personality of the teacher may be at fault, and a mutual dislike based on prior experiences may be at the root of personal attitudes which are no small obstacle to better behavior on the part of the child. How often have we heard, "That crazy teacher, how I hate her!" "That hard-faced teacher, it makes me nervous every day to be in her room!" "That sarcastic teacher, you can never do anything to please her!" Imagine a sensitive child being obliged every day to face a situation which is so distasteful. With all the admiration which I have for the teaching profession and for most members of it whom I know, I sometimes am compelled to believe that the greatest requisite for good teaching is the fine personal influence that can come only through understanding the natural history of the child, and this must include appreciation of the needs and responses of the overly sensitive, the unstable, the psychopathic personality.

Personality Traits of Parents and Teachers may Influence Delinquency

After all of the foregoing we must assert again at this point that most people who are confronted by the problem of treating of delinquency in children have to do with mentally normal offenders. It is perhaps not strange, in the light of the overstatements which have been made in recent years concerning the relationship between delinquency and mental abnormality, particularly mental defect, that relatives sometimes bring a thoroughly normal child for examination and begin by asking whether or not he is normal mentally. This is much as it was a little earlier when there was considerable newspaper talk about delinquency being caused by some pressure of the skull on the brain. Parents used to convince themselves that they knew what particular knock on the head did it in the same fashion as some parents nowadays come to a clinic attributing a paralysis or other ailment to some fall or head accident which could not possibly have caused the trouble.

Most Delinquents Normal Mentally

247

Now, a great deal already stated in this chapter about the inner mental life, educating to self discipline, change of environment, etc., for delinquents who are not normal mentally, can be applied just as well in a discussion of the treatment of those who are quite normal mentally. And, also, not a little that one may say about misconduct in the mentally normal applies equally well to those who are abnormal.

First Generalization: Importance of Origin of Idea of Delinquency For the purposes of this chapter, which must necessarily deal with the subject in brief and cannot possibly include many items which a more professional monograph would require, I shall attempt to give some generalizations which will embody fundamentals. Earlier in the chapter I insisted that I knew of nothing which was more essential to sound procedure in the treatment of a delinquent than getting at the particular ideational life which leads to delinquency. The first of the generalizations, then, may well be the statement that of all the inquiries which one can make concerning the delinquent and of all the questions which one can put directly or indirectly to the delinquent himself, nothing is so important as those which have to deal with how the ideas of delinquency gained entrance into his mind. In thinking of any special thoughts or special ideas which may possibly stand in the most immediate relationship to delinquency, as cause to effect, it is knowledge of their origin which will be most likely to give us an understanding of what they are. And without understanding this feature of the background in origins one is quite apt entirely to miss the dynamic center of the whole situation and to make a botch of the treatment. In order to illustrate this and a number of other points in the treatment of delinquency, I offer an illustrative case study.

Case of a Chronic Delinquency A young man of twenty-one has lived for years in a city in New York State, where he has had all the advantages that a particularly wholesome environment offers. My information comes from the intelligent father and mother and from a friend, the family physician. All these and other relatives have attempted to check this boy's tendencies toward delinquency, but without avail. After lapses into dishonesty for a dozen years, he has recently been in a very serious affair involving, through forging and misrepresentation, the bank account of a relative. Quick settlement with the bank prevented the matter from coming to court, but the parents are now in desperation. It is the old story: early misrepresentations and pilfering leading on to larger stealing; much lying at first in obvious self defense, later larger fabrications.

And yet one finds that the delinquent presents a pleasing personality, having good looks, good bodily structure, good address, and mentality in many respects considerably above the average. Morover, he is much concerned about himself and readily acknowledges his own weaknesses and transgressions. Indeed, this has been characteristic of him all along. Naturally, one is interested to know what sort of treatment such an apparently rational and responsive individual has received. Early he was reasoned with and punished by deprivations and whippings; more recently there have been the usual mother's tears and pleadings and the father's stern admonitions, with more deprivations which the boy has always accepted in stoical fashion. The physician and others have gone with him into the question of his habits and his companionships, and have unearthed various details, the boy always manfully maintaining that the trouble was with himself and not with his companions, and nothing came of it all. It should be added that there has been harmony in the household and about methods of discipline, not, however, to the extent that the mother has always been made acquainted with the extent of her boy's misdeeds.

If one could give a good picture of the surprise of these parents when they learned the true facts of the case,

His Pleasing Personality Reasonableness; His Treatment

Ignorance of
Intelligent
Parents

so easy for us to ascertain, it would do much to enforce the value of this chapter. The mother, an unusually intelligent woman, said, "How can it be that parents can be blind in their working toward an end at which they have so earnestly aimed. Why aren't we better educated concerning causes and about what goes to make conduct. If years ago we had only known more!"

Not one of those who had tried to take a hand in the guidance of this boy seems to have made the sort of rational inquiry that investigation into àny other natural phenomenon would surely involve. During the long years of his delinquent career, and this has been true in many another case we have seen, no one obtained from the boy the story of beginnings, learning under what circumstances and through what incentives he began his lying and stealing. And yet these facts concerning origins are very often just what are necessary to a correct understanding of a case and to formulating rational plans of treatment.

Ineffective-
ness of
Direct
Inquiry

No doubt the question was oftentimes asked the boy, "What makes you do such things?" Or even, "How did you get such ideas into your head?" And the answer to this type of question practically always is, "I don't know." Nor in the consulting room is there any better response to such direct questionings. In fact, the delinquent very seldom reasons out the basis of his own conduct well enough to be able to state causes. His delinquent tendency is a fact to him, perhaps a distressing fact, one that stands in the way of larger pleasures and successes; and yet to himself it is not altogether explicable.

Dynamics of
Hidden
Mental Life

Moreover, one finds sometimes that the child all along has an underlying feeling that he is not understood. "They don't know what I've been up against," is the sort of comment on parental treatment that I have heard over and over again. To have continually in the background of consciousness unfortunate ideas which have not been shared with advisers often produces a perniciously active and continuing source of energy making for misconduct. It may not always be clear just why this is so, why what is hidden is so dynamic, so urgent, and yet the history of many cases proves that it is a fact.

In the case I am relating one felt it useless directly to inquire about the source of the trouble or advisable to ask *who* had influenced the delinquent for the bad; indeed the young man quickly said he had been going with a "bunch of boys and girls that were not too good, and yet weren't so bad either." He added, "I've always told my father he needn't blame anybody else for anything I did." Now that is an attitude that is frequently taken in the first statement toward companions, perhaps logically, perhaps manfully or generously, or in evidence of desire not to be considered foolishly weak willed.

Loyalty to Companions

But approaching the matter by a different method, historically, as one might say, and more impersonally, and inquiring about incidents and interests and companions at this or that age, and about what sort of children the various companions were and what were the activities engaged in with them, we may, and oftentimes do, get a very clear statement of essentials. Our young man suddenly said, after we had him placed in memory amid a little group of children when he was five to seven years of age and in the town where he then lived, and talking about their playtimes and other features of their comradeship, "I'll tell you, doctor, that's where it began, right there. I began lying so they wouldn't know when that boy and girl came over to my house when my mother had gone out in the afternoon. I learned to lie and to steal right there. I remember the bag of candies I bought with the first money I took from my mother's purse." He told how that sort of thing with the little group of three went on for some time and that he lied much so that his mother should not know that the others had come to their house. There was

The Historical and Impersonal Inquiry

more to it of course; the group had spoken together of some bad things and engaged in some bad sex practices. And what he now remembered as his peculiar emotional reaction to the affair was his discomfiture and shame and feeling of inferiority at so breaking with family confidences and standards of honesty, however indefinite his appreciation of such things may have been at that early age.

The Golden Moment for Treatment Now, whatever the outcome will be in this case, after all these years of habit formation and whatever there may be in the way of peculiar personality traits on the part of this young man which has led him towards misconduct, back at the beginning was the golden moment when his parents might have learned much and prevented much. That is the point to be stressed here. They did discover something of his lying and pilfering tendencies then, even though they knew nothing of the source or extent of it. They merely punished him for it and he at once became cowardly about the punishments, he says, and lied all the more. Thus the treatment was not at all directed at the cause of the trouble.

At the time when a child is first detected in delinquency, even in lying, then is the time to dig deep into every possible motivation or into every association or source from which the idea of the specific misconduct may have been gained. In most cases, I find, it is some personal association or experience which is at the source or root of the misbehavior and the child is not going to tell what has happened unless confronted by the specific and detailed but sympathetic inquiry which he can respond to without damage to his sense of childish propriety, whether that be loyalty to comrades, shame about the affair, unnecessary exposure of himself to punishment, and so on. But too much suggestion which might elicit false accusations or false confessions must be avoided; tactful indirectness is required.

By way of a second generalization I would stress the

value for treatment of considering the matter of delin- Second Generalization: Importance of Special Time Relationships of Delinquency quency in its chronological aspects. During what weeks, on what days, at what hours are the tendencies to misconduct displayed? In few cases is there continuous exhibition of bad behavior. All study of a case is designed, of course, to dig out the relation of cause to effect. Does it take place, this misconduct, on special occasions or at special hours, and if so, why?

Today a father comes in with his little boy who has A Case in Point been pilfering from his pockets and money drawer, having taken probably over a hundred dollars during the last half year. The boy knows now when the stealing has been done—always in the early morning. The father has lectured and whipped the boy, remaining bound to the idea that he would not lock up all the household cash,—it was too disgraceful and troublesome. But he has never put two and two together in time relationships, although in answering questions about the boy's habit he tells how early he wakes up. The boy, in turn, under simple questioning tells of a companion who likewise steals and how they share this as a great secret, how the early waking hours are filled for him with wishing half-dreams and how he then plans getting out quietly before the others are awake to get at his father's pockets or purse. Indeed this boy of nine years goes on to say that he does really want to do very differently and that he is sure he can if he can keep away from the other boy of eleven, which is easy enough to accomplish. He says especially that if he can keep from having these morning wishes and temptations he can do differently—he never has them for a minute at any other time. And this second problem seems easy enough to solve, for the boy goes to bed at seven and goes right to sleep; he is all slept out long before the others are awake.

It is just by such a change in habits and management of a child that we have seen many a case cured. A boy

Other
Special
Time Re-
lationships returns from school glum, defiant, hateful, mean to the pet animals on some days. The question is not what is wrong in general, but what is there specifically behind the time relationships? We have in mind a boy who was studied on account of such behavior from a general medical standpoint by very good physicians but without any beneficial result. It proved to be a companionship affair on certain days when there was exchange of obscene conversation which the boy hardly understood but hated himself for; and to this dissatisfaction with himself he reacted, as many people do, by taking it out on his surroundings.

And other cases, where at intervals and only occasionally there are outbreaks of misconduct of any kind,—do these come after some certain visit or special experiences, or as related to some holiday or hours of idleness? One could bring many case studies to bear on these matters of time connection in delinquencies. But the time feature of a case (this is a point that must not be forgotten) should be related to the possibility of special inner as well as outer experiences that are contributing factors in causing delinquency.

Very much delinquency has its inception during hours of idleness, in bed as well as out of bed, and during times when pernicious day-dreaming is possible. (Of course, day-dreaming may be of fine ambitions and wishes.) To trace misconduct to this inner source and to these times is to do more toward getting a clue to rational and efficient treatment than almost anything else which may be done. It is possible to safeguard the young individual by preventing the occurrence of such times and seasons when delinquent thoughts develop much more easily than it is possible to prevent opportunity for the delinquent acts themselves to follow.

And this naturally leads us to consider another point which is important enough to be made a generalization:

It is of great importance for treatment to understand the special conditions or circumstances under which a boy or girl develops any recurrent idea of delinquency. Is it in relationship to any locality or companionship, to any school, or playground, or home situation, to any recreation or place of recreation, or any employment? One may often get at this through studying time relationships. But again, the special condition often involves mostly the inner mental life. Those who have studied our published case histories will be familiar with the various aspects of the life of the mind that have to do with reviving an idea of delinquency. The phenomena are, for the most part, based on the laws of mental association; one idea follows another because they were earlier linked together. Vivid instances occur. One little girl, when she read the name George, especially in school, thought of what George her schoolmate had said that was bad, and one thought would lead to another till she would be spurred on to the actual misconduct, stealing, that they had talked about. And the thought of certain pictures seen at the time of definite suggestions toward delinquency, or of tabooed words (obscene or related to sex), because these had been uttered by others at the time of delinquent acts, may arouse chains of thought that end in the performance of misconduct.

Third Generalization: Importance of Knowing the Special Conditions under which Delinquent Ideas Recur

These special conditions may be met by way of treatment not only by vigorous, wholesome, constructive measures, but also by learning of and breaking up old associational thought processes by the formation of new and better chains of association. This requires skill, but it is entirely possible and by the use of common-sense methods.

Nothing that needs change in the outer circumstances of the child is more difficult to achieve than breaking up of bad neighborhood companionships. Under the ordinary conditions of life, it is asking a great deal, sometimes too much, to have a child utterly refuse to associate

Suggestions for Treatment of Environmental Conditions

with the other children who live near him. Nor is it usually effective for anyone to attempt to reform the crowd as such unless the children have a great deal of time and oversight given them. A single child or a group of children will need new interests to command them either through change of residence or change in recreational or other activities in connection with which the delinquency has developed. We find ourselves in this matter drawing particularly on the following conception of possibilities: change of family residence or placing the child with relatives; putting him in touch with entirely new centers or features of recreational life; "placing out" for a longer or shorter time by child-helping agencies; change of schools or of teachers or of the curriculum to fit the child's special abilities, disabilities, interests, or needs; attacking the problem of group misconduct by the appeal of probation officers or others to guardians of a child's wayward companions, or through juvenile court action; and finally, change of various living conditions or habits if these appear to play some part in developing delinquent tedencies.

Attack Upon Conditions (a) Directly Causing or (b) Affording Opportunity for Bad Ideas

The reader can see running all through these suggestions that the attack is really always upon (a) those outer conditions which may be influencing the child's mental life by directly suggesting ideas of misconduct, or (b) upon those conditions which afford an opportunity for the child of himself to cherish, or consciously or subsconsciously to re-awaken, the ideation or imagery that creates the impulse to misconduct.

A Case in Point

A case comes to mind as I write these last paragraphs— a boy brought for study from a country home in another State, a "placed out" boy, eight years old, who is showing some peculiarly vicious tendencies towards cruelty, obscenity, and sex habits (although the little fellow is reported in many ways to have good traits and he is intelligent and truthful). With very little effort it was found that his troubles are always secondary to his thoughts and that these are awakened by very definite opportunities and external associations, always when he is alone, generally when he is in the barn, and then only when he begins to think of his cousins, now in an institution, who taught him much of this when he was not more than five years old, and about whose misdeeds he has heard much from the other boys. Can there be any doubt, in the light of what we have said heretofore, about how to go ahead in the treatment of this case?

Since so much has been made in preceding paragraphs of the mental life, there should be some enumeration of the measures for treatment that directly influence such thought processes of the child as tend to produce delinquent conduct. With both the normal and the defective, if any special abilities are discovered one may well consider giving healthier satisfactions and new interests through chances for developing activities which may command the child's vigorous attention. And in this attempt at forming new adjustments we should aim to develop in the child a better feeling of his being somebody of worth in the world, counteracting in every way possible the inferiority feeling which is so frequently discovered among delinquents. And then there is the matter of confidences with parents. These should be rated very high as influencing the child's mental life, but they should not be carried to the extent of allowing the psychopathic young individual to over-exploit his feelings and desires for recognition—there is some strength in mental reserve. Incentives toward better conduct undoubtedly may be received through good reading—have we not all experienced this?—or by bedtime or other appropriate suggestions. And need we say anything about the high value of religious and ethical instruction, although we are rather afraid of preachment to those who are already delinquent, because we have so frequently seen cases

Suggestions for Treatment through More Favorable Opportunities for Growth of Better Mental Interests

Rationale of Discipline and Punishment

where the religious approach was unavailing on account of the underlying facts not being understood. Then we frequently advise meeting the child on the level of his perplexity concerning tabooed words, setting him right about them and particularly about his sex ideas, making plain the biological truth and the essential purity of sex relations. Other measures that have to do with the modification of the thought life have been hinted at heretofore, but again we would insist upon this whole matter not being taken in too general a sense but that there be realization that what is most required is special help at special times.

No part of this chapter is to be construed as argument against either discipline or punishment, which, to my mind, play a part in every well-ordered life of old or young. The discipline of work, of doing right, and of many other necessities in adult life, as well as the discipline of education and right conduct in childhood are very real. Punishments in various forms come to adults who fail to play the game of life well, and the child needs to realize this so that he will not think that he alone is subject to guidance, obedience, and retribution.

But every bit of the regulation of a child's life should be aimed at the development of the power of self-discipline. Even punishment well administered has this as its end. If punishment of any kind, particularly corporal punishment, is poorly adapted so that a bad spirit in the child is engendered, then it defeats its own best end. We find that delay in the procedure of punishment, whether in family life, as when it is promised that the father will whip the child when he comes home at night or returns from a trip in a few days, or when delinquents are held in a court detention home, encourages the growth of an entirely pernicious spirit, whether of fear or of vindictiveness in the child. I earnestly counsel the adoption of measures of discipline carefully calculated so that no bad spirit on the part of the child, whether developed from his own inner feelings or from the suggestions of others concerning the discipline which he should have, will be permitted or encouraged to develop.

Just exactly what forms punishment should take is beyond the province of this chapter to discuss, because such immense variations are advisable according to the habits and customs of the community, of the institution in which the child may be, and of the school and the home. What has a good influence on one child may turn out badly with another, not only on account of variation in innate emotional response, but also in the ideas which the individual has imbibed from his environment. What is perniciously humbling to some children may not be so to others; while rabid vindictiveness may be aroused in one child by some form of discipline that another has been accustomed to take without notice. We may go to novels as well as to real life for stories that bear this out. Again, this is a matter of adaptation of measures of treatment to the child's peculiarly personal needs. *Individualization of Punishment According to Customs and Personal Needs*

In the treatment of delinquency both the child and the environment have to be considered. *Summary*

The best method of procedure is always through getting at a fundamental understanding of the trouble.

There are various physical defects and ailments which may be conceived of as needing treatment in the delinquent child, but mainly from the standpoint of offering the best possible basis for reformation rather than as directly causing delinquency.

The mental life of the child is the most important for consideration; delinquency arises directly from the character of the child's ideas.

Mental defect is a matter that has to be considered, and also lack of good mental balance, whether as actual mental disease or as showing itself through a psychopathic personality. All these form well-known, immediate backgrounds of delinquency.

But the vast majority of delinquent children are quite normal mentally. With these the most direct approach to the whole problem of delinquency is through their ideational life—(a) the origin of their delinquent ideas, (b) the special times and periods when these especially recur, and (c) the essential conditions or circumstances under which delinquent ideas recur. The investigation of these points gives a most valuable short-cut to the treatment of any case, and indeed sometimes is an absolute requisite to the cure of the delinquent trends.

There are many suggestions for the treatment of external circumstances and of mental life that should come through common-sense observation and reading, but no feature of the situation should be left out of account.

Disciplines and punishments are frequently advisable and sometimes necessary, but they should be very well directed so that they may not influence the individual in any unfortunate way. They must be well considered and well adapted to the personal needs of the child.

XIII

The Care of Intellectually Inferior Children

THE exact scope of the problem indicated by the title of this chapter is difficult to define. There is no universally accepted official definition even of the term "mental deficiency." Some would broaden this term sufficiently to include merely backward and retarded children. It is not our purpose, however, to discuss the problem of the merely dull child, who is laggard in school but who gives promise of becoming an altogether normal, self-supporting, self-controlling adult. We shall use the term in its more restricted meaning to apply to those children who, because of subnormal mental endowment, will not be able to adapt themselves to an ordinary environment or to maintain existence independently of some external support and guidance. We shall, however, lay special emphasis upon that group of mentally deficient children who approximate the normal in their general capacities and outlook, because it is this group which is most numerous and, in many respects, most important both from the social and the educational point of view.

For purposes of clearness, it is necessary, however, to recognize at the outset that there are different degrees of mental deficiency just as there are different degrees of normal and superior intelligence. Many classifications have been proposed to differentiate and describe these varying degrees of mental deficiency but in many respects the most satisfactory classification is that contained in the Mental Deficiency Law of England. This law defines idiots as "persons so deeply defective in mind from birth, or from an early age, as to be unable to guard themselves against common physical dangers."

Imbeciles are defined as "persons in whose case there exists from birth or from an early age mental defectiveness not amounting to idiocy, yet so pronounced that they are incapable of managing themselves or their affairs, or, in the case of children, of being taught to do so."

And morons are defined as "persons in whose case there exists from birth or from an early age mental defectiveness not amounting to imbecility, yet so pronounced that they require care, supervision, and control for their own protection, or for the protection of others; or, in the case of children, that they, by reason of such defectiveness, appear to be permanently incapable of receiving proper benefit from the instruction in ordinary schools."

The Distinction between a Dullard and a Deficient Child

What is the difference between a dullard and a deficient child? It may not be altogether scientific to make a rigid distinction between them. It has been maintained that grades of intelligence fade into each other like day, dusk, dark and dawn; and that it is arbitrary to draw sharp lines between the grades. For practical reasons, however, we insist that a clear-cut distinction should be made between the dullard and the deficient child. And the distinction should be made in favor of the dullard. A dullard is not a very high-grade moron; he is not a super-moron. He is to be regarded as a definitely normal individual, whose general alertness is simply below the average. He is organized along normal lines. He may be slow witted; but he is not weak witted. He has considerable mental stamina and stability. When we describe him psychologically as a low-grade normal, we do it in no derogatory sense. He may be backward in school; he may be rather obtuse in abstract, academic subjects; but in his natural sphere he succeeds. He makes his way in the world, because he has enough mother wit to do so. This is more than we can say of the moron; for, as Tregold has pointed out, even the highest-grade moron is lacking in "that essential to independent existence, 'common sense'."

The above definitions and distinctions are placed frankly before the reader in order to avoid undue confusion. It is very important, however, to caution the reader against placing normal children and the mentally deficient children in absolutely different categories. The mentally deficient child is not a separate and peculiar species. He belongs to the human family. His educational, if not his developmental psychology, are of the same general character as that of the normal child. In many respects he may very closely simulate a normal individual. He may need specialized educational procedures, but in general he must be approached as though he were a normal child with certain limitations and handicaps.

We do not treat the blind child and the crippled child as though they were apart from the human family. We ought to acquire a similar attitude and philosophy with respect to the mentally deficient child, even if his handicap is in the field of intelligence. It may be said that the recent developments in the study and treatment of mental deficiency have tended to emphasize the normal rather than the pathological aspects of mental defect. The whole problem appears less forbidding and more manageable from every point of view than it did even a decade ago.

At this point we may take a glance at the progress which our knowledge has made in this field. Only a little more than a century ago, medical writers were still confusing the concepts of insanity and idiocy. Esquirol made a distinction between these two conditions. The progress of modern medicine in the fields of neurology and physiology and endocrinology (the study of the internal glands) have helped us considerably in under-

Medical Knowledge of the Problem

standing the physical basis and physical characteristics of mentally deficient children. In a relatively few instances, such as cretinism, this medical knowledge has suggested the possibility of curing certain developmental types of mental deficiencies. Cretinism, however, is a relatively rare form of mental deficiency and it must be diagnosed in early infancy if the administration of thyroid tablets is to accomplish fully curative results.

We mention this fact because parents and teachers are still too prone to look hopefully toward glandular extract thereapy for the cure of mental deficiency. Medical knowledge in its present state emphasizes the incurability of feeble-mindedness, but it has thrown considerable light on various causes of feeble-mindedness and indicates how the community, through proper preventive measures, may reduce the number of feeble-minded in the population. All eugenic measures which insure soundness of stock will, in the next generation, increase normality and reduce subnormality. There are, however, numerous cases of mental deficiency in which no hereditary factor is demonstrable and in which the causative factor is a disease or damage which curtails the development of the brain. All medical and public health measures which promote maternal hygiene, which improve obstetric and midwife practice, and which control infectious diseases will, in the aggregate, materially reduce the number of feeble-minded. Moreover, in spite of the fact that medical science is unable to cure mental deficiency, it must be insisted that the advice of the physician is necessary at many points because of the physical complications involved.

Psychological Studies of the Problem Our understanding of the problem of mental deficiency has been both broadened and deepened by the development of educational and child psychology, particularly during the last fifty years. The child study movement which was so prominent in the 1890's concerned itself chiefly with the psychology of normal children but it gave an impetus to the study of subnormal and handicapped children. Experimental and educational psychology likewise made contributions to a better understanding of the limitations and characteristics of subnormal minds. In 1896, Lightner Witmer, professor of psychology at the University of Pennsylvania, established at Philadelphia what is reputed to be the first psychological clinic for the diagnosis and treatment of mentally exceptional and atypical children. In 1899, the Board of Education of the City of Chicago, established a department for research into the problems relating to educationally exceptional children. In 1898 the Faribault (Minnesota) School for the Feeble-Minded established a department of research. In 1906 a similar research department was established at the Vineland Training School, in Vineland, New Jersey. These are a few of the early indications of the more scientific interest in the problem of the care of mentally deficient children.

Somewhat more extended mention must be made of the work of Alfred Binet, who, in 1904, was appointed by the Minister of Public Instruction in France as a member of the commission which was charged with the study of measures to be taken for insuring the benefits of instruction for defective children, and whose services in mental measurement were referred to in Chapter VII. This eminent psychologist was appointed because of his investigations and interest in the general field of child study. He had made significant studies of mental development in his own children.

The Contribution of Alfred Binet, in France

The commission decided that "no child suspect should be eliminated from school and admitted into a special class without first being submitted to a pedagogical and medical examination from which it could be certified that, because of his state of intelligence, he was unable to profit by the instruction given in the ordinary schools."

This practical situation revealed to Binet the necessity of establishing a more scientific diagnosis of inferior states of intelligence. He met the problem by devising what he called a measuring scale of intelligence which graded children according to their mental age. Binet did not pretend that this scale has the accuracy of a clinical thermometer, which reads to the tenth of a degree, but he called it a scale because it is made up of standardized units or tests. Five or six simple tests for each age from three to twelve or sixteen years of age furnish the basis of measurement. What is normal or characteristic of a given age being known, we can determine roughly whether a child tests above age, below age or at age and we can tell how much he deviates from his chronological age. The mental age of mentally deficient children, therefore, gives us some idea of their retardation.

Binet's researches led to a stupendous amount of investigation relating to the problems of subnormal mentality. Particularly was this true in America where hundreds of articles and scores of books indirectly owe their inception to the suggestive writings of Alfred Binet. In a measure this is true even of the vast psychological enterprise of the World War, in which 1,700,000 soldiers were tested by graded intelligence scales.

American Investigations The psychological investigations in this field, both in England and America, have followed closely the conceptions of Binet. Professor Lewis Terman of Stanford University made a revision and extension of the Binet Measuring Scale which has come into wide use. This version of the Binet Measuring Scale expresses a mental rating by means of an "Intelligence Quotient" or IQ., which is derived by dividing the ascertained mental age by the chronological age. If the numerator (mental age) and denominator are equal we have a quotient of *1*, or expressed on a percentage basis of 100. If the numerator is 2 and the denominator is 3 we have a value below 100; if the numerator is 3 and the denominator is 2 we have an IQ of 150. It has been suggested that an IQ of 70 or less must indicate mental deficiency, but this is not a safe rule to follow because there are too many exceptions. A large amount of error and confusion has been caused by the uncritical use of mental measurements. Still the mental age is an objective measure of mentality, and as such it is a good point of departure for estimating the capacity and educational treatment of a subnormal child.

The convenience and apparent precision of mental measurement methods led originally to an exaggerated emphasis on the factor of intelligence in the problem of the care of mentally deficient children. In many cases the classification, and even the training of backward and defective children were too exclusively determined by mental age ratings. Psychiatrists have called attention to the danger of exaggerating the purely intellectual factor in the study and treatment of handicapped individuals.

Personality Traits as well as Intelligence of Importance in the Case of Feeble-Minded Individuals

The psychiatrist, by training and professional experience, is accustomed to take into account the total individuality and to emphasize the significance of personality traits. Recent literature and practical work in this field alike have placed increasing stress on the personality factors. Numerous case studies have shown that the mental age and IQ of an individual are not all-determining with respect to his vocational capacity. In some instances, a youth with an intelligence age as low as five years has done surprisingly well industrially, because of favorable personality endowment. Mental surveys of the after-career of mentally deficient pupils discharged from special classes and similar surveys of former inmates of institutions for the feeble-minded have revealed a relatively high degree of earning power on the part of individuals who had been diagnosed as feeble-minded. The experiments of progressive institutions in the colony care of the feeble-minded have also revealed in a new light the vocational possibility of subnormal individuals.

The most important investigation and demonstration in this direction has been made by Dr. Charles Bernstein, superintendent of the State School (for the feeble-minded) at Rome, New York. His vision and constructive efforts in this work have demonstrated that the higher grade of feeble-minded individuals can be trained for productive labor in industrial, agricultural, and domestic fields. It has also been demonstrated that a small group of forty defectives, after preliminary training, can be placed in a rented house, presided over by a matron and her husband and, with this dormitory serving as a home and recreation center, these defectives can go out and do house work, farm work and shop work. There are over thirty of these extra-institutional vocational colonies in New York and they are being operated at a great economical saving to the State.

A recent New Haven experiment to determine the vocational possibility of subnormal girls in factory work, showed that even a girl of a mental age of six years could earn nine dollars a week, under specially favorable conditions. A boy who was a member of a vocational colony for mental defectives in the Adirondacks one year received the prize for planting the largest number of trees planted by any one person in the United States.

These successful efforts in the vocational community control of mentally deficient individuals are mentioned here because such demonstrations have almost revolutionized our conception of the feeble-minded individual and have made our whole attitude toward him more constructive and hopeful. Our educational procedure with reference to mentally deficient children should take into full account their many vocational possibilities.

Practically all cases of mental deficiency are recogniz-able and become established before the age of six years. The adequate training of the deficient child can not, therefore, be postponed to the time when he is of school age or of wage earning age. His training can not begin too early and here, as elsewhere, there is danger in ignoring the importance of the pre-school period of his development. There is also danger that the deficient child will, during this period, be sadly misunderstood and even imposed upon. I have seen many instances in which a defective child was punished severely because he seemed unduly troublesome and unreasonably obstinate. Sometimes these situations drift into unconscious forms of cruelty to the child and extreme vexation for the parent.

The Pre-School Care of the Deficient Child

It is necessary to realize from the outset that the deficient child will be slow in his learning and that in no way can he be forced beyond the level of his capacity. He may even be slow in learning to walk and to talk; he may be slow in acquiring habits of cleanliness; but within his limits he will yield to judicious discipline and to systematic training. This training must, in the beginning, concern itself with the very simplest matters, such as putting on shoes, buttoning blouse, using the handker-chief properly and a multitude of simple acts in the field of his every-day life. Great patience and tolerance must be exercised in this period when normal children develop with such striking speed.

There can only be vexation and disappointment if the child is continually compared with his normal peers, but if the parent can assume the courageous and scientific attitude of treating the defective child in terms of his actual mental maturity the whole situation will tend to become more tolerable and more constructive, because within his sphere the child has considerable learning capacity. It will also make the atmosphere of his upbringing more wholesome and reduce the tendency to nervousness and irritability which sometimes actually undermine the health of the mother. The writer has seen too much of this whole problem to be blind to the disappointment and difficulties involved, but he has noted that the parent who is able to take the most rational, that is, the most psychological, view of the educational problem is most likely to secure results and to maintain a wholesome atmosphere in the domestic training of the child.

The Laws of Habit Formation Apply to the Mentally Deficient Child The ordinary laws of habit formation which are discussed in this volume (Chapter VII) apply with equal force to the mentally deficient child. A great deal of his education must come, as we say, thru the force of habit. We can not rely too much on his initiative and personal judgment because it is in these directions that he is most impoverished. Habit formation, however, does not depend altogether upon drilling and repetition. Even a mentally deficient child is largely governed by motives and emotional considerations, just as you and I are. He thrives best in an atmosphere of happiness, and wonders can be accomplished thru the liberal use of encouragement and praise. In fact it might almost be made an unqualified rule that mentally deficient children, either at home or at school, can not be praised too often. To be sure, this commendation must be made with certain pedagogical skill but the rule should be,—"praise too much rather than too little." Scolding has a very small amount of value even when skilfully done. We recommend a policy of encouragement with respect to the feeble-minded largely because we wish to strengthen their own personality sense and to increase their self-respect. Many a deficient child behaves more defectively than he needs to because he is enmeshed by certain feelings of inferiority. The inferiority complexes, so called, are by no means limited to normal and psycho-neurotic individuals.

The chief objective in the home training of the pre- school deficient child should be school entrance. The parent should so far as possible train him so that he will adjust himself reasonably well to other children. When the deficient child should enter school is a question which can not be answered arbitrarily. In some instances school entrance will be postponed until the age of eight or nine years because the child is better adapted to home than to school life. On the other hand, there are many deficient children who would profit, at least by kinder-garten experience, as early as the age of three, four, five or six. Other things being equal, it is desirable to give the deficient child the benefits of the social training and handwork which are characteristic of a modern kinder-garten. The kindergarten teacher can not be expected to make extreme adjustments in behalf of a deficient child, but she will usually be found ready to coöperate if the child is at all amenable.

School Training

The public school systems of our larger cities have established special classes for educationally exceptional children. In some instances such classes have been created for the blind and semi-blind, deaf and semi-deaf, for the speech defectives, and, in New York, even for cardiac defectives. In the same spirit, public schools have set aside special classes and special teachers for the training of mentally handicapped pupils. The intelligent parent will ordinarily regard these provisions as in the nature of special advantages for the deficient pupil. Enrollment in these classes is rarely above fifteen, and the equipment is usually more expensive than that in ordinary class rooms. The special class teacher also has special professional training for her work. These favorable conditions permit a great deal of individual attention to each child. They also make possible a flexible program which emphasizes physical and motor and personal training as well as the academic subjects. Although the special class, with all these facilities is unable to accomplish a complete cure, it is able in many instances so to organize and stabilize the mentally deficient pupil that he has a much greater prospect of happiness and usefulness in the world than he otherwise would have.

Generally speaking, the three R's are of very secondary importance in the educational treatment of the mentally deficient pupil. Most high-grade defective children learn to write and to read simple letters and they should not be denied these accomplishments even if they can put them to very little practical use. The three R's at least have a certain cultural value for the mentally deficient child, but his educational welfare is prejudiced when a disproportionate emphasis is placed upon the three R's. In former years it was sometimes argued that a drill in arithmetic would have a tendency to strengthen the feeble mind; this is faulty psychology. We can only strengthen the minds of mentally deficient children by organizing their behavior into habits of healthful and useful activity.

Increasing the Moral and the Personality Sense of the Mentally Deficient Child

All academic work such as drawing, handicraft, modeling, weaving, sewing, basketry, woodwork and dancing, plays, games and physical education have a certain strengthening effect because they increase the morale and the personality sense of the mentally deficient pupil. These activities, when well conducted, also have a certain pre-vocational value. Special class provisions in our large cities have helped to define the nature of the problem of mental deficiency and incidentally they have had a beneficent, liberalizing effect upon the education of normal children. These classes have also demonstrated to the community the measures which it must take if the feeble-minded are to remain with security and comfort within its boundaries.

Moreover, the special class has demonstrated how we can meet the needs of the deficient child who can not have the benefits of special class instruction. It must be admitted that the great majority of mentally deficient children are in village and rural schools or in regular class rooms where they cannot be assigned to special classes. It does not follow, by any means, that the deficient child in these circumstances should be either excluded from public school or treated as though he were an ordinary, normal child. It is always possible, whether he is in a crowded class room or in a small rural school, to institute some special educational adjustments in his behalf. Such an individual program should resemble the methods which are used in the special class. It will not take an undue amount of the teacher's time or energy to institute such an individual program arrangement, especially if she enlists the aid of some of her brighter pupils or some one in an upper class, and makes the work a kind of domestic problem in which the others are encouraged to help. Naturally the deficient pupil will be permitted to share in the regular school work when he is able to do so, but during certain periods of the day special forms of activity should be arranged for him. The teacher may start with only one special period, but gradually she may develop a special program which will keep him busy and content during most of the school day.

Individual Special Program for the Deficient Child

The problem of mental deficiency, like a great many human problems, finally reduces itself to economic and vocational considerations. Chronologically, the feeble-minded child matures as quickly as the normal child, but once in his teens the question soon arises,—"what can he do when he must leave school?" Some years ago the stock answer to this question was "send him to an institution," but this answer is little short of absurd, for the simple reason that we can not build institutions enough to house all of our defectives; and still more because it is neither humane nor wise to attempt to send all of them to such institutions, even if the provisions were available.

Vocational Guidance

The notable work of Dr. Bernstein has shown that a large proportion of high-grade mental defectives, under the proper safeguard, can be adjusted to community and industrial life. The leisure and free time of these defectives must be securely protected, particularly in the case of girls; but given such protection, it is possible for the community to solve a large part of its own problem instead of assigning it all to some state institution for solution. Dr. Bernstein states the case in these words: "We are convinced, as result of our experience for fourteen years in colony and parole work with boys, and six years with girls, that where such boys and girls can render themselves self-supporting, even to the extent of paying for their own supervision and where girls can earn, as many of these girls do, as much as $14.00 to $21.00 a week in mills, . . . society has no moral right to deprive the individual or community of such opportunity or service."

The keynote, therefore, of the educational treatment of the mentally deficient child should be vocational training. Even during the pre-school period, the parent should begin to envisage a youth who, although he may not be able to compete on equal terms with his fellows, may still work side by side with them under favorable conditions of guidance and oversight. This is a legitimate expectation except, of course, in more pronounced cases of deficiency and those higher grade cases which are complicated with highly unstable personality traits. But for the vast majority of mentally deficient pupils, there is a simple vocational outlook of some kind which keeps life worth living. Wholesome personal habits, a career motive and practical vocational skill constitute the major educational objectives in the training of the deficient child.

Once a child has left the protection of the public school, he becomes a vocational problem and he is potentially a social problem. Frequently parents, teachers, and relatives can in a large measure solve this problem for themselves, thru common sense measures. There is, however, abundant room for effort on the part of social agencies and welfare organizations. Careful social case work pays even with the mentally deficient. The finding of proper employment, the safeguarding of conditions of employment of a feeble-minded youth, is a constructive form of social service. Private individuals, professional social workers, local committees, "Big Brothers," "Big Sisters," have here a concrete field for coöperation, accomplishment, and civic inventiveness. We have not yet unlocked all the local community resources which will really solve the human problem of the feeble-minded but we are finding the way in the new kind of education which is being provided through special classes and individualized special programs.

1. Strictly interpreted, the term "mental deficiency" **Summary** applies only to those children who cannot profit from ordinary methods of instruction and who will need a certain degree of external guidance and oversight on reaching maturity.

2. In a medical sense, mental deficiency is incurable; but in a psychological sense, it will respond very definitely to treatment. All but the lowest grade of mentally deficient children are educable, trainable, improvable. We can not make over a mentally deficient child into a normal child, but we can organize and condition his behavior in constructive ways.

3. The education of the deficient child should begin in infancy. Training in personal habits is of primary importance. Academic training is of secondary importance.

4. From the beginning he should be trained with the hope of ultimately making him happy and useful in some employment. A career motive should be developed.

He should be encouraged whenever possible and be made to feel that he is of some importance in the world.

5. His pre-vocational training should be provided by a special class where this is feasible. When it is not possible a special program should be planned for. Parents, older pupils or sisters or brothers, and teachers can coöperate in building up such a program for his individual benefit.

6. When he reaches wage earning age, vocational guidance becomes of supreme importance. Every effort should be made to find a simple job; or to make a part time vocational arrangement of some kind which will enable him to remain in the community.

7. Not only social agencies, but relatives and self appointed friends can coöperate in maintaining a supervision and guidance which will make his life in the community relatively contented and safe.

XIV

PROVISIONS FOR INTELLECTUALLY SUPERIOR CHILDREN

I T WAS formerly believed, and many people believe it
still, that at the beginning of life all children of the
nation are equally well endowed with capacity for
learning. In the United States, at the present time, the
educational philosophy of the people at large takes little
heed of the form in which human ability is actually distributed. The forefathers declared that all men are
created equal. In what respect this equality prevails
was not stated, but later generations seem to have assumed that all were thus declared to be equal in ability.
Therefore, in regard to penal procedure, political power,
educational administration, and other important human
functions, little or no recognition of individual differences
in ability appears.

Individual Differences

Beginning about 1885, with the efforts of Francis
Galton in England, psychologists have been gathering
measurements of mental capacities. Especially within
the latest decade, much new knowledge has accumulated,
showing how greatly human beings differ in mentality.
The measurements show, also, that these differences
exist in childhood, and can be determined with a high
degree of reliability, even by present imperfect methods,
as early as the sixth year of life.

It is easiest to think of the facts about individual
differences at first in terms of physique. Everyone can
see for himself that a thousand ten-year-olds in a city
school system vary greatly among themselves in height.
Furthermore, if these could be grouped along a street
according to their height, beginning with the shortest and

How Individuals in a large Group are Distributed

ending with the tallest, it would be easy to *see* that the differences follow certain laws. By far the greatest number of the children would be clustered at the *center* of the group. These would be very much like each other,—neither very tall nor very short, but *medium* in height. As the children, in the order of arrangement, became shorter, they would also be fewer; and the same thing would hold, at the opposite extreme, for the tall. We should see what experts in measurement call *a curve* or a *surface of distribution*, with a great many individuals falling near a central (median) point, and yet with a few children deviating from the central group, toward two opposite extremes.

These *facts of distribution* hold throughout organic nature, and the study of them is called the study of individual differences. When the traits involved are mental, we speak of the psychology of individual differences. It is a marvelous principle of biological nature that human beings are endlessly diversified in mental endowment. A mental ability is distributed in the same form in which height is distributed, though the range is greater in the case of mental traits. For instance, no child is two hundred times as tall as any other child of his age, in terms of any unit; but some children are two hundred times as keen in certain mental performances as others are, in terms of the units of measurement employed.

Figure 1, page 279 shows the form which is approximated, when a great many children of the same age are measured in mental capacity. In order to clarify its meaning, we may recall what was said of the distribution of height, and we may also look at Figure 2, page 280, which shows a familiar instance of these phenomena. Birds distribute themselves against the sky in the familiar form, when they·undergo the test of flight. We wish to discuss in this chapter that part of the distribution which is approximately indicated by the mark drawn across

FIGURE 3.

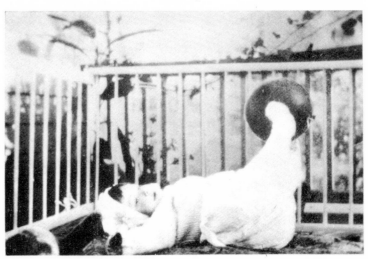

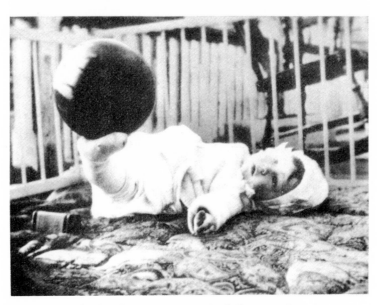

Showing the power to use and coördinate muscles.

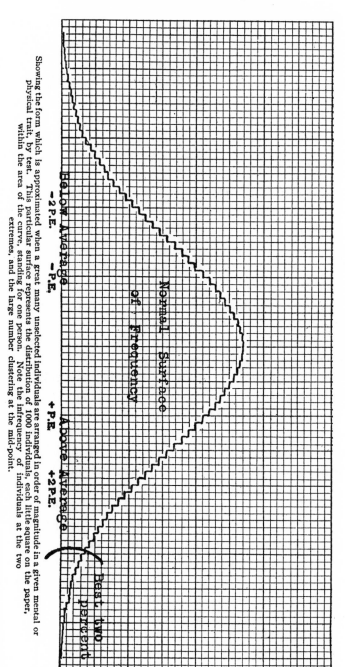

FIGURE 1

Showing the form which is approximated when a great many unselected individuals are arranged in order of magnitude in a given mental or physical trait, by test. This particular surface represents the distribution of 1000 individuals, each little square on the paper, within the area of the curve, standing for one person. Note the infrequency of individuals at the two extremes, and the large number clustering at the mid-point.

Below Average   Above Average
-2 P.E.   -P.E.   +P.E.   +2 P.E.

Normal Surface of Frequency

Best two percent

Figure 1, page 279, the best one to two percent,—in this instance, as respects intellectual power. These individuals, in whom we are now interested, are, therefore, as far above the average as the so-called feeble-minded are below.

FIGURE 2

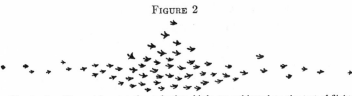

Showing how Figure 1 is approximated when birds are subjected to the test of flight (Schematic).

History of the Study of Ability The major part of our discussion will be devoted to the generally competent,—those who, as we say, are of very superior *general intelligence.* Psychologists have learned that there is a *coherence of capacities* in persons, so that one who is above average in one performance is able to surpass the average in most other performances, also. It is this fact of human nature which gives rise to the term, *general intelligence.*

The history of the study of superior as contrasted with average individuals is very interesting. It dates back into the nineteenth century. As there were then no quantitative methods of measuring intelligence, the approach was through the study of notable achievement in the world's work. This, of course, limited the study to adults, so that the early accounts have little to say about childhood. It was ascertained that eminent persons constitute a definite, small percentage of the population; that they are most often born in cities or on the estates of nobles, in long settled countries; that they have many more distinguished relatives than people ordinarily have; and that they originate usually in families of superior social-economic status.

Although little of importance has been reported concerning the childhood of eminent persons, still one student has made this his theme. In 1894, Yoder published a study of the boyhood of great men. Fifty individuals are included in this survey, concerning whom it appeared that they were, as children, healthy and interested in play; that they had been born over a very wide range of years in the reproductive life of parents; that many of them were "only" sons; and that a decided majority were derived from well-to-do families.

The methods of mental measurement now make possible the identification of superior intelligence, during childhood. We can approach the study of competency more directly, and at an age when education is doing its work. General intelligence in children is classified in various terms. Most often, perhaps, this is at present done in terms of IQ (intelligence quotient), which is the ratio of birthday age to intellectual development, already referred to in Chapters IV and XIII. That a child scores at an IQ of 100 means that intellectual development is that of the average child of the given birthday age. An IQ of 100 represents "par", as regards intelligence. A ratio of less than 100 means some degree of inferiority to the average, while a ratio above 100 means some degree of superiority. The best one per cent of children, as respects intelligence, test at or above 130 IQ, approximately. It is in such children that the interest of this chapter centers. It is not known just how widely intelligence can vary in terms of IQ. The most intelligent children reported up to this time test between 180 and 190 IQ, and are, of course, very infrequent.

The Modern Approach

Persons who have no organized knowledge about children, nevertheless use typical phraseology in speaking of the gifted. When we hear repeatedly, from various people, that a given child is "old for his age," "so reliable," "very old-fashioned," "quick to see a joke," "youngest in his class," or that he has "an old head on young shoulders," or "such a long memory," we usually find him to be highly intelligent, by test. The phrases used do not

Symptoms of Ability in Children

necessarily indicate any actual appreciation of the child's quality, but are used merely to describe present performances. That the child who is "old for his age" stands, and will continue throughout life to stand, among the highly intelligent of his generation, is not usually in the thought of those using the phrase. Also, other important symptoms of superior intelligence, such as very early interest and success in learning to read, are not popularly recognized.

Even teachers, who are no doubt among the best judges of children, have very indefinite knowledge of what are the important symptoms of intelligence. Very often they fail to think of the traits just mentioned as significant, and make the mistake of judging as "most intelligent" the children who are doing good school work in the grade where they happen to be placed. In this way teachers not uncommonly may judge as "most intelligent" very dull, over-age children, doing good work in the lower grades. Thus, for instance, they may not realize that being "youngest in the class" is an important symptom of superior ability. Teachers, of course, differ very widely among themselves in the reliability of their judgments. It has been shown that they are more accurate in their judgments of the stupid than they are in their judgments of the bright.

Unintentional Segregation of the Able The methods of mental measurement have demonstrated that in this country and abroad certain schools have long been segregating bright children, for instruction, without explicit recognition of the fact. In England, Burt has shown that boys attending a famous preparatory school are intellectually gifted above the average of the juvenile population. In the United States, children attending private schools, where tuition is paid, are rather highly selected for mental endowment. Mental tests show that in many such schools the pupils have a median IQ of near 120, instead of a median at par (100

IQ). These are surprising, rather than expected, findings, as it had been inferred that private schools might be hospitable to the stupid, in consideration of tuition fees. It seems clear that parents who are able to pay tuition charges have few dull children to present for schooling; so that wherever tuition is paid, immediately a selected group is obtained.

These facts were unrealized by educators until very recent years, as was also the fact that pupils who succeed in high school are of superior intelligence. These unintentional selections of the able are not, however, as severely restricted as those which we wish to consider here. They include children from the best fifty per cent of the juvenile population; whereas we wish to consider especially those who constitute the very best one to two per cent, i.e., those who test at or above 130 IQ. In terms of school work, this means children who are potentially able to pass with credit through a first-class college; and all who can surpass them in achievement, including those capable of winning highest honors in college and in the professions. (It is now recognized that to perform college work with credit requires a very high degree of intelligence.)

How do very bright children compare with unselected children, in disposition? Terman has given us the most reliable evidence at present available on this point. He obtained independent ratings by parents and by teachers, of the character traits of bright children in California. The rating scale used was in five degrees, so that a rating of 3 would be just average, 1 being the highest rating possible. Consensus of parents' opinions gave a rating of about 2, while teachers gave an average rating slightly higher for the bright children. Thus the intellectually able are judged by parents and by teachers to be above average in character. The children thus rated were those designated by Dr. Terman to be judged for character,

Character and Temperament

after they had been selected as superior intellectually, *by test.* They were not *selected as bright* by teachers' or parents' ratings (though such ratings subsequently made showed that teachers and parents judged them to be above the average in intellect, also).

It is of incidental interest that teachers rate bright children higher in all respects so far reported than their parents do. This is because teachers know a great variety of children, including the incompetent; whereas parents know well only their own children and those of their own friends, constituting usually a very restricted range of competency. A parent of a superior child, asked to rate the child in any respect, will very often give a rating of "average." When asked why he thinks the child is average, the typical reply is, "Because he is just about like the rest of the family."

Expressions of opinion by other special students of the gifted are in agreement with Terman's findings, with one exception. Miss Gillingham, of the Ethical Culture School, in New York City, studied twenty-five bright children, many of whom reached the top intellectually, and she concluded that they were, on the whole, lazy, inaccurate, and otherwise inferior in character. It is possible that this group represents a selection on some peculiar basis, which would cause it to differ from other groups reported; or that the judgments expressed are on the basis of some unusual criterion. The only unusual feature of selection which appears is that the children were almost all Jewish, the attendance at the school studied being largely of Semitic origin. However, other groups of Jewish children have been studied (see reference 15 in the bibliography of this Chapter) with conclusions which differ from those of Miss Gillingham.

On the whole, present evidence indicates that superior intelligence is accompanied by superior temperament in children, and by superior stability and stamina of character.

For about twenty years it has been clear that children who do well in school work are larger and stronger than those who do poor school work, age for age. This fact is susceptible to more than one interpretation. From it we might infer that superior physique is a determinant of school standing. Or we might infer that the intellectually gifted are large and strong, as a group.

Very recently by the method of mental tests it has been established almost certainly that children of superior intelligence are commonly large and strong for their age. Baldwin measured children in private schools some years ago, and found that they exceeded the norms formerly secured for children in general. Since that time it has been demonstrated that pupils in the schools studied by Baldwin are of distinctly superior intelligence. Also, superior children in the public schools have been shown to be larger and stronger than their schoolmates of equal age.

In New York City, in 1923 (see bibliography for this chapter), 45 children, all testing in the highest group for intellect, were compared with an equal number of children from the middle fifty per cent, and likewise with an equal number from the lowest group. Age, race, and sex were kept constant in all groups. The medians for the three groups ran as follows:

	Very Bright	Of Ordinary Intelligence	Very Dull
Height (inches)	52.9 ± 1.6	51.2 ± 1.2	49.6 ± 2.1
Weight (lbs.)	74.0 ± 9.4	63.9 ± 5.2	59.5 ± 6.5
Wt.-Ht. Coeff. $\frac{(Wt.)}{(Ht.)}$	1.31 ± .13	1.19 ± .10	1.14 ± .12

As regards the two extreme groups, the bright are 3.3 inches taller than the stupid, as a group, and 14.5 pounds heavier. It should be added that there is nothing in such results to indicate that the degree of intelligence *depends* upon the physique, or that either could be altered

285

Size and Strength

by altering the other. Also, it must be especially stressed that the figures pertain to the *mid-point of the group*, in each case, and that there are several individuals among the bright who are smaller than the median stupid child. These facts of *overlapping* between the groups preclude the feasibility of judging intellect from size, in an individual case.

The present writer has made measurements of physical size on five children, who test above 180 IQ, and who are among the most gifted ever reported in the literature of child psychology. The measurements are in agreement with the trend just cited, and stand as follows:

	Age Yrs.Mo.	Height (In.) (Norm)*		Weight (Lbs.) (Norm)*	
Child I	8–8	52.0	(50.1)	64.7	(55.9)
Child II	9–4	55.3	(52.0)	102.0	(61.5)
Child III	9–7	53.2	(52.2)	56.5	(62.1)
Child IV	10–2	64.0	(57.7)	76.0	(82.8)
Child V	13–4	63.5	(58.2)	162.0	(89.5)

These five children aggregate 17.8 inches more in height than would five representative children of their respective ages, chosen from good private schools, and 109.4 pounds more in weight.

Measurements of power to grip with the hand show that the bright children involved in the above comparisons are as strong in the left hand, and stronger in the right hand, than children of ordinary intelligence; and that they are stronger in both hands than the stupid.

Figure 3, opposite page 278, illustrates the power to coördinate and use muscles, of Child I, described above, in infancy. At the age of 11 months, this child (IQ 187) would amuse himself by balancing large, soft balls on his feet and on his hands, as he lay in his crib. The physical sturdiness of the child, which is typical of the bright, is illustrated in Figure 4, opposite page 294, and his physical

*Baldwin's norm, to the nearest half year.

appearance and his play interests, in Figure 5, opposite page 294. Such children commonly learn to walk and to talk at a conspicuously early age.

Although children of superior intelligence are usually superior in motor ability as well, teachers often rate them as "below average" in this respect. This illusion is due to the fact that the very bright, being youngest in their classes, are thus contrasted with older children in motor performances. Since coördination, speed and accuracy in movement depend much more closely on physical development than they do on mental development, the young child appears awkward in contrast with his less gifted, but physically more mature, classmates. A seven-year-old who stands in the top quarter of seven-year-olds in muscular control, will nevertheless stand low among eight- or nine-year-olds in penmanship, industrial arts, or athletic games.

As regards health, Terman again furnishes us with the most extensive evidence. The bright children rated at his request for character, were rated also for health, with the result that both parents and teachers rated them above average, as a group.

Does a child who scores high in intellect in the early years of life, continue to score high as he grows up? There has been a widespread superstition that gifted children become dullards, or at most end as mediocre men and women, as they mature.

Do Superior Children Become Superior Adults?

Psychologists have now re-tested many children of all degrees of mental ability, over periods in some cases as long as ten years. The outcome of these researches is that individuals maintain very nearly the same relative positions during mental development, and at maturity. The dull remain dull, the average continue to be average, and the gifted maintain their superior status, as they grow.

Figure 6 shows mental growth curves for superior children, as contrasted with average children. These curves result from repeated annual tests made by the Bureau of Child Welfare Research, at the University of Iowa:

FIGURE 6

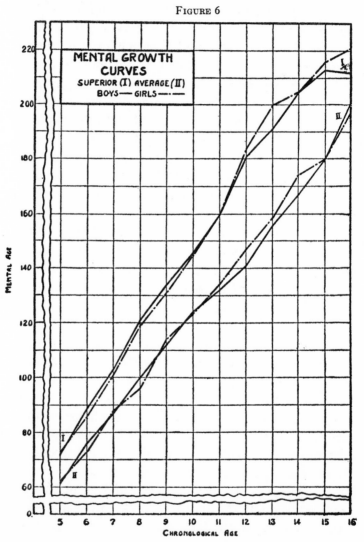

Showing intellectual growth of superior children, in comparison with average children, year after year. (Reproduced by courtesy of Dr. B. T. Baldwin and Dr. L. I. Stecher).

It is possible, even by present imperfect methods, to identify at the age of six years those who as adolescents will stand in the highest quarter of their group for general intelligence. There is every indication that superior children grow up to be superior adults. It is the dull children who become our adult dullards.

There is a set of circumstances, incident to selection during school life, which creates an illusion of decreasing brightness in superior children, as they grow older. In the primary grades the whole range of school children of an age is present, and the bright seem very bright in contrast. As children go on up through the grades, however, the dullest are constantly "left back"; so that by the time high school is reached all of the extremely dull children have been eliminated from the comparison. A child of 130 IQ is a very bright member of his group in kindergarten; a rather bright member of his group in high school; and but an average member of his group in a first-rate college. His intellectual quality does not change, but his group of competitors becomes more and more highly selected, creating the illusion of retrogression on his part.

As we proceed with this chapter, it becomes increasingly evident that many popular notions concerning gifted children are contrary to scientific fact. The psychologist finds often the very opposite condition from that popularly supposed to exist. This is partly because those who have no exact knowledge of a subject always tend to found their beliefs on wishes, and partly because popular belief is always subject to illusions, like that described in the preceding paragraph.

Ancestry of Gifted Children

Thus, it is the popular belief that the children of poor and obscure parents, of manual toilers, and of "the lowly" are those in whom great gifts are likely to be found. If asked where to search for the most gifted child in this country, persons in general would doubtless suggest that one should look among the offspring of the humble, and especially of farmers in the country, sprung from poverty. The American idea that the children of the humble, and especially of farmers, are likely to become eminent, has its origin in the early history of this country. From two to three hundred years ago, nearly all children in America (including the gifted), were born of farmers, and in humble surroundings. The reason for this was that there were as yet no cities to exercise a selective influence, so that nearly all inhabitants lived perforce "in the country." This was still quite true even down to a hundred years ago.

Prolonged studies of the origin of very gifted children in this country, born since 1900, have been confined largely to cities. They have shown repeatedly that the great majority of these children originate in families where the father is a professional man, an owner or executive in business, or a clerical worker. Only a small minority of children testing in the highest group for intellect, originate among the manual workers in cities, in the United States (where the social-economic competition is relatively free for all). There are various possible interpretations of this fact, but the inference most favored by all subsidiary facts is that the very intelligent are those who rise in the world by competition, and who are also able to produce children like themselves.

In fact, it has been proved again and again that ability "runs in families." There is a marked resemblance among brothers and sisters in mental tests, and a still more marked resemblance between those who are twins. The brothers and sisters, or the siblings, as they are sometimes called, of gifted children are themselves very superior, as a group. As an illustration of this fact may be cited an investigation recently made in New York City (see reference 11 in bibliography). The brothers and sisters of the bright children, whose physical measurements we have described, were given mental tests. The children originally selected by tests had an average IQ of 151. Their brothers and sisters yielded an average IQ of 128. All but two of them tested above "par," and of those one tested just at "par" (100 IQ), and the other close to "par" (96 IQ). This is a very striking result when we remember that of unselected children, half of the brothers and sisters will fall at or below "par" in mental tests (see Figure 1, p. 279). Mental tests of twenty first cousins of these same children yielded an average IQ as high as that of the siblings. Their parents, too, have met with sagacity the mental tests administered by life, as is proved by their excellent social-economic status.

Furthermore, gifted children have a disproportionately large number of eminent persons among their adult relatives. For instance, among the close relatives of the five children, to whom we have already referred as testing above 180 IQ, the writer of this chapter has counted forty persons, who were writers, judges, inventors, founders of institutions, governors, noted scholars, officers of high rank in army or navy, distinguished surgeons, priests, or rabbis. The chances are very slight that a child picked at random from the population will have even one adult relative of the distinction of the forty attached to the family trees of these very gifted children.

It remains to be added that the parents of superior children produce very small families. Apparently the extremely able will not choose the biological and economic burdens of repeated reproduction. This is a psychological fact which is interesting for the national future.

It has been stated that the census of the gifted has so far been confined largely to centers of population. We do not know to what extent children in the top quarter of intellect are to be found on farms in this generation. We do know, however, that where rural children have been tested at random, in this country, they yield a somewhat lower average intelligence than city children yield. From this fact we should expect that the country now yields relatively few very gifted children to the thousand. From tests made in the county of Northumberland, in England, Thomson concluded that "the highest ability appears to be found *close* to the cities and *far away from* the cities, the intermediate areas having fewer cases of high ability, as though they were drained by selection."

Some Individual Cases

In order to make our discussion somewhat more concrete at this point, it will be useful to consider a few individual examples. The following are cases chosen at random from a great many on record:

A is a little girl ten years of age. Her IQ on repeated annual tests has stood at 140, 148, 145. Her school work has been excellent, from kindergarten onward. At the age of five years she entered the first grade on her own initiative. Children are expected to be six years old before entering first grade, but A, who had entered kindergarten at four years of age, presented herself to the teacher of first grade at the opening of the following school year, with the statement that she had finished the kindergarten. She was taken on trial, and made one of the best records in the class during the year. A has always gone to private schools. Her father is a university professor, and her mother is a college graduate. She has one brother, whose school record is superior.

B is an eight-year-old boy. He has a serious defect of the eyes, as a result of which he has never had more than a small fraction of normal vision. Parents and teachers wondered how he could learn so much when he could see so little, and brought him for examination. His IQ was found to be 156. Both the mother and the father of B are college graduates. His brothers have school records which indicate that they are of superior intelligence. But none of them has shown the "mental grasp" which characterizes B, despite his visual handicap.

C is a girl ten years of age, first recognized as bright when a survey was being made in a certain school district, to discover children of exceptional intelligence. Her IQ has stood at 164 on two tests made several years apart. Neither of her parents is educated, the father being employed in a tailor's shop. They are immigrants. C's home surroundings are those of a typical tenement, in the city slums. Her sister and two brothers all test above the average intellectually. This case represents the few instances in which an extremely gifted child is found with uneducated parents, in a poor home. Such children prove that the intellectual ability revealed by tests does not come from home surroundings. It is not possible to observe the family in this case beyond the parents, as other relatives live in Europe.

D is an eleven-year-old boy, who tests at 167 IQ. He is very large for his age, and of exceptional firmness and stability of character. His father is an army officer of high rank, and his mother is a college graduate. He is one of seven children, only one other of whom has had mental tests. This sister's IQ has stood at 189 and 188 on two tests made a year apart. There are many eminent relatives on both sides of D's family. His parents had not thought of him as very exceptional.

These cases serve to represent the group of gifted children in our schools. Since about one in every 250 children is as bright as Child A here described, it is evident that among millions of school children there are many of this calibre to be found. The higher the intelligence, the rarer the child, of course, as may be recalled by glancing back at Figure 1, p. 279, in this chapter. Of the cases described, A, B, and D are typical of the bright, as regards occupation of parents, and other social conditions. Child C is very exceptional in this respect. Child B is exceptional in having a severe visual defect, and has been mentioned here especially to show that intelligence does not depend upon perfection of the special senses.

Experimental Education of Gifted Children in the United States

For a considerable number of years there have been consciously attempted selections of the most capable children in our schools, for purposes of education. In 1919 Freeman sent a questionnaire to all cities in this country of 25,000 population or over, inquiring as to special provision for the gifted. He learned that a considerable number of school administrators recognized the existence of gifted children, and attempted to provide for their special needs, usually by establishing special classes for rapid advancement. In several instances the work was on a sufficiently modern basis, so that mental tests were used to select the children. Most recent information on this point will be found in the forthcoming publication of The National Society for the Study of Education (see reference 11, Chapter XIV, Bibliography).

Among the first of the classes to be selected by mental tests was that reported by Race in 1918, from Louisville, Kentucky. Here several young children with a median IQ of 137 were segregated, and made very rapid progress, covering the prescribed curriculum of the elementary school at about twice the ordinary rate, without more than ordinary effort. Race found them to be healthy, well-balanced, and capable of work much beyond the average.

In the years following 1918, several detailed reports of similar work appeared, among which those of Whipple, of Specht, and of Coy are of particular interest. All of these class-room experiments showed that children selected as very intelligent by mental tests are capable of much greater progress in school than is possible for them under ordinary conditions. The influence of such studies is already felt to some extent, in educational administration. For instance, at the Conference on Educational Research and Guidance, held at San Jose, California,

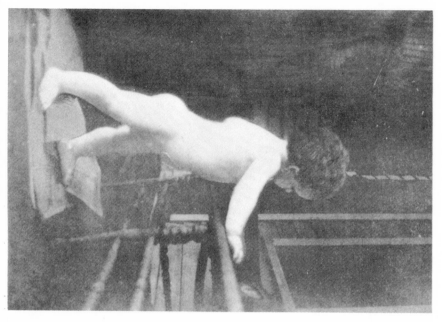

FIGURE 4.

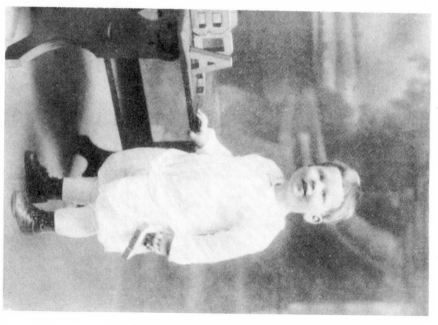

FIGURE 5.

in 1922, Dickson stated that during the year just passed, about 11 per cent of children in the elementary schools of Berkeley and Oakland had been given special opportunity suited to their superior endowment.

Class-room experimentation with highly endowed children has been reported since 1916 in Germany from Berlin, Hamburg, Breslau, Mannheim, Leipsic, Frankfort, Charlottenburg, and Göttingen particularly. In Germany, as in this country, this work has gone forward in cities, because it is only in centers of population that a sufficient number of the very gifted can be found conveniently located to form special classes. The desirability of identifying the gifted who live in rural communities has been discussed with urgency in Germany, where the need to foster that nation's mental power is now very great. No solution of this administrative problem has yet been found.

Experimental Education of the Gifted Abroad

After the World War, republican Germany abandoned the policy of educating children according to the social-economic status of their parents. To find and to train the gifted, wherever existing, was seen to be a primary condition of national rehabilitation. As there are many educational psychologists in Germany, the work of selecting the *Hofnungskinder* (children of promise) has proceeded rapidly and systematically. It is probable that to-day Germany is giving more official administrative recognition to special education on the basis of innate mental endowment than any other country.

In the majority of reports it appears that the selection of pupils is made by mental tests, supplemented by teachers' judgments as to strength of character and physical stamina. Germany cannot afford special education for those strong in intellect only. The child must be strong in every way to warrant the investment. Children annually or semi-annually selected thus from the *Volksschulen*, are given a special course of study in the last years of the elementary school, to articulate with the higher schools. Both boys and girls participate in these special advantages, but in some cities only half as many girls as boys are permitted to be chosen. The psychologists, Peter and Stern, have pointed out that in the tests used for selection, the girls equal the boys in performance, and that this raises questions of policy concerning the education of girls, which are, perhaps, especially distressing in view of German traditions of education.

Countries abroad other than Germany seem to be doing little or no class-room experimentation to find the best education for the gifted. At any rate, such experiments are not reported in their literature.

Special Talents

It was said previously in this chapter that the multitude of man's abilities for performance cohere as regards amount; there is no biological law of compensation, whereby a person who is gifted in one respect is usually inferior in other respects. People like to suppose that there may be such a law, because if there were, the human idea of fair play in nature would be satisfied. Biological nature, however, does not behave according to our ideas of justice. The mentally superior person tends to be superior in all respects (even in physique, as shown in preceding paragraphs in this chapter), but there are a few exceptions to this rule of coherence among abilities. Psychologists have discovered at least two talents which do not seem to have much relation to ability in general. These are talent for drawing and talent for music. A child stupid in other respects may excel in music or in representative drawing, and similarly a child who is very bright may be specially defective in these respects. Talent in representative drawing apparently arises from a happy combination of a great many variable functions which are specialized. Likewise, musical talent arises from a fortunate combination of highly specialized abilities, which may occur in children otherwise dull, or may be deficient in children of superior intelligence.

Few surveys have been made to show how ability in drawing and ability in music are distributed among school children. Such as have been undertaken in music yield the familiar form (see Figure 1, page 279), and show a very great range of musical sensitivity. The most extensive work in this field has been done in the State of Iowa, by Seashore and his students.

A few surveys of ability to draw have also been made. In Berlin, at the present time, when the semi-annual *Begabtenprüfung* is held, a test of talent in drawing is also made, so that children gifted in this special way may receive training in the school of design.

The most conspicuous problem of those interested in rational education for exceptionally intelligent children is now, perhaps, that of the curriculum. What should they be taught? By whom? With what goals in view? The problem is no longer one of selection primarily, but of instruction. Should all children who test very high as regards intellect, be educated for science, for the professions, and for the direction of industry? Should society induce some of them to join the manual trades, as hand workers? Should unskilled labor be drained by educational policy more thoroughly than it now is drained by competition, of all first-rate intelligence? These are disturbing questions of consequence, which affect the educator.

Present Problems in the Education of the Gifted

Questions somewhat more immediate, and less completely philosophical in nature, concern the relative claims of rapid advancement as against enrichment of curriculum for the gifted. These questions are in some of their aspects susceptible to experimentation, but they have not been so approached as yet. Educational speculation seems, on the whole, to favor enrichment of the curriculum, but there is no agreement as to what the additional subject matter should be. In 1923 a report appeared (see reference 1, bibliography) of the selection of a class of young children, organized for the purpose of experimenting in the class room with curricular material adapted for the needs of the very intelligent. This class is being continued at the present time.

The objection is sometimes raised that special education for the bright is not suitable in a democracy, where all are equal. The obvious reply to this is that all are not equal in capacity. The biological truth is that all are unequal. Schools cannot equalize children; schools can only equalize opportunity. It may well be thought to be highly undemocratic to provide full opportunity for the exercise of their capacities to some, while to others the same offering means only partial exercise of their powers. It is hard for a psychologist to define democracy, but perhaps one acceptable definition might be that it is a condition of affairs, in which every human being has opportunity to live and work in accordance with inborn capacity for achievement.

Summary   For convenience, we may now recapitulate briefly the important facts which have been established during the past twenty years, concerning intellectually gifted children. Mental tests, given to large numbers of unselected children, yield always a few who attain superior rank. In various localities studies have been made of those ranking in the highest percentile, that is, of "the one child in a hundred," by test. These studies show that such children are usually youngest in their classes, though still much below the point where they could readily function, in the ordinary graded school. They learn very rapidly, and progress more than twice as fast as average children can, when they are segregated in special classes. They are large and strong for their age, as a group, and are superior in character and temperament. They maintain their superior status, as they develop, and do not tend to become mediocre, as has been popularly supposed. The majority of them originate (in America, where social-economic competition is relatively free for all) in families where the fathers are professional men, clerical workers, or business executives, and they have many more distinguished persons among their relatives than chance would allow. Very few extremely gifted children originate among manual laborers, in cities where investigation has gone forward.

Educational policy in the United States at present gives scant consideration to these children, because the current social philosophy of the people denies the existence of innate, permanent, hereditary superiority. To them are assigned, in general, the same tasks as are assigned to average children; with the result that they manage, on the whole, to win an occasional extra promotion, though practically never to an extent that would permit them to work at full capacity.

As the new knowledge gleaned from mental tests becomes gradually diffused, the social philosophy which disregards the existence of the superior will undergo changes. Already progressive educators here and there are applying the new knowledge in educational administration. They are experimenting with new methods of teaching the gifted, and are trying to formulate additional studies for them,—trying to provide genuine opportunity for these children. As a result of such psychological and educational research, we shall soon have as much accumulated knowledge about the gifted as we have about the deficient, and shall be in position to do justice to the competent as well as to the incompetent.

THE ADOLESCENT PERIOD; ITS PROBLEMS, REGIMEN,
AND HYGIENE

The Onset
of
Adolescence

THE period of adolescence is the period during which a child is developed into an adult. This period is variable in length and in the age of its onset or beginning. Some children manifest the beginnings of adolescence as early as the tenth year, while others show no signs of the onset until they reach the fifteenth or sixteenth year; but these are extremes. A great majority of children show the beginnings of adolescence at twelve, thirteen or fourteen for girls; or at thirteen, fourteen or fifteen for boys.

There is a marked difference in this matter of the time of onset of adolescence in different races. The Mediterranean nations show a distinctly earlier beginning of adolescence than is found among the Nordic nations. For instance, girls of Italy may enter puberty as early as nine or ten years of age, and usually begin adolescence definitely as early as the eleventh year; while girls of the far north in Europe seldom enter adolescence before the age of thirteen, and most of them do not become adolescent before fourteen or fifteen.

In America there is such a mixing of peoples through intermarriage of Nordic and Mediterranean nationalities that one is not surprised to find that a large proportion of girls the country over enter puberty during the thirteenth year.

As to boys, there seems to be a similar difference in the age at which puberty begins in those of Mediterranean as compared with those of Nordic nations. However, the definite date of beginning of puberty in boys is more difficult to determine, because they do not experience any definite, easily-apparent function like the menstrual period of the girl.

While Italian, Greek, and Spanish boys become adolescent at twelve to fourteen and Scandinavian boys at fourteen to sixteen, the mixed nationalities in America show an average age of onset of about fourteen, and a large proportion of American boys enter puberty during the fourteenth year.[1]

In the above paragraphs the terms puberty and adolescence have been used apparently interchangeably; but while the onset of puberty and adolescence coincide in time, the term puberty is properly applied to the period of three or four years during which a youth becomes thoroughly established in the development and functioning of the sex apparatus. This period of puberty occupies the first three or four years of the adolescent period. The terms puberty and adolescence are therefore not synonymous. Adolescence is the longer period and includes the three-year period of puberty as well as a four or five-year post-puberty period. The following diagram indicates the age limits of the five "ages" or periods from birth to maturity:

				Post-Puberty
		Pre-	*Puberty*	17 - Young Men - 22
	Early Child-	*Adolescence*	14 - Youths - 17	16 - Young
	Hood	10 — Boys — 14	13 -Maidens -16	Women - 20
Infancy	3 — Boys — 10	9 — Girls — 13		
0— Boys — 3	2½— Girls — 9			ADOLESCENCE
0— Girls —2 ½				

The post-puberty phase of adolescence is devoted to the maturing physical organs and tissues and the training of their powers; so that by the time a young man reaches twenty-two and a young woman reaches twenty we expect them to show full maturity of every organ and of every physical and mental power.

[1] G. Stanley Hall gives thirteen as the age at which most girls enter puberty and fourteen as usual for boys. P. 415, Adolescence, Vol. 1.

It will contribute much to the clearness of our understanding of adolescence if we have a clear picture of the boy and girl before they cross the threshold into adolescence.

Pre-Adolescence

There is a well-defined period or stage of development preceding adolescence that is called the pre-adolescent or pre-puberty stage of development. The period lasts three or four years and extends, roughly speaking, from ten to fourteen in boys and from nine to thirteen in girls.

It seems to be a general law of nature that the transition from one stage or phase of life to the next is never a sudden one, showing rapid and extreme changes; rather nature's transitions are almost always very gradual. We can, therefore, get a clearer picture of the typical pre-adolescent by picturing a boy of twelve and a girl of eleven than by picturing a boy of fourteen and a girl of thirteen, or a boy of ten and a girl of nine. In other words, we get the most accurate picture by selecting a subject from the middle of the period.

Differences between Boys and Girls

The boy of twelve is usually not appreciably larger than the girl of eleven; and as was demonstrated by H. P. Bowditch, of Harvard University Medical School, about 34 years ago, the measurements and general appearance of the boy and girl above mentioned are strikingly alike. They are quite apt to be interested in similar sports and games and to enter vigorously into them without any marked differences between the two as to activity and efficiency. The twelve-year-old girl is almost sure to be superior to the twelve-year-old boy in active sports and larger than he in all her physical measurements.

However, despite physical and functional similarities between the boy and girl of the mid pre-adolescent period, there are some interesting temperamental differences. Boys are almost sure to be interested in pets;—as rabbits, guinea pigs, dogs, goats, ponies, etc. Girls are much less interested in live pets; their interest is in dolls. The boys are interested in such activities as scouting, fishing, trapping, camping—in short, in woods-lore and water-lore in general. Girls of this age are far more interested in playing house, "going calling" and in giving doll parties.

One interesting phase of pre-adolescence is that while there is a definite sex consciousness there is not a reciprocal sex attraction. The boy thinks of the girl as "girl," but he does not seek close social relations; in fact, both boys and girls of this age are very unsocial toward each other. If one wishes to spoil a boy's birthday party just invite some "nice little girls" to come. By the same mark, if one wishes to spoil a little girl's birthday party, just ask some "rough, blundering boys" to come.

Boys of this age are almost sure to exhibit thoughtless cruelty, as, for example, pulling the wings from butterflies to see how they can navigate without them, or pulling the legs from grasshoppers with a similar object in view, or robbing a bird's nest to add the eggs to their collections.

Furthermore, boys of this age are very likely to drift or to be led easily into vulgarity. As the cruelty of the boy is due to his thoughtlessness, similarly his vulgarity is due to ignorance. He is not inherently either cruel or vulgar; he simply does not think things through. In short, the boy is a young barbarian. As to morals, he is *unmoral*, rather than *immoral*. As to social instincts, he is *unsocial* rather than *anti-social*.

Having sketched the outlines of a picture of the typical pre-adolescent, let us now do the same for the adolescent. **Adolescent Traits** As there was an advantage found in selecting a mid pre-adolescent for our picture, so it will be advantageous to select a mid-adolescent, say a seventeen-year-old youth and a sixteen-year-old maiden. This youth and maiden are probably in the third or fourth year at high school. Physically, the youth has made a remarkable growth in the five years since we last observed him. He is perhaps five feet and eight inches in height, broad-shouldered, deep-chested, hard-muscled and fiery-eyed,— a good all-around athlete. He must use a razor at least three or four times a week to keep his beard in order. He is much more likely than his sister to be interested in mechanics, electricity, radio, and in the mechanism and running of autos and motor boats, in canoeing and sailing, in hunting with gun and dog and in fishing with rod and reel.

He is socially not only quite conscious of the femininity of his girl classmate and associate in school, but he wishes to associate with her. This wish is evidently reciprocated. There is at this age not only sex consciousness but also reciprocal sex attraction.

Morally the mid-adolescent youth has experienced an awakening; he is no longer unmoral; either he is definitely and positively moral and ethical or he is definitely and positively immoral and unethical. The reason for this moral consciousness is in all probability due to the fact that the youth of seventeen is beginning to be thoughtful, and in his thinking of things that he observes, he reaches logical (or near-logical) conclusions; and he is acquiring a tendency to shape his line of action in accordance with the conclusion which he has reached.

The maiden of sixteen is now quite definitely a young lady. Her figure is attractive as a rule and she is graceful in her movements. Her measurements, as shown in the study by Bowditch referred to in a foregoing paragraph, and also demonstrated by W. W. Hastings (Manual of Physical Measurements, 1902), show a remarkable modification. She is perhaps five feet, three inches in height; her pelvic measurements are, relative to her other girths and diameters, much increased. Also the girth and depth of chest at the fifth rib level are greatly increased relatively because of the development of the breast. Her head is adorned with a wealth of glossy hair.

Mentally, she is likely to be especially interested in

music, art, and the domestic arts and crafts. Morally, she is likely to have high ideals and altruistic motives. Socially, she is sensitively conscious of her femininity and the virility and manhood of her young men acquaintances and friends, and is happy to meet with them socially.

Contrasting the typical mid pre-adolescent with the typical mid-adolescent of each sex, we note that a remarkable change has taken place. The boy has become a young man, and the girl a young woman. The young man is typically *man*; the young woman is typically *woman*. The young man could father a child, the young woman could mother a child. Each one is sexually mature.

What has wrought this remarkable change?

It has been known for thousands of years that if the sex glands be removed from a young male of any of the higher mammals, the male so treated does not develop the physical and psychical qualities typical of the male. In the orient in ancient times, most of the males of the domesticated animals were castrated or surgically deprived of the sex glands,—of the testes or gonads. The reader is probably familiar with the frequent references in history and literature to the eunuch, who is simply a male from whom the gonads have been surgically removed.

One would think that in the long ago men would have thought the matter through and would have concluded that the gonads must produce some substance which, absorbed into the system and distributed through it, cause the development of the qualities and attributes distinctive of virility. Removing the gonads, thus depriving the organism of the influence of the glands, would profoundly influence development. But if anyone thought the matter through he did not make any experiments and describe them; for it was not until late in the nineteenth century that it began to dawn upon the minds of

What Has Made the Boy a Man and the Girl a Woman

biologists and physiologists that glandular tissue prepares, not only the external secretion with which everyone is familiar, but also a secretion that is poured back into the lymph and blood and distributed throughout the body to exert an activating and controlling influence upon organic development and function.

It would take us too far afield to detail the epoch-making pioneer work of Brown-Sequard[1] in France, of Poehl[2] and Zoth[3] in Germany. The best summary of the earlier investigations of internal secretions from the gonad glands came from the pen of Prof. Francis H. A. Marshall[4] and is entitled the *Physiology of Reproduction.*

It was early discovered that there are several glandular bodies that prepare internal secretions; for example, the thyroids prepare such a substance, early called *Iodo-Thyrin;* the adrenals prepare *Adrenalin;* the pituitary gland prepares *Pituitrin.* The literature has become voluminous and scores of investigators for two decades have devoted much of their time and the resources of great university laboratories to discover the wonderful secrets that lie at the foundation of life.

Prof. Shaefer,[5] the English Histo-Physiologist, wrote the best summary of these researches that had appeared to date (1914).

We now call these internal secretions *Hormones.* They are thought of as "Life-ferments". These Hormones are very complex nitrogenous bodies. Poehl's second publication, 1894, gives the composition of Spermin, which was thought to be the Hormone of the testes, as $C_5 H_{14} N_2$; and Dr. G. Stanley Hall[6] remarked about it in 1904,—"Spermin is perhaps the most complex of all things in the organic world"; but we have found that these Hormones are very much more complex than

---

[1] Brown-Sequard, "Internal Secretions" Archives de Physiologie, 1889.
[2] Poehl "Spermin" Berliner Klinische Wochenschrift, 1891. "Spermin" Zeitsch. f. klin. Med. 1894.
[3] Zoth, in Pfluegers Arch. f. Physiologie, 1896.
[4] Marshall, "Physiology of Reproduction," Longmans Green & Co., London, 1910.
[5] Shaefer, "Endocrine Organs," London, 1914.
[6] G. Stanley Hall, "Adolescence," Vol. 1, 1904.

Poehl's formula would suggest. As a matter of fact it is now quite certain that Poehl's method of analysis decomposed the Hormone from the testes, and that spermin, as he wrote its formula and as he isolated it from testicular extracts, is only a small portion of the real Hormone.

What does this all mean? Simply, that recent researches have demonstrated that the gonad glands of both male and female prepare a Hormone or "Lifeferment" that, absorbed into the lymph and blood, distributed by the lymph and blood all over the body, causes the development of all those physical and psychical qualities distinctive of virility or femininity, as the case may be. This being true, the removal of the gonad glands (the testicles or the ovaries) deprives the body of the Hormone that is necessary for its typical development and we have the fatted steer instead of the fighting bull; the plodding gelding instead of the prancing stallion; the cringing, flabby-muscled eunuch instead of the courageous, hard-muscled man.

Removal of the ovaries of a young girl causes her to fall short pitiably from the development of ideal, typical womanhood. The effect of castration of the female is as profound and far reaching as in the case of the male.

Having now determined the cause of the remarkable development of the youth or maiden into the typical adult, let us note the outstanding features of that development. At the threshold of adolescence, the boy of fourteen begins to receive this Hormone above discussed from his gonad glands. No one has yet determined the amount of the Hormone that is taken into the blood from these glands, but certain it is that there is only a small quantity, perhaps a drop or two in a twenty-four hour period. We have every reason to believe that this Hormone passes into the blood continuously, night and day, from the onset of the period of adolescence or the threshold of

Physical Development of the Boy

puberty to the beginning of senescence or old age.

The first noticeable result of its influence on the boy's development is conspicuous increase in height. If he has been growing, say two inches a year during pre-adolescence, he is likely to add three or perhaps four inches in one year to his stature and an equal amount to his stretch of arms. This increase of stature is fairly symmetrical and there is a proportional increase in all his skeletal dimensions. Similarly, there is a rapid growth noticeable in his muscular system. This growth makes itself evident in the girth of his arms and legs especially.

It was discovered some thirty years ago by those who were making a careful study of physical growth that this growth presents two interesting features. First, the increment of growth presents a rhythmic advance; for example, the boy who during his fifteenth year adds three inches to his growth is practically certain to add a smaller increment during his sixteenth year (say two inches) and a larger one again during his seventeenth year, perhaps another three-inch growth, then to drop to a one or two inch addition to his stature during his eighteenth and nineteenth years. This rhythmicity of growth was demonstrated by the writer in a long series of observations of boys of an eastern school, through a number of years, taking two measurements a year of the same boys; many hundreds of the boys having presented themselves for as many as six or eight successive measurements during the years of their most rapid development.[1] Another feature that has been discovered is that during the period of especially rapid height-growth, there is a distinct relative decrease of girth increment. This phenomenon was discovered during the study of the school boys above referred to. In popular terms, one might say that boys shoot up and then spread out, only to shoot up a second time and spread out again, there

---

[1] W. S. Hall, "Changes in the Proportions of the Human Body during the period of Growth," Journal of the Anthropological Institute of Great Britain and Ireland, 1895.

being two definite waves of growth in both frame and muscles during adolescence, the crest of the skeletal wave alternating with the crest of the muscle increment wave.

As a part of the physical development of the adolescent youth, there is a proportionate growth of all the internal organs and systems of organs, as for example, the lungs and respiratory system, the heart and circulatory system, the liver, stomach, and digestive system. The rapid growth of these internal organs fills the trunk, which has naturally greatly increased in all its dimensions.

In the realm of physical development there is a remarkable increase in hair-growth. This manifests itself not only in the growth of the beard which, by the way, is likely to be in evidence only slightly before the end of puberty; but early in puberty the pubic hair as well as hair in other localities comes clearly into evidence.

Another noticeable change that comes at the threshold of puberty is the change of voice. The high-pitched, thin treble of the boy becomes the deep, sonorous base or the clear, ringing tenor of the man.

At the threshold of adolescence, the girl of thirteen begins to receive from her gonad glands (ovaries) the Hormone distinctive of the human female. Her response to the influence of this Hormone that is circulating throughout her system is parallel, step by step, to the response which the male of the species shows, as described above. By the time she is sixteen, we expect her to show the physical and psychical characteristics that were described above for the mid-adolescent girl. In the maiden as in the youth, physical development predominates during puberty, while psychical development, maturity, and training predominate during the post-puberty stage of adolescence. By the time the young woman is twenty years of age we expect her to be mature in all those qualities that are distinctive of typical womanhood.

The Development of the Girl

Nature's General Plan

Nature is preparing in the adolescent a home builder. She is preparing in the young man an individual who can support and protect not only himself but also a family. She is preparing in the young woman, one who possesses the charm requisite for society and the skill and resourcefulness necessary for a wife and mother in a home.

As a part of nature's plan, the typical adolescent begins early in that period of development to experience *sex urge*—i. e., a strong desire to possess and to mate with one of the opposite sex. The purpose of this sex urge in the economy of nature is evident. But for sex urge the young male of the species would not seek to mate with the female and similarly the female of the species would not accept the advances of the male or wish to mate with him. Apparently, this sex urge is a primordal necessity and we see it manifested among all higher animals, especially in mammals and birds and it may exist in lower ranks of animals.

Now, if the youth and maiden experience sex urge and are conscious of this desire years before it will be feasible and proper, in our present social structure, to wed and start their home-building and family life, how will this influence their lives and how will it influence society?

Manifestly, the youth must from the first control this sex urge. Failure to control would lead to unwholesomely early mating or to illicit sex relations out of wedlock, either of which would be sure to lead to unfortunate results. It is perfectly evident as we study nature that the youth and maiden must control their sex urge. They must live in purity and chastity—*the continent life.* This is the ideal condition which we should seek to bring about. During unmarried youth the ideal life is continent life.

After maturity is reached the ideal social relationship of the sexes is *monogamous* wedlock, to which relationship both parties should live in absolute fidelity.

Failure to control sex urge has led to what we recognize as the *social evil*. Social wrong living may manifest itself in various ways. For example, in illicit relations;— in libertinism, in prostitution, in adultery, in fornication, etc. The result of illicit and promiscuous sex relationships is a tragic spread of venereal disease which destroys the health and efficiency of individuals, chokes the family happiness, and leads often to degeneration and death, blotting out more families than any other cause of family extinction.

Departure from Nature's Plan: Falling Short of the Ideal

One of the sad results of illicit sex relations is the birth of children out of wedlock, which introduces into society the problem of *the illegitimate child* and the *unmarried mother*.

Still another phase of lack of control of sex urge is seen in the habit which is widespread especially among early adolescents, namely, the habit of *self-abuse* or *masturbation*. This habit, as a matter of fact, is very frequently begun in the period of pre-adolescence and not a few cases come to the attention of physicians in which even little children indulge the act. The writer is led to believe from his long study of these problems of childhood and youth that the activating motive of self-abuse in the child is quite different from that in the youth. The two most prevalent causes of self-abuse in children of the pre-adolescent or earlier age are: first, *uncleanness of the person*. Mothers and caretakers of little children frequently neglect the proper care and attention that should be given to insure the absolute cleanliness of the sex apparatus. The male child particularly is not at all easily kept in the condition desirable unless he has been circumcised. The writer has for many years urged parents to circumcise every boy during his infancy. If the baby boy is not circumcised, accumulating secretions are likely to cause local irritation and discomfort. The child instinctively attempts to allay the local discomfort by rubbing his organs. In that way many boys drift into the habit of self-abuse. Little children of both sexes must be kept clean and must be taught cleanly habits.

The second prevalent cause of this unfortunate habit is to be found in the deliberate *teaching* of the habit to innocent little children by older associates, either playmates or sometimes nurse girls. The wise mother may protect her child against this wrong teaching only through a most vigilant watching and supervision of the child's associations and play; and even despite a great vigilance it is not at all infrequent for children to be led into the habit.

One element that should be considered in this problem is the fact that during pre-adolescence the child is going through a period of vulgarity. Vulgarity seems to be a part of our heritage from barbarism. The barbarian boy seems to be inherently vulgar; or if not precisely that, we all must admit that if ever a boy may easily drift into, or be easily led into, vulgarity in thought, language, and habits, those are the crucial years. It is because of this mental attitude more than anything else that the pre-adolescent child, perhaps especially the boy, is so extremely likely to acquire the habit of self-abuse. The writer is convinced from a study of responses to a questionnaire which he sent out among college men fifteen years ago, that at least 90% of the boys from even our most careful families indulge for a shorter or longer time, perhaps for a few weeks only, in this habit.

Whether the habit is as prevalent among pre-adolescent and early adolescent girls as among boys the writer does not know positively from reliable researches; but he has been led to believe that it is far less prevalent among little girls who live the ordinary, family life, as members of a typical home than among boys. However, matrons of institutions for girls say that from time to time, that is, every few months, or every year or two, the coming into their circle of a girl who has the habit will lead to a rapid acquiring of the habit by several or many of the girls of the institution.

In the adolescent the habit may be started to satisfy sex urge, or it may be continued from childhood as a habit, in which latter case the hold of the habit is made very much firmer by the sex urge of adolescence.

Those of us who have given years of study and atten- **Hygiene of** tion to these problems of the life of the individual, the **Adolescence** family, the community and the State, come early in our study to be convinced that the social problem—the problem of right social relationships between men and women in human society—will never be solved and society brought back to or brought up to the condition which we recognize as ideal until children and young people are taught in home and school the sacred truths of life. The writer would formulate two general principles that may well govern us in this instruction of youth.

1. The instruction that is to form the basis of habits during adolescence and subsequent years must be begun in early childhood and in pre-adolescence, and should continue during puberty.

2. The instruction must be positive and constructive; —i.e., it must be such that high ideals of life will be firmly established. In other words, if nature is to score a great success in her preparation of the home-builder and family maker, this preparation must begin in early childhood, must be continued as a definite unfolding of life lessons, and must establish right habits, high ideals, and aspirations.

Some of the fundamentals that must be established are:

1. A recognition of the sacredness of life; **General**
2. A recognition of the sacredness of motherhood; **Principles**
3. A recognition of the sacredness of the family circle, and of fatherhood;

4. A recognition of the sacredness of the body as the temple of womanhood or of manhood.

5. Establishing wholesome thought, habits,—modesty in our daughters,—chivalry in our sons;

6. Establishing hygienic habits which will be conducive to the development of perfect physique and the maintenance of perfect health.

The fundamentals above enumerated should be established in the order in which they are written, the first two imparted during early childhood, the second two (3 and 4) during the pre-adolescence period, and the last two (5 and 6) during puberty.

The Life Story The child of five to seven years is almost sure to go to mother with a question about life,—the origin of life, asking: "Mother where did you get me,—where did I come from?" Or, "Mother how did the baby come?" The mother must answer it truthfully. Let her tell nature's plan, in a *spirit* of *reverence;* and in telling how the new life comes, the mother should reveal to the questioning child the fact that the *mother sacrifices much* for the new life. The child will be impressed with a feeling of the sacredness of life and of motherhood, and will be held to mother by a bond of confidence and love. This bond between mother and child will insure to the mother the leadership of the child during all the years of early childhood and pre-adolescence.

The Story of Manhood, —and of Womanhood When the child reaches the age of nine or ten, the second group of life lessons should be instilled. In the ideal family life the mother will instruct her daughter and the father will instruct his son. But if the father fails to do his duty by the boy the mother should lead both daughter and son into a knowledge of the origin of life.

As we have seen, the boy goes through the wood-and-water-loving period of pre-adolescence; this is the period when he is especially interested in scouting, in camping, in hiking through the woods and along the water courses. All these activities are of the out-of-doors and are adapted especially to the needs of boys and men; for that reason the father and son should be pals and chums for years. In their hikes afield the father will have frequent opportunities to explain life in its various phases to his son. Among the life lessons, the father must explain to his son nature's method of developing manhood in the youth.

The father should explain how at the threshold of puberty the testicles of the boy begin to do two very important kinds of work,—they begin to prepare a wonderful "elixir of life"—the Hormone—which is absorbed immediately into the blood, is carried to every active tissue of the body and causes the development in the youth of all those qualities which are distinctive of ideal, virile manhood. It should be explained that these qualities are maintained throughout life, to the beginning of old age, by the influence of the "elixir of life"—the internal secretion from the testicles—the Hormone from the gonad glands. The father also should explain how the semen, or seed, begins to develop slowly in the testicles early in the period of puberty; also that the semen is a fluid, possessing wonderful qualities. This highly potential semen should not be wasted. The father should, in a spirit of reverence, explain nature's plan for the starting of a new life—*fatherhood*. The boy's knowledge of the life history and family history of pets and domestic animals will make this easy to explain. With such instruction the boy will easily acquire high ideals of manhood, of the family, of life, and of life-relationships. Having accomplished this, the father can lead his son to observe absolutely correct habits in his personal life. The boy will certainly have the natural feeling of reverence for his mother further strengthened and firmly established. This attitude toward his mother is destined at the threshold of adolescence to form the basis of his attitude toward womankind in general, his attitude of *chivalry*.

The Story of Womanhood In a similar way the mother may lead the pre-adolescent daughter to look forward to life with high ideals and unfaltering confidence. Let her teach the little girl of ten or eleven that in nature's plan for her developing womanhood she will begin at the threshold of puberty to receive into her blood from her ovaries an "elixir of life," a Hormone. This "elixir of life"—this internal secretion—carried to all active tissues by the blood will cause the development in her of the qualities distinctive of ideal womanhood. When the child is so taught she acquires high ideals of life and of womanhood. She will instinctively feel that her person is sacred to her future womanhood, and to her future wifehood and motherhood. A girl so instructed by her mother will never acquire distorted viewpoints of life, or the unclean personal habits referred to above. Girls so mothered naturally become modest, idealistic, and above reproach in their thought-life and habits.

After such a course of preliminary instruction during early childhood and pre-adolescence, the instruction in adolescent hygiene is very simple and certain of the best results.

Protection Against Bad Habits The principal reason for telling the child of pre-adolescent age the story of manhood or of womanhood is with the definite end in view of impressing the child with the feeling of the sacredness of the body so that such an unnatural act as self-abuse will seem revolting. If the parent has really done effective teaching the child will need only a few words of admonition after he has heard the story of manhood to make him at once and forever stop the habit of self-abuse, if he has already learned it; or to be effectively protected against being led into the habit if he has not already learned it.

The parent might mention, perhaps rather incidentally, the fact that children that become addicted to the habit are in great danger of seriously marring their budding manhood or womanhood. No detailed, gruesome descriptions of "insanity and human wreckage" should be portrayed. Even if it should be demonstrated as true that self-abuse may cause insanity, much the strongest motive for right living is to be found in painting the glories, wonders, and beauties of ideal and perfect manhood and womanhood, and simply warning the child that indulgence in the wrong habit will mar this beauty and perfection, and cause him to fall short of the ideal.

At the threshold of puberty, preferably just before crossing it, the parents should explain to their children— mother to daughter, father to son—about the matter of periodicity. The mother should explain to the daughter, nature's plan in the life of woman. When the mother explains that this experience to which the girl is introduced at the threshold of womanhood is nature's method of preparing for future motherhood, the girl, budding into womanhood, is quite reassured and acquires the right mental attitude toward life and its experiences. Any efficient mother will, of course, instruct her daughter regarding precautions which should be observed in order that the young woman may be regular and in uniform good health. *Periodicity*

Similarly the father should explain to his son that soon after the crossing of the threshold into puberty he may expect an occasional *nocturnal emission,* or loss of a fluid which collects in two little bladders (vesicles) that make a part of the internal sex apparatus and are located back of the urinary bladder and next to it.

In nature's plans, this albuminous vesicular fluid is provided to furnish nourishment for the sperm cells or spermatozoa of the semen. But these sperm cells of the semen are supposed to remain dormant for months during continent-living, athletic youth. There is, therefore, no immediate need for the vesicular fluid. Consequently, when the vesicles become filled and distended they simply empty. This usually happens at night—we call it a nocturnal emission, and look upon it as representing nature's method of relieving the tension in the sex apparatus—her method of taking care of the continent-living young man.

Dr. G. Stanley Hall, after a study of the world's medical literature on the subject of spontaneous emissions (noctural or diurnal) was led to remark, "Spontaneous emissions are probably as universal for unmarried youth as menstruation for women" (Adolescence, Vol. i, p. 453). In checking the medical literature with his own findings in thousands of interviews, with college men especially, the writer is inclined to modify the rather sweeping statement of his colleague quoted above. The writer has found a considerable proportion of youths and young men of high school and college age who claim to be seldom or never conscious of a spontaneous emission or to have noticed the marks of such that may have occurred during sound sleep. Of course, if a young man is resorting to the act of self-abuse even as infrequently as once in two weeks, he would be quite unlikely to experience any spontaneous emissions. It is easily conceivable that a young man may be living clean and continent and still not experience a spontaneous emission, because the vesicular fluid may be reabsorbed or may be voided along with the urine at the time of the morning micturition once in two, three, or four weeks.

The regularity of this function, if it may be so called, may be disturbed in four different ways. First, frequent emissions may be caused by an inordinate drinking of water in the evening, thus filling up the system with water which in turn will overfill the bladder by two or three o'clock in the morning, causing that organ to press against the vesicles, thus evacuating them. Second, frequent emissions may be caused by excessive albumins in the diet; for instance if a youth eats three eggs every morning he would facilitate the secretion of the albuminous vesicular fluid, which increased secretion would be voided with increased frequency. Third, increased frequency of emissions may be caused by faulty position during sleep. We are mammals. The mammal does not sleep on its back, but midway between side and belly. The man should sleep on his side. If he sleeps on his back the weight of his bladder resting upon the vesicles may evacuate them. Fourth, the most prevalent cause of frequent emissions is to be found in the sex excitement incident to the modern close-up dance and the "petting party" or spooning. This proximity of the body of a girl or a woman is practically sure strongly to excite sexually any red-blooded young man. As a result of this sex excitement, semen pours up from the testicle into the ampullae and vesicles, filling them to the limit. Following such an experience the vesicles are very likely, in fact almost sure to evacuate in the early morning hours. Incidentally the spontaneous emission which follows a strong sex excitement is accompanied by a draining off of semen and the young man addicted to this folly will feel the depletion of his manly vigor just as surely as the youth who is addicted to the habit of self-abuse.

When a young man understands nature's plan in a man's life, he can be led easily by his father, or other leader whom he respects and trusts, to adopt the continent life—the life of no sex indulgence of any kind— as the only regimen that will keep him perfectly fit physically, and the only program of life that will keep him worthy of the pure girl whom he hopes some day to wed.

Any wholesome-minded young man hopes some day to win and to wed a chaste, healthy, efficient young woman. If he is trying to play the game of life fairly and on the square, he will recognize that the young woman has a moral and ethical right to demand of the young man who is to be her life partner, the same qualities that he is demanding of her: clean life, health, and efficiency. This means that we have reached a stage of social development where we recognize that there should be one and the same standard of living for the man and the woman:—*The Single Standard.*

Summary   The typical *pre-adolescent* boy is egoistic, thoughtless, blundering, rough, noisy, rude, unmoral, and unsocial. He is interested in woods and water, and in live things. There is sex consciousness but no reciprocal sex attraction between boy and girl.

The typical *adolescent* youth is thoughtful and considerate. He has had a moral awakening and begins definitely to show the beginnings of altruism. He enjoys camping, hunting, and fishing. He is virile and aggressive, but not selfishly so. He is athletic and coöperates effectively in team work. There is not only sex consciousness but also a mutual and reciprocal sex attraction between youth and maiden.

The remarkable transformation—boy to man, girl to woman—is due to the influence in them of a Hormone from the *gonads*. This recently discovered "life ferment," entering the blood from the sex glands, causes the development of typical male qualities in the youth and of typical female qualities in the maiden.

One phase of the sex development is the experience of *sex urge* on the part of the adolescent. Uncontrolled sex urge has led to a train of evils—unhappiness, weakness, disease, degeneration—which we call the *social evil*. The cure of the social evil can be accomplished only through establishing right mental attitudes and habits in the adolescent.

The thought habits and mental attitudes and physical

habits of the adolescent are much influenced by the experiences of the preceding period—pre-adolescence. It is therefore strongly to be recommended that the instruction of the young begin early and that it be given by the parents, so far as that is feasible.

A fundamental principle to be followed in the instruction of youth concerning social relationships and personal attitudes and habits is that the instruction should be idealistic, positive, and constructive—not negative or morbid or fearful.

PART III

PRESENT STATUS OF OUR KNOWLEDGE
OF EDUCATION

Another important function of the public school in a democracy is the discovery and development of the gift or capacity of each individual child. This discovery should be made at the earliest practicable age, and, once made, should always influence, and sometimes determine, the education of the individual. It is for the interest of society to make the most of every useful gift or faculty which any member may fortunately possess; and it is one of the main advantages of fluent and mobile democratic society that it is more likely than any other society to secure the fruition of individual capacities. To make the most of any individual's peculiar power, it is important to discover it early, and then train it continuously and assiduously. It is wonderful what apparently small personal gifts may become the means of conspicuous service or achievement, if only they get discovered, trained, and applied. . . . . In the ideal democratic school no two children would follow the same course of study or have the same tasks except that they would all need to learn the use of the elementary tools of education—reading, writing, and ciphering. The different children would hardly have any identical needs. There might be a minimum standard of attainment in every branch of study, but no maximum. The perception or discovery of the individual gift or capacity would often be effected in the elementary school, but more generally in the secondary; and the making of these discoveries should be held one of the most important parts of the teacher's work.

—*Charles W. Eliot*

CHAPTER XVI

The Need of Bridging the Gap Between Our Knowledge of Education and Our Educational Practice

THE public school is designed to develop the pupil, but it is readily agreed by all that the needs of the individual pupil change with the social and community needs. Society is an organism. Social and community needs are therefore continually changing. It follows that the science and practice of schools must change. As a rule both social and educational movements require time and changes take place slowly. Educational science and practice do not keep step. One necessarily lags behind the other and, even if it were possible to keep knowledge and practice in education abreast of each other, there would be the necessity of constantly adjusting the schools to a changing social order.

The School and Its Aims Constantly Changing

The institutions of a democracy are changed with the consent of the people and depend upon popular enlightenment and control. The institutions of an absolute government are modified by one or by a few usually without the consent or knowledge of those governed. It was the consciousness of this fact that inspired the American Declaration of Independence. As might be expected, it requires a longer time to modify institutions which depend upon popular control than those which are autocratically controlled. The observation of this fact has brought many Europeans, particularly monarchists, to believe that a democracy is clumsy, unwieldy, and inefficient as compared with monarchies and autocracies.

The Modification of Institutions in a Democracy is Slower than in an Autocracy

325

This was a leading factor in Germany's attitude in the recent World War. Those of us who have faith in democracy believe that there is a greater measure of safety in popular control. This idea was advanced by the New England statesman, Fisher Ames, quoted indirectly by Emerson in his essay on Politics: "Fisher Ames expressed the popular security more wisely when he compared a monarchy and a republic, saying that a monarchy is a merchantman, which sails well, but will sometimes strike on a rock and go to the bottom; while a republic is a raft, which would never sink, but then your feet are always in water."

Those of us who are sometimes impatient with progress in our Republic should remember that the very thing which provokes our impatience protects us from rash and precipitate action which might incur disaster.

Our Educational System Shares the Characteristics of Our Form of Government

Our American public school system, like our government, is an institution of the people, by the people, and for the people. In America, education emanates from the people. In Europe, it emanates from the government. In America, the school system originally was controlled entirely by the people residing in a very small district or locality. Gradually a certain degree of control has been vested in counties in some sections of the country and everywhere certain powers of school regulation, particularly the establishment of standards of attendance, teaching and organization have been ceded to the States. The first State Superintendency was established in New York in 1812 and, by the time of the Civil War, all the States of the North had similar officers, but such an office did not exist in the States of the South until after the Civil War. Prior to the War only twenty-four cities had superintendents. No power of controlling education in the States has ever been ceded to or exercised by the Federal Government. The transition from the district system to the city, township, or state system of

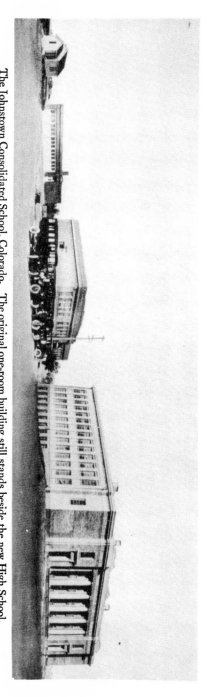

The Johnstown Consolidated School, Colorado. The original one-room building still stands beside the new High School.

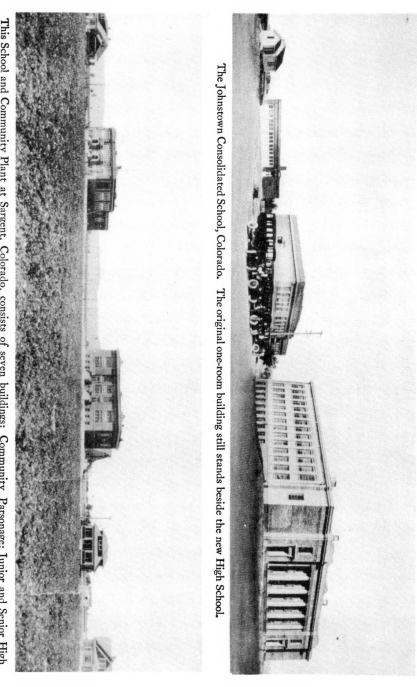

This School and Community Plant at Sargent, Colorado, consists of seven buildings: Community Parsonage; Junior and Senior High School and Community Center Building—used as educational, social, civic and religious center; Grade Building; garage with twelve motor trucks; home of mechanic and janitor; home of superintendent; Women's

control does not mean taking education out of the hands of the people, but simply a more efficient administration by officers who are nevertheless responsible to the people and are either elected by the people or appointed by the representatives of the people. There is no tendency in America to take the control of the schools from the people. Usually in a European country, as for example in France or Germany, the entire control, organization, and administration of the schools are vested in a minister or ministry. Those who complain that progress is slow in American schools in some respects as compared with European schools, should remember that we have the same protection from exploitation and disaster in our school system which we possess in our political system.

Education has existed in the world in some form or other for thousands of years. Science or the treatment of phenomena in a systematic manner by the discovery and presentation of truth in an orderly process of classification is quite modern. More science has been developed and applied to man's use in the memory of persons now living than was produced in the entire previous range of history.

The Greatest Obstacle in Bridging the Gap between Knowledge and Practice in Education has been the Absence of Scientific Method in Education

Natural science, or that mass of knowledge dealing with things, plants, and brutes, such as geology, physics, botany, and zoölogy, developed before social science or that mass of knowledge which pertains to man and his moral, political, and intellectual relations. In fact, these latter branches of knowledge are largely in the process of being born and developed at the present time. No attempt to attack problems of education from a scientific basis had been made until the last few decades. True, there have been before this those who, like Pestalozzi, Herbart, Froebel, and others, attempted to establish educational methods on experiments of one kind or another, but not until the twentieth century did anything appear worthy of the name of science in education.

Education, when first subjected to careful study, was called philosophy, then pedagogy, and only quite recently has it been called science.

For centuries education continued as a matter of tradition and opinion, and because of the recentness of the scientific method, most of our educational knowledge and practice is still based upon traditional beliefs. In consequence, a major part of educational practice is unsupported by scientific experiment and still is a matter of controversy, debate, and arbitrary decision. The lack of a scientific method of attacking education has probably been the most outstanding difficulty in harmonizing knowledge and practice in education.

Education is Now Established as a Science Education is now generally regarded as a science, but this recognition has only recently been won. Education has suffered an experience similar to agriculture. In 1857 a group of men went to the University of Michigan seeking to have agriculture taught there. They were regarded with skepticism as no one at that time considered agriculture as a science or capable of systematic instruction. That group of men left Ann Arbor and founded an institution for teaching agriculture at Lansing, Michigan. In 1862, the Federal Congress passed the first Morrill Act granting land to institutions which proposed to teach agriculture and mechanic arts. Other institutions were established similar to the one at Lansing, and other acts were passed by Congress extending Federal support to them, until we have agricultural and mechanical colleges, together with experiment stations for the scientific investigation of agriculture and kindred subjects, in every State in the Union.

Formerly, the term "farmer" was a derisive synonym for ignorance. Agriculture was based upon opinion and oftentimes superstition. Failure of crops was frequently attributed to planting in the wrong phase of the moon, or even to the vengeance of God. To-day agriculture is

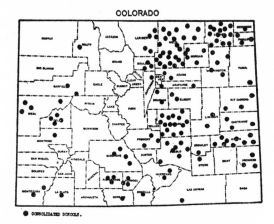

COLORADO

● CONSOLIDATED SCHOOLS.

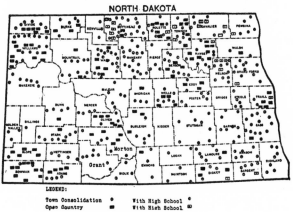

NORTH DAKOTA

LEGEND:
Town Consolidation ●   With High School ◉
Open Country ■   With High School ▣

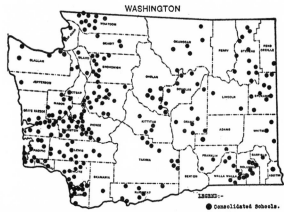

WASHINGTON

LEGEND:-
● Consolidated Schools.

The consolidation of one-room rural schools is making rapid headway throughout the country. What is shown on these maps of Colorado, North Dakota, and Washington is similar to what is taking place in other States.

329

a science. Practice is based upon actual experimentation and results. Even productivity of soil and water supply are being changed by scientific planting, rotation of crops, soil analysis, fertilization, and irrigation. Crops are no longer dependent upon opinion or the providence of a beneficent God, but upon the knowledge and ignorance of men.

It has been only a few years since a small group of men, the pioneer among whom was Edward L. Thorndike, began to contend that mind and its products could be subjected to careful scientific measurement, qualitative and quantitative. They encountered skepticism and some ridicule, but they persevered. To-day, education has secured the same recognition as to scientific treatment that has been accorded to agriculture, though that recognition may not be so general among the people outside the educational world. The establishment of scientific method in the field of education should be the means of bringing educational knowledge to a more general and unquestioned acceptance and therefore make possible some abridgment of the gap existing between our theory and practice in our schools.

Sometimes Knowledge Outruns Practice, and Sometimes Practice Outruns Knowledge

It should be noted that a gap exists between our knowledge and practice in education, both because in many instances we know a great deal that would improve the schools that we do not or can not put into practice, and because we practice a great many things in the schools about which we have little or no knowledge. Sometimes knowledge is ahead of practice, and at other times practice is ahead of knowledge. We shall proceed to discuss these two general phases of the problem with which this chapter deals and illustrate with concrete examples.

Previous to the establishment of education on a scientific basis, there was a possibility of deriving knowledge for the improvement of schools because each school was after all a kind of experiment or laboratory in which children were being taught. There existed also the opportunity for mutual discussion and comparison among those responsible for the management and direction of schools. Although the measurement of results and the evaluation of methods and materials were largely matters of guesswork, opinion, or rough estimation, there were many things that came to be generally recognized as true because of the nature of circumstances or the general consensus of opinion arrived at by a great many working independently of each other. And thus there existed a body of knowledge about education which was outside the pale of mere opinion or controversy before there was a scientific treatment of education. At the present time, most of our knowledge about education is of this kind because scientific methods are so recent that very little information of a scientific character has yet been derived. In recent years, experimental methods have been employed on a large scale and schools have been established for testing principles of organization and types of instruction, such as the Lincoln School in connection with Teachers College, Columbia University, the Gary schools, and others, but as yet we have not had the time to evaluate these and little scientific knowledge has yet been accumulated.

There was Knowledge of Education Before Education Became Scientific

Although we have had some generally accepted knowledge about schools, we have always experienced difficulties in attempting to get it into use. There are numerous reasons for these difficulties. We shall mention only some of the more important ones and treat them under the following headings: Conservatism in Education; The System of Popular Control; Changing Conditions Outside the Schools; Control of Education on Political Rather than Professional Basis, and Necessity of Training Teachers.

Some of the Reasons Why Practice Lags Behind Knowledge in Education

Schools and school people have always been regarded

as conservative. Ideas and traditional thinking are not
easily changed. American educational ideals are very
largely the result of Greek thinking before the time of
Christ. Plato, Aristotle, and others are largely responsible
for our cultural scheme. The thoughts of these ancient
Greeks completely dominated European thought even
after the downfall of Greece. Greek culture conquered
Rome when Roman arms conquered Greece. After the
middle ages, Greek culture was revived all over Europe.
The Greek philosophers and thinkers became arbiters in
all matters of learning. A question arose about the
existence of spots on the sun. It was concluded after a
search through all the works of Aristotle that there could
be no spots on the sun because Aristotle made no mention of them anywhere.

"The conservatism of men in education is nowhere
demonstrated more clearly than in their clinging to educational principles long after the reason for doing so no
longer exists. No one will doubt the advances that have
been made in the scientific world as a result of the Bacon-
ian philosophy. In fact, since Bacon's time, the world
has been made over. We have entirely cut loose from
the past in medicine, physics, chemistry, and the other
physical sciences, and no one would think to-day of
basing research in these sciences on deduction. We gain
our knowledge of them from a study of things. What the
ancients gave us in them has been brushed aside as worthless rubbish. But in education we still cling to the past,
although there is every reason to brush it aside that
there was in the case of scientific knowledge. In fact,
educational principles must go hand in hand with scientific principles, or they are worthless. Plato said, 'All
the useful arts are degrading, and the end of education is
to cultivate the thinking powers,' and we are willing to
risk all on his judgment. At the time of the Renaissance,
when men were digging from their hiding places the

manuscripts of the Greeks, some fellow happened to dig out this philosophy of Plato, and it has had such a tremendous influence that to-day we are unable to break loose from it."[1]

We have already referred to the fact that the American school is controlled by the people and we have pointed out that this has a virtue in that it prevents rash and precipitate changes. Changes cannot be made as readily as in European countries where the system is controlled by the government. Every voter in America shares in the control of schools. Progress in educational practice can only be made after an idea has been presented by educational leaders to the public in such a measure as to convince at least a majority of the voters that it is desirable. For this reason, if for no others, educational practice would have to lag behind educational knowledge. A certain period of time is necessarily required to convince the public with reference to an educational need even after it becomes obvious to those who have the schools directly in charge.

The System of Popular Control

This is such an important element in the conservatism of tradition in our schools that I think it will be worth while to discuss it a little further. It should be remembered that many voters have attended school at a time when the school was quite different from the present or the time at which they are called upon to exercise the ballot in school matters. For this reason, almost any man or woman thinks that he or she can judge school needs without any assistance from the professional school man. Editors do not hesitate to write very positive editorials about what the schools should have and should not have, even though they attended an old-fashioned district school and have never visited a school since. It is just as if those who had never traveled in anything except stagecoaches would undertake to-day, without having seen a modern train, to discuss the railroad and

[1]See W. B. Bizzell and M. H. Duncan "Present Day Tendencies in Education," p. 26.

its needs. Nearly everybody has gone at some time to some kind of a school so the public has an assurance about its knowledge of schools which it does not have about law, medicine, or any other matter of public concern.

This attitude of the public makes it exceedingly difficult for school leaders to get their knowledge of education into practice. As we have already pointed out, it has the virtue of protecting the schools against anything that has not already been thoroughly discussed and demonstrated to the public if not tested by scientific method. On the other hand, school leaders have not in the past shown the degree of interest in educating the public about school matters that is desirable. Educators are too prone to discuss their problems among themselves in a technical way unintelligible to the public. It should be remembered that if sometimes the public may seem stubborn and intolerant in voting on bond issues, consolidation, and other school measures, educators are inclined to appear at times intolerant to the public. It is true that a great many agencies are now operating to bring schools and school administrators and school teachers into contact with the public, such as Parent-Teacher Associations, women's and men's clubs, and others, but the lack of this kind of program for informing the public about schools has made the gap between our educational knowledge and practice much greater than it should have been.

Changing Conditions Outside the Schools

Another prolific source of difficulty in keeping our schools abreast of educational knowledge is found in the changes outside the school of a social, economic, industrial, or political character which are unforeseen and beyond the control of those who are responsible for the schools. We have already pointed out the fact that society is an institution which is organic or constantly changing. In consequence of this fact, no educational problem can ever be settled with finality. We are just now passing through a period of violent upheaval and readjustment in social, economic, and political affairs. The World War involved us in revolution and reconstruction in many directions. All of this has a vital and profound effect on schools and education. This same problem of readjustment has always existed and will be necessary in the future development of schools though, of course, not in the same degree as it exists to-day as a result of the war. This general trend is admirably set forth by J. L. Horn:

"Again, this development of mass education has been taking place during a period which is itself a transition in the history of humanity. The development of the sciences; the establishment of cities; the political revolutions and the resultant changes in the form of government and of social concepts; the industrial revolution and its far-reaching changes in economic and social relations; the abolition of many well-established relations such as those which inhered in the institution of feudalism; these changes, as history goes, are so recent as to be practically contemporary.

"The very fundamental motives underlying mass education have been changing within the period of its institution. Beginning as we did with the purely religious motive, followed by the political motive inherent in democratic government under universal franchise, the motive of the moment must take into account the increasing complexity of modern life, requiring as it does many skills, abilities, and capacity to adjust, all of which implies ever increasing equipment, and an ever longer period of training.

"Public education has gone through an evolution comparatively easy to trace. Beginning as a luxury reserved for those of high station it became, through the accident of the point of view of the Reformation, a religious need

to be supplied by the State or church or some philan-
thropic agency. With the development of political democracy, it has become a definite secular function based
on political motives; and finally in America it has become
an institution of which every one is required to avail
himself by compulsion of law to an ever-increasing age,
and almost everywhere beyond the age of twelve."[1]

**Control of
Education
on a
Political
Rather than a
Professional
Basis**

Administrative positions in education were political
in their origin and professionalization has been slow.
This presents at the same time one of the outstanding
causes as well as an example of our difficulty in bringing
educational practice in accord with our knowledge. Certainly no one believes that partisan politics should have
any relation to schools. Education is no more a matter
of partisan politics than religion or morals. No political
party could be interested in an issue which would tend
to hamper public schools or their improvement. And
yet, in the case of the chief educational officers of the
States, most of them are elected upon a partisan ticket
in a political campaign. There has been a long and persistent agitation by school leaders against this practice,
but in thirty-four States the State Superintendent of
Public Instruction or similar officer is still elected in this
way. This position was not generally recognized or
established until the period just before and just after the
Civil War. At first there was no conception of the position as a professional occupation. It came into existence
in many States as a clerical function exercised by some
other state officer. Since its recognition as a separate
office, it has been often regarded as a political reward.
Generally the voters are much more interested in the
candidates for Governor or other state offices than for
that of State Superintendent. The tendency to vote the
party ticket has prevented much consideration being
given by the average voter to the educational or professional qualifications of those running on the state

[1] J. L. Horn, "The American Elementary School," pp. 274, 275.

ticket for the most important educational position in the State. At the present time, only six States have the chief educational officer appointed by the Governor, and only eight States have them appointed by the State Board of Education.

What has been said about state administrative officers also applies to other administrative officers to a greater or lesser degree, particularly county and district super-intendents. There is an exception in the case of the city superintendency. This position has come to be almost completely divorced from partisan politics and, uniformly, city superintendents are selected by boards of education or other bodies which usually seek to find persons with the proper professional training. But even here politics cannot be completely eliminated, because candidates for these boards frequently run on partisan tickets and sometimes reflect their sentiments in their attitude on the matter of an administrative or executive officer.

A very important and difficult problem which makes accommodation of educational practice to knowledge a slow process is the necessity for training teachers which arises when new forms of organization or methods of teaching are attempted. Some educational reforms re-quire a long period to become effective because a new generation of teachers must be trained who have the technical and professional knowledge necessary to carry the proposed changes into effect. William McAndrew puts this in a very effective phrase when he says, "Teach-ers have a vested interest in certain subjects and meth-ods." By this he means that because certain persons have learned to teach certain subjects in the curriculum and have learned in the normal school or by experience to employ certain methods of instruction, it is difficult to change the curriculum or methods of instruction be-cause some people will have to lose their jobs. In any

Necessity of Training Teachers

case, it always takes time to train either the same teachers or new ones who will have the technical knowledge and skill to teach the new things or teach in a new way. An example of this difficulty is found in the attempt to develop vocational education in the United States. Since the passage of the Vocational, or Smith-Hughes, Act by Congress in 1917, appropriating money from the Federal Treasury for the stimulation of vocational education in the States, the greatest difficulty experienced in setting up a program of vocational training, which was undertaken in each State after the passage of the Federal Act, has been that of securing those who had the necessary professional and technical knowledge and training in agriculture, trades and industries, home economics, and commerce, to undertake the direction of this work.

Teacher training is still an unsolved problem in American education and most of those teaching in our schools do not have the proper professional preparation. This fact accentuates the difficulty of bringing the school in line with the best educational knowledge because those charged with the instruction of the youth do not have the professional skill to employ modern or new methods. Horn cites one phase of the difficulties arising from the teacher training problem when he says, "One of the most potent factors tending to hold the American school system and its divisions in a grip of rigid immutability, has been our double system of teacher training. In their efforts to recruit teaching forces for the elementary schools, the early school men established training schools—our normal schools—institutions where training was given in methods; where just enough was taught to provide for the immediate need of securing teachers for the schools. On the other hand, teachers for the secondary schools have naturally been recruited from the colleges; and so the double system took root. A vicious circle was established. The normal school, originally a most useful institution, has by the very fact of its growth and development, at the same time that it has always limited its functions to the training of elementary-school teachers, fastened the rudimentary inevitableness of the elementary school upon the American system; for the teachers trained for that school have ordinarily not been equipped to enrich its curriculum by the introduction of secondary-school subjects in the earlier years."[1]

We have attempted to present a few of the obstacles in the way of a closer adaptation of theory and practice in our schools. There are other factors equally as important as those we have presented and many minor considerations which would require much space to present.

The Need of Reorganization of the School Curriculum

It is not the purpose of this chapter to point out the present practice of schools or show just how far this practice lacks unity with our present knowledge, but it would seem worth while to show in a broad way just what is the general situation as a result of the retarding factors just described.

About thirty years ago leaders in education began to realize that our school curriculum in America, particularly in its elementary stages, was outworn and urgently in need of reform. It was pointed out that as elementary education, secondary education, and higher education had all historically developed independently, there was no real articulation in the curricula of these important divisions of our school system and that, as a consequence, there was much wastage in pupils dropping out of school at an early age and, among those who continued, in the actual time required to pass through the system from kindergarten to college or university. Our college graduates were found to be two or three years older than those of European institutions and an agitation for reorganization was started. At the beginning the discussion was precipitated largely by Charles W. Eliot, then President of Harvard University, and William R. Harper, then

---

[1]J. L. Horn, "The American Elementary School," p. 20.

President of the University of Chicago. President Eliot, interested largely in reducing the age of college graduates, raised the question as to how the school curriculum might be shortened and at the same time enriched. The discussion quickly became general and aroused much interest among all types of school men. The agitation has continued since that time. Many conferences have been held, important committees have been appointed and have made valuable studies, numerous volumes have been written, and a great deal of experimentation has been done. All of this has shown to the general satisfaction of school men that a complete reorganization is badly needed, and yet the conditions to-day are very largely as they were when the agitation began.

Our Elementary School System Borrowed from Germany, and Our System of Higher Education Arose Independently

Our elementary school system with its "grades," was borrowed from Germany. Some have doubted this, but a careful investigation will establish the fact. A bulletin of the United States Bureau of Education says: "In America, during the period when our schools were being molded into the semblance of a system, German influence in shaping the structure was much more direct and potent than has been generally recognized."[1] Charles Brooks, the forerunner of Horace Mann in Massachusetts, is quoted in the same bulletin as follows: "From what I have learned, it is my opinion that the Prussian system is to make a new era in the public education of the United States."[2]

Likewise, the college and university in this country originated as an agency for higher culture and the so-called "learned professions." In the German system, the elementary school of eight grades did not prepare for anything above it. Students passing through the elementary school could not enter the gymnasium, which corresponds to our high school, much less the college or university. The masses passed through the elementary

[1] See Reorganization of the Public School System, United States Bureau of Education Bulletin, 1916, No. 8, p. 20.
[2] Ibidem, p. 22.

school into the common occupations and industry. The only way they could get any more education was in the "continuation" school. Those who expected to go into the professions or "higher walks" started at the same age, generally six years, as the masses began the elementary school. After three years of special training they passed into the gymnasium, from which they could enter the college or university. The German system of education was therefore the counterpart of a social and political caste system.

Unfortunately, the American school system was largely affected by the German. Hence the lack of articulation of its parts. The American high school was a comparatively late afterthought, attempting to furnish a route from the elementary school into the college in response to a demand that came from the democratic ideals of America.

In the circumstances, it is not strange that our system should have turned out to be wasteful and poorly articulated. The loss of students dropping out of our system and the tremendous loss of time by those remaining in it have been abundantly shown. **Waste in the American School System**

Under our system the pupils generally remain in school fairly well until the fifth grade. F. E. Spaulding has called us a nation of "sixth graders." After the fifth grade, there is a tremendous leakage. The United States Bureau of Education made a study of what becomes of the fifth-grade boy and girl. The study showed that of 1000 pupils in the fifth grade, 830 pass to the sixth grade, 634 of them enter the eighth grade, 342 of these reach the high school, but only 139 graduate; and while 72 of the original 1000 enter college, just 23 finally finish.[1] **Loss Due to Pupils Dropping Out**

President Eliot proved at the outset of the discussion that an enormous amount of time was wasted by the pupils remaining in the elementary school. Concerning

---

[1] United States Bureau of Education Bulletin, 1920, No. 34.

Time Wasted by Those Who Remain in the School

this experiment he wrote: "I procured two careful estimates of the time it would take a graduate of a high school to read aloud consecutively all the books which are read in this school during six years, including the history, the reading lessons in geography, and the book on manners. The estimates were made by two persons reading aloud at a moderate rate, and reading everything that the children in most of the rooms of that school have been supposed to read during their entire course of six years. The time occupied in doing this reading was forty-six hours. The children had, therefore, been more than two solid years of school time in going through what an ordinary high-school graduate can read aloud in forty-six hours."[1]

Experiments and Practice Have Shown that Elementary Curriculum Can be Shortened

It has been conclusively shown that the elementary curriculum is too long and that the upper grades do not hold the pupils, especially the bright ones, because of the deadly and formal nature of much of the subject matter and because so much of it is a mere repetition of subject matter in the early grades. There was once a time, when a few parents thought children might skip grades or pass on without completing all the work, but teachers were shocked at such a suggestion. It has now been conclusively demonstrated that bright pupils may be pushed ahead into higher grades and soon do just as well or better. Even repeaters have been found that would do better in the grade above, than in the one in which they have failed.

Furthermore, in many places the elementary curriculum has been shortened a year or more apparently without any actual loss in educational advantage to the pupils. Many cities and some States have a seven-year elementary course instead of the old eight-year course, giving the same amount of material in seven years as is usually given in eight years. Kansas City, Missouri, has had this kind of seven-year elementary schools since 1867, and

---

[1] Quoted by R. L. Finney, The American Public School, p. 227.

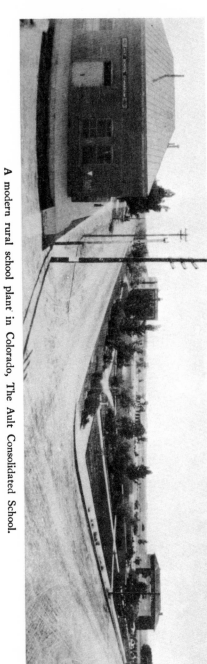

A modern rural school plant in Colorado, The Ault Consolidated School.

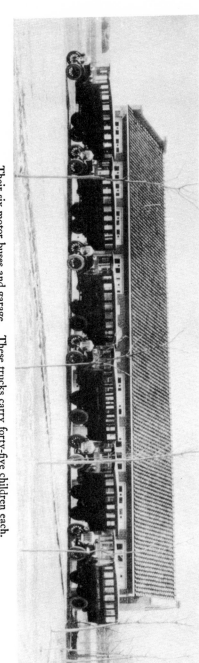

Their six motor buses and garage. These trucks carry forty-five children each.

in 1918 forty-eight cities had it. Louisiana has used it throughout the State for years and studies have shown that the pupils have held their own with those who have completed the eight-year course elsewhere.

It has been shown with equal clearness that the courses of study, particularly in the last grades of the elementary school, can be enriched and reorganized so as to deprive them of their deadly formalism and furnish motivation that will stimulate pupils to continue in school. The Junior High School is a solution of this problem. The Junior High School has demonstrated its success beyond peradventure and has revitalized the curriculum in the seventh, eighth, and ninth grades where the traditional curriculum was so deadening; and further, it helps to bring into articulation the elementary school and the secondary school. It does this by offering a course of study in the seventh and eighth grades, which anticipates the high school curriculum in specialization and by a kind of exploration discovers the aptitudes of pupils, so that they can later follow a course in the high school which is adapted to their temperament, abilities, and needs.

It Has Been Demonstrated With Equal Clearness that the Curriculum Can be Enriched

Notwithstanding all that has been demonstrated with reference to the inefficiency and waste of the traditional curriculum, it still remains in use in most places to-day. The attack upon the elementary curriculum is still being carried on with vehemence and the effort is still being made to accomplish an articulation between the elementary and high schools.

In Spite of What Has Been Demonstrated About Waste and Other Shortcomings, the Traditional Curriculum Still Remains in Most Places

"The American public school system now stands, after three centuries of growth, complete in form only. Its three divisions, elementary, secondary, and that embracing higher education, are joined together, end to end, forming a lineal whole. . . . In organic relation, in sharpness of province, and in distinctiveness of function, these divisions are not yet satisfactorily articulated."[1]

In 1920, J. L. Meriam offered objections to the tradi-

---

[1] U. S. Bureau of Education Bulletin 1916, No. 8, pp. 1-2.

tional elementary school curriculum, still generally in use, and characterized it as:

"Aimless; it does not function in the lives of pupils.

"Lifeless; mere form subjects predominate.

"Disconnected; fourteen school subjects are treated as unrelated except when arbitrarily and superficially correlated as school room arts.

"Congested; the crowded situation is due to the treatment of empty details.

"Wasteful; 'Progress through the grades' consists of 'marking time' and 'busy work.'

"Untimely; the traditional curriculum is not apace with the vital issues of the day."[1]

Many Instances Where Practice Outruns Knowledge

We stated that lack of unity in educational knowledge and practice is occasioned both by the fact that knowledge sometimes outruns practice, and also by the fact that practice sometimes outruns knowledge. We have shown concretely how we continue in practice much that our knowledge has shown undesirable. Much more could be said about that great unexplored field of education, where lack of experimentation or even empirical knowledge makes it necessary for us to practice without knowing. This gap, however, will be gradually closed as our application of scientific experimentation enables us to discover what the facts are and removes practice from the sphere of opinion and guesswork.

The Lincoln School

In 1917 Abraham Flexner published a paper under the title "A Modern School" which has recently been republished in a volume with another paper on "A Modern College." Flexner's "Modern School" called for a very radical reorganization and, when published, was based largely on opinion. The General Education Board, however, provided Teachers College of Columbia University with the funds to establish a school in which Flexner's ideas could be tried out. As a result we have had the Lincoln School for the past six years, running largely as

[1] J. L. Meriam, Child Life and the Curriculum, p. 52.

344

an educational laboratory and experiment. In this way, it will be possible eventually to determine in a scientific manner how far the practice of the Lincoln School is sound and how far Flexner is correct in his opinions. This is only one of many similar, though perhaps less important and less extensive experimental studies of educational theory and practice.

No matter how much progress we make in educational science, we shall never be able to keep practice from outrunning knowledge to some extent. New and attractive materials and methods will be constantly appearing through discovery and invention, and there will be those who will try out these new things, and naturally so, prior to any educational experimentation to determine the proper methods for the best results. An illustration of this is afforded at the present time in the increasing introduction into the schools of motion pictures in the absence of any knowledge about their educational value, methods of use, and proper modes of presentation.

Practice Will Always Outrun Knowledge to Some Extent

They are being introduced because of the general appeal that they make, the vitality and interest that they inject into the course, and the convenience that they offer in presenting much that was presented formerly in other ways. It will require long and careful experimentation to determine how much more effective these pictures are than the old methods, what material should be presented in this way, the devices that should be employed to secure the best results, and other questions of similar nature which readily suggest themselves for answer.

The absence of scientific method in the treatment of education is one reason why it has been difficult to bridge the gap between our knowledge of education and our practice of teaching. However, education is now becoming established as a science, and it should be possible in the future to achieve more success than we have had in

Summary

the past in keeping educational practice abreast of our knowledge of education.

Again, practice has lagged behind our knowledge of education, partly because of the conservatism which has been so persistent in education. Men cling to educational practices longer than they do to practices in almost any other field of human interest and activity. Another reason why practice has lagged behind our knowledge of education is because in our country there is popular control of the schools. A certain period of time is required to convince the public with reference to an educational need, even after it becomes obvious to those who have the schools directly in charge. Practically all our people think they are competent to render a decision regarding any phase of educational practice.

Still another source of difficulty in modifying practice to keep abreast of developing educational knowledge is found in the social, economic, industrial, and political changes which take place outside the school and which make it impossible to settle any educational problem with finality. The control of education has been largely on a political rather than on a professional basis, and this has retarded the development of educational practice as compared with the development of the science of education.

Again, it has been extremely difficult to provide adequately for the training of teachers so that they could keep abreast of our advance in the development of educational science. Further, teachers have had special interests which have made it difficult or impossible for some of them to see education as a whole in an unprejudiced way. The normal school system of the country has tended to perpetuate traditional educational practices without due regard to the increase of knowledge respecting educational values and methods.

It is now realized that there is an urgent need for the reorganization of the school curriculum. Our elementary school system, was borrowed largely from Germany, while our system of higher education was developed independently. There has not been proper articulation between the different parts of our educational system. As a result, it is generally believed that there is needless waste in our educational work. There is waste due to unnecessary elimination of pupils from school. There is also needless waste on the part of those who repeat grades in the schools.

Experiments and practice have shown that the traditional elementary school curriculum can be shortened. It has also been shown that the curriculum can be enriched by the addition of subjects which would have value in contemporary life.

While emphasis has been placed in this chapter on the failure of practice to keep abreast of scientific knowledge respecting education, still it should be said that in some ways practice outruns accurate knowledge. We still teach certain subjects and employ certain methods without knowing whether they are the most valuable and effective subjects and methods that could be employed. However, experimental schools are being established to investigate and test educational doctrines in the hope that all our practice may eventually be based upon adequate and accurate knowledge, although we must perhaps expect that in some respects practice will generally outrun accurate and adequate knowledge of educational values and methods.

XVII

CHANGING OBJECTIVES IN AMERICAN SCHOOLS

The Establishment of Free and Compulsory Schools

OUR early forefathers engaged for many decades in vigorous and often heated debate over the question of establishing free and compulsory education for all children, regardless of their social, economic, or racial status. There may be some readers who can remember the time when the schools were not free; every parent paid for the tuition of his children. It was quite generally believed in our country in former times that it would be unjust for a community to make every citizen contribute to the education of all the children of the community, because it was held by many, though not by everyone, that schooling was of benefit only to the children who received it. But even in the first period of our history, it was urged by some persons that the training at the public expense of all the young would be of advantage to all the people, since an ignorant person would not be able to comprehend the requirements in order to become a decent and law-abiding citizen. It was asserted by a few that every adult who had had no schooling would become a menace to the peace and welfare of the community, and that therefore every child should be *compelled* to acquire the rudiments of knowledge so that he could at least read.

In 1642, the Massachusetts Colony enacted a law *compelling* parents to have their children taught to read, and enforcing fines if they neglected this duty. In 1647, the same colony enacted a law requiring that every community having as many as fifty householders should appoint a teacher of reading and writing and should provide for his wages in any way they deemed best. This law also required that every community having as many as one hundred householders must provide a Latin grammar school to prepare youths for the university. Nevertheless, the majority of our forefathers believed that an educated adult would have an advantage over an uneducated one because he could make his living in an easier way, would have more leisure for enjoyment, and his education would improve his social status; but these benefits would be of value solely to the individual and not to the community. Since most of the people held this view in earlier times, the schools were originally private institutions for the most part, and were supported by those who could afford to pay tuition fees. In those days, few persons would have thought of suggesting laws compelling all the people to pay taxes for the support of public schools, for the reason that it was not generally believed that a person who could not read or write or use figures would imperil the economic, social, or moral welfare of the community.

Any reader of these lines would be impressed by an examination of the arguments for and against the establishment of free schools and compulsory education laws, which arguments extended over a considerable period in our early history. As one traces the discussion down through the years, he can see how those who maintained that the schooling of *all* children—at least in the rudiments of education—was essential for the welfare of *all* the people in the community, continually gained force and adherents, until finally the balance of power swung over from the opponents to the advocates of universal free education. The proposition that made the strongest appeal and that ultimately determined positive action was that every person who could read, write, and calculate according to the needs of daily life, and who had learned something about religion and the founding of our government and the principles of freedom upon which it is maintained, would make a better citizen than one who could not read or write and so who would have to depend upon others for information regarding the nature of our government and what is demanded of every individual in order that it should continue to be strong, stable, and prosperous. In the discussion of this matter, statements were frequently made to the effect that autocratic and monarchical forms of government exist where a large proportion of the people are ignorant. Just as frequently one reads that in a government like ours all the people must possess the rudiments of knowledge or else our democratic institutions cannot survive; if only a few are educated while the many are ignorant, the former will in time take unfair advantage of the latter, and democratic government will perish.

These propositions were presented so vividly and forcefully by the early friends of universal free education that they were at last successful in overcoming the opposition to the maintenance of a school system which required that all the citizens in a community should contribute to the education of all the young, even though some of the people had no children themselves to take advantage of the schools. There were a few persons in every community who protested as vigorously as they could that it was an injustice to make a family in which there were no children help pay for the education of other people's children. Those who clung to this view were upheld by intelligent and leading men in other countries; such men as Herbert Spencer in England, for instance, contended that a child who received an education gained benefit for himself individually, but that he did not contribute to the welfare of the people as a whole, and that therefore he should pay for his own schooling and others should not be required to assist him.

It should be specially noted that free and compulsory education was not established in our country for the

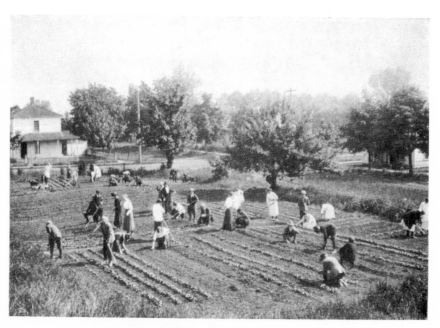

Every pupil ought to cultivate a plot of land.

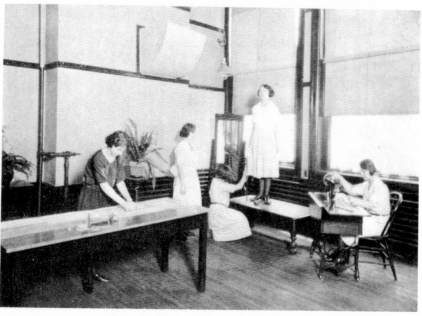

Dressmaking in a Chicago Public School.

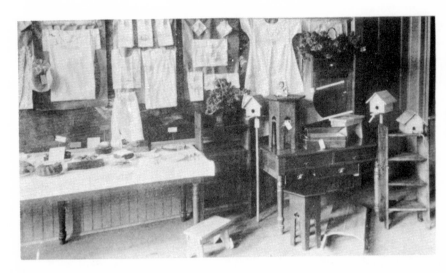

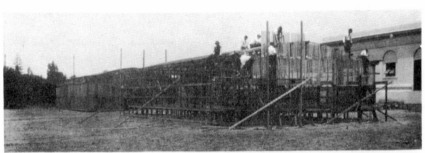

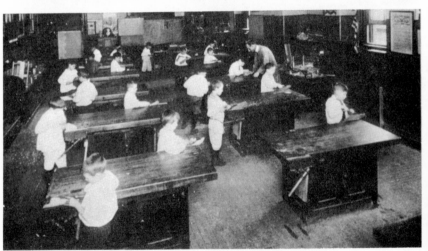

In a modern school pupils learn to do things which they will need to do after they leave school.

purpose of equipping the young so that they could get the most out of life individually; or at least individual betterment was regarded as incidental to the promotion of the general welfare. This view has persisted down to our own day and apparently is held at the present moment by most of those who are responsible for the support and administration of public schools. But there are among us persons who think that a graduate of a common school, a public high school, or a state-supported university, does not utilize his education for the promotion of community welfare so much as for his own material and social advancement, and they have recently expressed these views quite vigorously. The belief had become so widespread in our country that education is essential for good citizenship and that the better educated a person is the better citizen he becomes, that until recently one rarely heard a voice raised against this view. However, it was questioned actively and acutely by legislators in a number of States during the legislative months of 1923, and it is being questioned by boards of education as well as by laymen as these lines are being written. The occasion for questioning the value of education in promoting general welfare has arisen in connection with the discussion of bills for the appropriation of funds for the maintenance of state supported colleges and universities; and boards of education in some places are calling a halt to expenditures for public high schools. In some States, the funds asked for the support of universities were either not appropriated at all, or were greatly reduced; and the debates in the legislatures over the appropriation bills showed that there are persons among us who are sceptical concerning the advantage to the community of much of our present-day free higher education.

During the past two decades the expenses of high school education have increased several fold in our country. When public high schools were first established, only

Does
Education
Benefit the
Individual
or the
Community
Primarily?

an occasional pupil took advantage of them, but now the majority of pupils in many communities complete a high school course. This has required the multiplication of facilities for secondary education. Public high schools originally offered only one course of study; now the high schools in even the smallest towns offer several courses, and in the larger communities they offer many courses. The equipment in public high schools has increased enormously in quantity and cost during the past two decades, until to-day the typical high school in a city of twenty thousand or more inhabitants is better equipped in every department than was the typical college in our country five decades ago. As a result of the rapidly increasing cost of high school education, voices are just beginning to be heard in protest in some places. They have not yet made much impression upon the public and apparently they are not retarding the progress of secondary schools, for every day one reads of the building and equipment of magnificent new high schools, in small as well as in large communities. Further, elaborately equipped junior high schools in which the methods of senior high schools are introduced—at least in part—are being established everywhere. More will be said about junior high schools at another time; they are mentioned here simply as an illustration of the fact that while a few persons in many communities think we are doing an injustice to some taxpayers in providing expensive free secondary education for all the young who wish to take advantage of it, still the majority of our people firmly believe that any boy or girl who completes a high school or university course will be of greater service to the community than one who terminates his education with the completion of the eighth grade or earlier. It should be mentioned in this connection that the Carnegie Foundation for the Advancement of Teaching has taken a stand in its last report, just published, against public high schools as they are at present organized and administered, maintaining that they are far too expensive and that it is not just to tax a community so heavily for such costly education as is being provided in most communities.

It seems certain that the proposition that the education of all the young contributes to the general welfare, increasing as the education is increased and the educational period prolonged, will be critically examined during the next decade, both by the advocates and by the opponents of free higher education. The present writer has already heard a number of influential persons express approval of the views of the Carnegie Foundation for the Advancement of Teaching, referred to in the preceding paragraph. There are a few students of public education who are beginning to express doubt regarding the fairness and wisdom of multiplying educational facilities at public expense for all the young who wish to take advantage of them. Just recently, the present writer heard a prominent dean of a college of education say in an address at a large educational convention that our schools are becoming top heavy; that they are being overloaded with boys and girls who should be engaged in some practical work rather than attending school. He maintained that it was not worth while for more than fifteen or twenty per cent of the graduates of the elementary school to go forward into the secondary schools, and that not more than five per cent at most of the graduates of high schools should go on into colleges or universities. He argued that secondary and collegiate education is becoming so expensive that the educational system will break down, at least unless we can think of some new way of raising funds to support high schools, colleges, and universities.

It is significant that the dean's auditors seemingly did not sympathize with him in his doubts about the desirability or the possibility of continuing and extending our system of higher education. They listened to him in

How Can We Pay the Bills?

what appeared to be a hostile, or at least sceptical, attitude. They did not applaud his assertions. It was apparent that they regarded his views as reactionary. The people undoubtedly believe that the more education the better for the public good, and that there is no possibility, or at least no probability, of making our educational system too elaborate, too extensive, or too expensive. At the same time, the discussion of the address, after it was completed, showed that educational specialists are not unaware of the fact that some persons are beginning to ask for evidence that boys and girls who take advantage of free public education for twelve or sixteen years return to the community as much as they receive from it. During the next decade, questions of this sort will undoubtedly be asked freely and some plan will have to be devised to show conclusively to doubters, if it can be shown, that the more education a boy or girl receives at public expense, the greater service he can and does render to the community which supports the educational system.

It should be added that most of our people are not yet terrified by the increasing cost of our schools. It is readily granted that education is more expensive than any other public enterprise, and the end does not seem to be in sight yet by any means. Will we go bankrupt if we do not call a halt to educational building and equipment? To the increase in teachers' salaries? To prolongation of the compulsory school period? To the elaboration of the curriculum? To the appointment of school physicians and nurses? etc., etc. The friends of our public schools acknowledge that we cannot pay increasing education bills if we continue to pay as much as we have been paying for chewing gum, tobacco, gasoline, joy rides, motion pictures, women's clothing, cosmetics, jazz music, extravagant furnishings in our homes, and so on. Do you who are reading these lines appreciate that the nation's tobacco bill is greater each year than its bill for elementary, high school, collegiate and normal school education all combined? Do you know that there is as much spent for candy and chewing gum as for all our educational work, and that much more is expended for automobiles and gasoline for joy riding than is expended for school buildings, equipment, textbooks, teachers, health officers in schools, playgrounds, and all other items of school work combined? Do you know that baseball and the theatre cost as much as our total educational bill?

Those who approve our educational expansion and maintain that it should be continued claim that it really comes down to this: Is education of greater importance for national, state, and individual welfare than cigarettes, gasoline, confections, jewelry, silk stockings, movies, and the like? If we could spend as much money for education as we spend for luxuries—not depriving ourselves entirely of the latter but curtailing them a little—no nation in the world could keep in sight of the United States educationally. We could build up the minds, the health, and the character of our young people so that they would be equipped to meet the new problems which are sure to arise in our changing social and physical conditions. All we need to do, say the upholders of our educational system, is to shave off a little from our rouge bill, gasoline bill, movie bill, jazz bill, and automobile bill, and we will have adequate funds to pay all the educational bills. And the happiest outcome of this program will be that when we have more education of the right sort, we will be less interested in gum, rouge, jazz, movies, tobacco, baseball, and confections than we are now. It works out that way always; the interests developed in a sound education lessen the craving for physical and emotional indulgence.

Some readers may be asking themselves the questions: "Do all those who hold that public education promotes general welfare really believe this proposition? Do they

Why Do Parents Keep Their Children in Public Schools? keep their children in public schools because they think that if they are educated they can be of greater service to the community than if they are ignorant? Do parents urge their children to complete a high school and university course because they expect that by so doing they can advance the welfare of all the people in the community? Or do most parents keep their children in school as long as they can in the belief that the better educated they are the easier and better living they can make and the higher social position they can attain in the community in which they live? As a matter of fact, what objectives do American parents have in mind when they keep their children in public schools?"

Unquestionably the majority of parents believe that a boy or girl who is well educated will get on more easily than one who is poorly educated. The typical American parent thinks more of the prosperity of his own children than he does of the welfare of the community in which they live. One who has frequently to discuss with parents the question of what studies their children shall pursue in high school or in college becomes impressed with the fact that most parents do not consider whether or not a particular study will enable a child to understand the needs of and to serve the community in which he lives. It is quite rare to hear a parent say, "I would like to have my boy take such and such a course because he will receive training thereby which will help him to become a better citizen than he otherwise would be"; or "Unless he completes such and such a course he will not understand what the needs of the community are, and he will not receive any stimulus to use his talents to advance the welfare of the community"; or "I want my child to appreciate that the community has provided facilities for his education and so he must utilize what he gains in school for the benefit of all the people of the community."

Instead of such comments parents usually say: "I

want my boy to study geometry (for instance) so that he will gain good mental discipline, and then he will be able to handle himself successfully in situations in which he may be placed in daily life"; or "I want him to study bookkeeping so that he will know how to keep accounts accurately when he gets out into life"; or "I would like to have him study Latin so that he will receive culture and be able to associate with cultured people"; or "I wish he would study manual training so that he will be able to go to work at once as soon as he leaves school"; or "I would like to have him take a law course because I believe he could make a comfortable living in the law"; or "I don't want him to study teaching because this is a poorly paid profession and I think he can do better in something else." Not all American parents discuss the education of their children in such terms, but many of them do.

Fortunately, an education which will best promote the interests of the individual will, as a rule, be of greatest service to the community. An individual cannot make a good living unless he can serve people according to their needs. If he becomes a skilful surgeon at the expense of the State—many States are now supporting medical institutions in which training is almost or completely free—he will make a good living, but he will do so by serving the people who have made it possible for him to secure his education. Of course, he may take advantage of the fact that he is a skilful surgeon to overcharge those whom he serves, and undoubtedly this is the case in many instances; but nevertheless the community is vastly better off by making it possible for men to become skilful surgeons at public expense than if there were only such surgeons and as many of them as could afford to defray all the expenses of their education, both general and professional.

Again, one can make a fairly comfortable living who

The Interests of the Individual and of the Community are Reciprocal and Mutually Dependent for the Most Part has become an expert teacher entirely at the expense of the State, and he may take some advantage of the community in which he teaches because he is very able,— that is, he may secure a larger salary than he is really entitled to, considering that he is the beneficiary of the State, and that it would have been impossible for him to become a teacher if the State had not provided free training for him; and yet it is vastly better for the State to bear all the expense of training skilful teachers, even though they do not fully appreciate their responsibility to the State, than to depend upon the supply of teachers which could be secured if each one had to pay all the expenses of his preparation.

Even in the case of the individual who has at public expense pursued studies in the elementary school, in the high school, and in the university which do not fit him for any special service to the community—not even for teaching—it may still be said that he is of advantage to the community in that he disseminates knowledge as he moves about among people, and in his daily life he emphasizes the kind of conduct that the possession of knowledge confers upon one. If he has studied literature, mathematics, foreign languages, and the like, he will show some effect in his own behavior—in being more restrained in the indulgence of his impulses and appetites, and he will be able to throw light on problems which perplex people who have not had such training, and so he will be of service to the community even though he has no intention of serving it. His views, his conduct, his attitude in the face of intellectual and social problems will be emulated by the people with whom he associates; thus they will profit by his learning. It is probable that the way an educated man meets the situations of life is more to be desired than the way in which the uneducated man meets them, and so from this point of view as well as from the others mentioned, the influence of the educated man in a community will be more wholesome and beneficial than the influence of an uneducated man. The American people feel the force of this principle even though they cannot express it definitely; it is more a matter of faith with them than of explicit belief. This faith has been sufficiently strong to maintain courses of study in elementary and high schools and state supported universities that do not bear directly upon any of the material or social needs of life so far as the people can see.

The objectives which the typical parent has in view in keeping his children in school have partially, but not principally, determined the courses of study and methods of teaching and management in present-day American public schools. Parents have the bread-and-butter objective mainly in view in planning the education of their children. This does not mean that they advise their children to pursue studies which will prepare them directly for earning money when they leave school or college, though some parents do give their children just such advice. When they come to the school to talk with teachers regarding the work of their children, it is evident that they want them to study "practical" things; this is not true of all parents, but it is probably true of a majority of them. At the same time, they may be willing that their children should complete a course in algebra, for instance, not because they think it will be of direct service to them in making their way in the world, but they believe it will discipline the mental faculties; and one can make an easier living with a disciplined than with an undisciplined mind. Probably not more than five parents in a hundred chosen at random would advise their children to study algebra and geometry, for instance, merely in order that they may understand these subjects and gain intellectual benefits from them, even though they cannot apply them practically or gain mental discipline from them which they can use in the practical

The Objectives Which Parents Have in View

situations of daily life. As a matter of fact, astronomy has but few followers in present-day American education, and algebra is losing some portion of its once large following, even in the universities; and one reason why these branches are not popular is because they seem to be detached from the practical needs of life. Other subjects are offered in high schools and universities that are but little patronized for the same reason that astronomy and algebra are neglected.

The studies that are most numerously and eagerly pursued are those that apparently have direct reference to some profitable vocation or profession, or that have the reputation of being good subjects for mental discipline. During the past decade, there has been a shifting of emphasis in respect to studies in secondary schools, colleges, and universities. The experience of the World War gave tremendous impetus to applied science and economic subjects; but just now students are drifting away from these studies and electing others in their place, according as they hear that there are good opportunities in one or another calling,—in teaching, for instance, or in journalism, or in certain commercial fields. In the high school there has been a continual drift away from the so-called cultural studies into applied science and commercial and vocational subjects.

If left to themselves, and not taking account of the question of difficulty of mastery, pupils would, as a rule, choose the studies that their parents favor. They think of studies principally as means for advancing their material welfare and improving their social status. Studies that they believe will help them to make the most money and enjoy the greatest social prestige are the studies they will choose, as a rule, though individual interests and emulation play a rôle in determining their choices. The value of a study because of the social distinction which it confers upon its votaries plays a more important part in the southern and eastern than in the northern and western parts of the country. Latin, for instance, is more generally regarded in the East and South as the subject of chief value in the curriculum than is true in the North and West. The study of Latin in most high schools and colleges in the South, and to a lesser extent in the East, distinguishes a pupil from his classmates and sets him above them in culture and mental acumen. It is considered that one who pursues this subject is not so much under the dominance of practical needs as one who studies vocational, commercial, agricultural, or even scientific subjects. The pupil who pursues Latin is likely to enjoy more leisure and so-called cultured life than one who pursues other subjects. In the South and East the studies that are looked upon by a considerable proportion of the people as of least merit are those that relate most directly to the earning of a livelihood, while this is not the case, as a rule, in either the high schools or the colleges of the northern and western sections of our country.

The typical parent in every section of the country would like to have his children pursue studies which would enable them to get along well with the people among whom they must spend their lives. Even the parent who has given very little attention to the matter recognizes that certain studies are "fashionable" and that everyone must have some knowledge of them in order to avoid criticism by his associates. The greater his knowledge of them, the more highly he will be regarded by his friends. History, literature, music, and art are, as a rule, the subjects that the layman regards as essential in order that his children may avoid the criticism and secure the admiration of those with whom they come in contact. In most sections of the country, an adult who could talk glibly about current topics in literature would be ranked as a superior person in culture and people

Studies That Aid in Social Adaptation

would pay him homage. Even practical minded people place high value upon the ability to enumerate names and dates in history and to converse easily about the characteristics of books that are regarded as "significant".

The typical parent does not regard it as important that his children should study subjects that would help them to understand human nature in its deeper aspects in order that they may adapt themselves harmoniously to people. Psychology and philosophy would not prosper in any secondary school unless they were presented so that they would relate directly to teaching, and then those who were preparing for the teaching profession would pursue them while all others would leave them untouched. In the colleges and universities psychology is quite popular, but this is because it is regarded as essential in preparation for several vocations and professions,—journalism, teaching, medicine, and law. Courses in psychology that are designed to give an understanding of human nature without reference to any practical application are not largely elected in the colleges or universities. In other words, while parents wish their children to study subjects which will be of value to them in their intercourse with people, still they have in view superficial rather than profound social adjustment. We have not yet grown out of the practice which Herbert Spencer condemned ninety years ago in England,— parents wish their children to be educated according to the customs and fashions of the times. This is not altogether a disadvantage so far as the welfare either of the individual or of society is concerned, since taken as a whole, people appreciate knowledge of substantial worth, and they praise the individual who possesses such knowledge more than one whose knowledge is purely spectacular so that it cannot be used for the betterment of the community in any way.

The typical parent places some but not supreme

value upon studies that free the mind of a child from fear and superstition, but which do not relate in any way, so far as he can see, to the child's social or material advancement. To refer to the subject of astronomy again: the typical parent does not think that it would be worth while for his child to master this subject in order that he might thereby solve intellectual problems and increase the range of his mental vision. It does not seem to most parents that intellectual needs arising out of the complexity of the world in which one lives are as vital as physical needs; it is not generally considered that mental hunger is as pressing or as important as physical hunger. Indeed, the typical parent, in laying out a course of study for his child, takes slight account of intellectual needs as distinct from physical or social needs. He does not think that there can be intellectual pain from lack of understanding of the laws that operate in one's environment, as there may be distressing physical pain due to lack of harmony with the physical environment. *Studies That Dispel Fear and Superstition*

Finally, the typical parent does not strongly urge his children to pursue studies that enable them to discriminate between the things that are aesthetically admirable and those that are commonplace or ugly. The majority of patrons of the schools can hardly be convinced that a child has aesthetic needs that are comparable with his physical needs in their urgency and importance. Most parents would not of their own accord provide studies for their children which would enable them to reconstruct their environments so as to increase aesthetic objects and eliminate ugly ones, or to create aesthetic things appealing either to the eye or to the ear. The introduction of such studies into the elementary and high schools has, generally speaking, been opposed by parents in the belief that they are merely "faddish" and "freakish" as compared with the studies that have direct bearing upon the earning of money or *Studies of an Aesthetic Character* meeting the demands of the environment socially.

From this brief review it may be inferred that the objectives in present-day American schools are not being determined solely by parents or by pupils. If they were we would now have quite different courses of study from those we actually have in all our schools. The courses would be much less complex and highly differentiated than they are. They would relate almost entirely either to making a living in a profession or a vocation, or to acquiring attainments which are thought to be essential in securing social prestige. But if parents are not determining the objectives in our schools, then who is determining them? Teachers and students of education primarily. They have led and are now leading the way. They are accomplishing this through investigations in laboratory and classroom and discussion at educational meetings and in educational journals. And there is one objective that is becoming fundamental in American education, and that is,—preparation for all the needs of actual life. And what are these needs, as they are being agreed upon to-day and made the basis of the work in every phase of our educational system from the kindergarten through the graduate school of the university? First of all they are *social*, including personal, civic, and political relations. The leaders who are most frequently mentioned to-day in American education are those who are teaching that the chief need in life is harmonious adjustment to the people among whom one lives. Our educational psychologists maintain that nature has so constituted a human being that when his fellows show him honor, good will, and friendship he will be happy. On the other hand, when they are hostile toward him, when he is conscious that they are against him and not with him, he will be downcast and unhappy. Nature has established this as a fundamental law of human nature in order that people will be incited to live in accord with the demands of their fellows. If men had been so constituted that they did not care what their fellows thought about them, human society as we know it would be impossible. In developing human society nature had to equip a human being with emotions so that the indifference, hostility, or condemnation of his fellows would give him the keenest possible pain, and lead him to avoid the kind of conduct that brings condemnation and practice the conduct that wins approval and friendship. A human being not constructed on this plan is abnormal or degenerate.

We see now why the chief purpose of the school in America is to make an individual social. It is to teach him so that he will understand how he must live in order to dwell in peace and harmony with his associates. The school must, it is true, prepare him to make a living in a purely physical sense, but this is not the chief business of life at all. It is probably the chief concern of crude, primitive people who live close to the earth and whose chief need is to get enough to eat and to be protected from the elements; but the chief needs of one living in America today are very different from those of a savage in the forest.

How is this conception affecting the work of the schools in our country? We are coming to believe that a pupil should, above everything else, be trained to be a social being. He must learn to read, to write, and to spell, so that he may participate in what his ancestors have achieved, and what his associates are now achieving, and so that he may communicate his experiences to them. This should be the guiding aim always in the teaching of reading, writing, and spelling. A pupil should study history in order that he may learn the course over which the race has come, and so that he may understand the conditions essential to the welfare of human society in the present. The learning of dates and names in history, unless they help a pupil to understand modern society and adapt himself to it, is considered to be useless. The pupil should study geography in order that he may be a citizen of the world, and not simply of the street or town in which he happens to live at the moment. He should learn that human society to-day is bound together very closely, and while people may be separated in space they are, or should be, very close together in spirit;—we are all members of one body, and the conduct of one individual has an influence upon all his fellows. The pupil should study literature as a concrete presentation of social conduct. He should see that coöperation and altruism yield pleasure and happiness in the end, while antipathy and selfishness are certain to yield pain and unhappiness.

Thus American educational practice is being determined by the view that while the physical needs in human life are primordial they are nevertheless not of primary importance, for the reason that we have learned how to provide for our physical needs without devoting most of our attention or most of our energy thereto. By means of inventions we are making petroleum, coal, water power, electric power, and the winds do most of the work necessary to provide food, clothing, and shelter, so that we may be physically comfortable. The majority of the people in American life to-day devote only a small part of their thought and energy in any one day to providing for their physical needs. They devote a great deal more time and energy to the effort to solve the problems, first, of securing the esteem, goodwill, respect, and confidence of their fellows; and, second, of organizing and conducting community, state, and national life so that every individual may to the fullest extent possible receive all the benefits that flow from coöperative living in highly developed groups. There should be no misunderstanding here; it is recognized in educational theory to-day that everyone has physical needs and that these should be provided for in our educational régime. There should be studies that relate to the securing of food, clothing, and shelter, and the protection of health, but these should not occupy the most important place in the curriculum, either in the elementary school, in the high school, or in the college. But rather the educational materials that are concerned with personal, civic, and political relations, that show how people can live together in small and in large groups so as best to promote the interests and well-being of all, are regarded as of chief importance, and they are coming to play, if they do not already play, the chief rôle in our courses of study.

Acceptance of the social as the main objective of work in our schools has not been easy for parents and laymen, for the reason that it seems to them more or less visionary to maintain that the social need in American life to-day is greater than the physical or any other need. But educational psychologists are showing that the largest part of one's thoughts and feelings relate to his social adjustments. Most of his pleasures and pains have their source in his social contacts. The unsuccessful and unhappy individual is the one who is ill-adapted to the people about him because of temperamental, moral, or aesthetic deficiencies, rather than the one who does not have enough food, clothing, or shelter. There may be a few of the latter in every community, but the number is insignificant when compared with the total number of persons in the community. Further, the most stable and prosperous nation is the one in which the people are best organized and best trained in group adjustment and coöperation, rather than the one that is most prolific in material resources.

There is another objective which teachers and students of education have been pressing forward, and they have succeeded in securing an important place for it in the elementary and high school, in the college, and in the university, and this is the intellectual objective—enlarging the range of one's mental vision, pushing back the boundaries of knowledge and understanding so that one may know how the world in which he lives is constructed and how it operates. Educational psychologists are showing that one who does not understand the laws of the world in which he lives will be a victim to a greater or less extent of superstition and fear. Therefore, say the leaders in educational thought, all pupils should pursue studies that interpret the laws of nature, even though the knowledge thus gained cannot be applied to increasing one's material well-being or social prestige. Take physics or botany, for instance. These subjects may not have for the typical pupil any material or social value of importance, but they may have tremendous intellectual value in helping him to understand the phenomena of the world in which he lives. Every normal person, so it is urged, will come in contact constantly with these phenomena, and for this reason his education should assist him to comprehend them and to discover the laws that govern them.

In arranging the program of the schools so that they will prepare for the needs of life, teachers and students of education are laying stress upon still another objective. It is maintained that the welfare of every normal person is determined largely by the aesthetic or unaesthetic character of the objects and sounds he encounters in daily life. He cannot remain neutral in his environment. He either is pleased or is distressed by the sights and sounds that play upon him; some of them exalt the tide of life—increase his strength and pleasure—while others lower the tide of life and detract from his comfort and happiness. The latter objects and situations we regard as ugly or unharmonious, while those that increase our delight and stability we regard as beautiful or harmonious. So American schools have, after considerable opposition from laymen and parents, introduced into the curriculum subjects that teach the child how he can eliminate or modify the objects and sounds about him that cause distress and increase those that give him pleasure because of their aesthetic qualities. Singing, playing on musical instruments, drawing, painting, designing, etc., have come to play an important rôle in American schools, though some persons still condemn them by calling them "fads" and "frills". But the educational psychologist has been analyzing the sources of happiness and of distress in human life, and he has reached the conclusion that one's well-being is determined in an important degree by the aesthetic character of the things upon which he looks and to which he listens.

Finally, it is urged by teachers and students of education, as well as by parents and laymen, that one's well-being will be determined in a large measure by his fitness to perform some definite task which contributes to the welfare of society as a whole or one of its subordinate groups. In other words, most individuals must be prepared to practice a profession or a vocation which renders service to society. So our schools are shaping their programs so that they can attain the general objectives which are of importance for all individuals —physical welfare, social adjustment, intellectual understanding, and aesthetic appreciation and creativeness; then the objective of vocational or professional skill must be attained. This is the program which schools throughout America have entered upon and are trying to perfect, and which will be considered in detail in later chapters. It is as true of schools in rural sections as of those in towns and cities, that they are seeking to construct courses of study and to adopt methods of teaching and management which will assist the young to attain these objectives.

In the early history of our country, the schools were not free; parents paid for the tuition of their children.

The Professional or Vocational Objective

Summary Free and compulsory education was established only after a long struggle. It was believed formerly that education was of value primarily to the individual who received it; but the idea gradually grew in the minds of our forefathers that every person who could read, write, and calculate according to the needs of daily life and who had learned something about religion and the founding of our government and the principles of freedom upon which it is maintained, would make a better citizen than one who could not read or write and so would have to depend upon others for information regarding the nature of our government and what is demanded of every individual in order that it should continue to be strong, stable, and prosperous. The belief has now become widespread in our country that education is essential for good citizenship and that the better educated a person is the better citizen he becomes. Very recently voices have been raised against this view, but they have not yet shaken the faith of our people in the need of free and compulsory education for the welfare of the nation.

The expenses of education have increased fourfold in our country during the past two decades, and just now there is vigorous debate as to whether we can continue to support so expensive an educational system. The question is being asked widely to-day,—How can we pay the mounting bills for education? Many people are answering this question by saying that we must choose between education on the one hand and various luxuries in which we indulge, such as tobacco, automobiles, gasoline, motion pictures, expensive clothing, cosmetics, jazz music, and the like, on the other hand.

The majority of parents unquestionably believe that a boy or girl who is well educated will get on more easily in life than one who is poorly educated, and so they keep their children in school. The typical parent probably does not keep his children in school primarily so that they may become better citizens. Some parents send their children to school so that they may secure mental discipline in the belief that this will help them to solve successfully the problems which may arise in their daily lives. But fortunately, the education that will be of greatest service to the individual in fitting him for the needs of daily life will be of greatest value also for the community. A well educated person is an asset to the community even though he may not serve it directly. His views, his conduct, and his attitude in dealing with social and intellectual problems will be of value to the community.

The objectives which parents have in view in sending their children to school are not in all cases the same as the objectives which superintendents, principals, and teachers have in view in determining courses of study and methods of teaching. Parents generally urge their children to pursue courses that have direct reference to some profitable vocation or that have the reputation of being good subjects for mental discipline. During the past decade there has been a marked shifting of emphasis in respect to studies in elementary schools and colleges, due to the fact that new commercial and professional opportunities have magnified the importance of commercial and professional subjects.

The typical parent would like to have his children become adjusted harmoniously to the people among whom they live, but he does not, as a rule, advise them to pursue subjects that would help them to understand human nature in its deeper aspects. Psychology and philosophy would not prosper in any secondary school; and the latter subject, at least, is declining in colleges. However, psychology in its applied aspects is increasing in popularity.

Parents usually wish their children to pursue studies which are fashionable so that they may gain in prestige in the community in which they live. The typical parent does not appreciate the value of studies that dispel fear and superstitition. He does not value highly studies that cultivate a child's aesthetic appreciation and that give him skill in modifying the objects in his environment with a view to increasing their aesthetic value. Parents have generally spoken of the introduction of aesthetic subjects into the schools as faddish and ephemeral.

The chief objectives in American schools are not being determined primarily by parents but rather by those who conduct the schools, who are teaching that the first aim of the school should be to help pupils to understand and to adapt themselves to the people about them in harmonious relations. So the chief objective in our schools now is social adaptation, which includes personal and civic relations. The curricula, methods, and discipline in our schools are being determined largely in view of this chief objective.

It is recognized in American schools that each individual has physical needs which should be taken account of in his education, but these needs are not primary; or at least they are not of chief consequence in contemporary American life. They should not be ignored, but they should not be exalted to first place in our educational system.

It is becoming universally agreed by educational people that the school should enlarge the pupil's understanding of the world in which he lives so that he will not suffer from fear or seek superstitious explanations of the phenomena occurring in his environment. It is also agreed that every pupil should have training which will enable him to increase the aesthetic objects in his environment and modify or eliminate the objects and situations that cause discord and disharmony.

Finally, we are aiming in our schools to train pupils for some vocation or profession in the belief that he who is prepared to pull his own oar when he leaves school will make the best citizen and will get most out of life himself.

XVIII

CHANGING COURSES OF STUDY

R EADERS of this volume whose memory of school work extends back over a period of twenty-five years, and who are also familiar with the changes that are taking place at the present time in the curricula of the elementary and the high school, undoubtedly ask occasionally (the present writer has often been asked these questions):

"Why should there be such constant change in the branches that are taught in the schools?"

"What is the necessity for incessantly shifting emphasis, now on one branch, now on another; now introducing a new study, and again eliminating or curtailing an older one?"

"Would it not be possible, and if possible would it not be desirable to agree upon the studies of greatest worth in education and then stick to them?"

"Are not American teachers and school boards fickle and faddish in their educational notions?"

"Is it feasible to give pupils a sound education when those who manage the schools and teach pupils do not know what materials of education are of lasting worth?"

"Is it not true that the present generation of children do not possess the power of prolonged concentration on mental tasks which was possessed by preceding generations?"

"Is it right that every person in a community who has a freak idea about the training of the young should have an opportunity to introduce it into the course of study?"

Educational people in European and Oriental countries

Questions
Concerning
Our
Changing
Curricula

373

are continually remarking upon the rapid changes taking place in the courses of study in American schools. The writer has heard men in a number of foreign countries condemn our educational system because of its lack of stability. They have said that we do not know our own minds; we take up a fad in education, ride it hard for a few years, and then abandon it for another fad. It is a comment very frequently heard in most foreign countries, that so many subjects are taught in American schools that nothing is thoroughly learned by pupils and they acquire the habit of incessantly jumping from one topic to another, with the result that most of them become scatterbrained as compared with pupils in European and Oriental schools, who study only two or three or, at the most, four subjects at a time. It is charged that we do not train our pupils to be students or scholars; we simply entertain them with a great variety of superficial knowledge.

Why Are Our Schools So Different From Most European and Oriental Schools? One reason for the difference between the courses of study in American as compared with European and Oriental schools is found in the fact that in our country society is plastic and mobile, while in foreign countries it is fixed and unchangeable for the most part. We have no barriers which prevent the members of one economic or social group from emerging out of their group and entering another one. A father does not pass on his vocation, profession, or social status to his son; the son may engage in an altogether different occupation from his father, and occupy a very different social and economic position. But this is not the case in European and Oriental countries; or at least it has not been so until the present moment. As a consequence of the World War, the countries of the Old World may regain plasticity and mobility; at the present writing there are indications that the old order is changing—it has broken up completely in at least one nation, and it threatens to break at any

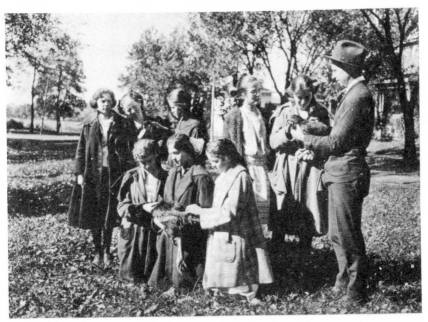

Learning to judge poultry in a rural school.

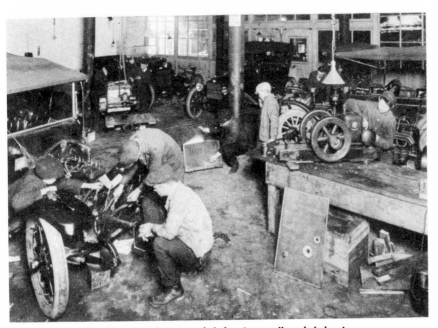

Pupils are taught to use their hands as well as their heads.

moment in other countries. But in most foreign countries society is still so non-plastic that social and political relationships do not change materially from one generation to another. An individual is born into a class or caste and is trained for his duties therein; and there is slight chance that he will shift from one class to another during his lifetime.

When there is hardly any change in social or political ideals or manner of life in a country from one generation to another, the training of the young in any one generation will consist in impressing upon them the ideals and practices of preceding generations. If a child is destined to become a member of the peasant class in a European or Oriental country, he will be trained therefor just about as his father, grandfather, great-grandfather, and on back for many generations were trained. There is no need to introduce anything very new into this system of education because there is little a child will have to do in his life that his ancestors did not have to do before him. It would disturb the social order if the members of the rising generation should be trained differently from the generations that preceded them. An American who keeps this fact in mind will not be surprised when he goes into a European or Oriental school to observe pupils pursuing practically the same course of study that had been pursued by their ancestors for centuries.

Just before the outbreak of the World War, the writer inspected Mohammedan schools in North Africa. Children were observed doing exactly the same kind of work and in just the same way as was done a thousand years ago, according to the records we have of early schools. The writer also inspected schools in a number of European countries, and he saw work going on in most of them that very closely resembled the description of school work given by writers several centuries ago. When asked why new studies embodying recent discoveries and extensions in our knowledge of man and nature and the development of the young were not introduced into the schools, teachers usually replied—"We think our children ought to study classical subjects—those that have permanent value and not the new and ephemeral subjects." And without exception teachers, and also laymen, when pushed for a justification of their narrow course of study— they did not themselves call it narrow—would say that the proper task of a school is to give children the rudiments of knowledge—mainly reading, writing, and numbers, to transmit to them the classical literature of the race, to discipline the mental faculties, and to develop good mental habits by difficult studies. According to this theory, two or three studies that rigorously discipline mental faculties are better than dozens of subjects that do not require severe application.

A Forward-Looking People Require a Different Curriculum From a Backward-Looking People

There is another principle which has played and still plays an important rôle in differentiating European and Oriental from American schools in respect to courses of study. We are living in the present more than in the past; we think more about what we are going to achieve in the future than about what our ancestors have achieved. Every day in our country we hear of new accomplishments in every field of thought and endeavor; and this has put us in a constantly expectant attitude. We anticipate that we will be better off to-morrow than we are to-day, because we will make improvements in every phase of our life. Since we are so well pleased with the present and are looking forward all the time for even better things in the future, we do not have a high regard, certainly not a reverence, for the achievements of the past. But it is exactly the reverse in many of the European and in all of the Oriental countries. The present and the future are of minor importance as compared with the past. This is not as true at the present moment of

Russia, England, and Germany as it was before the war, but it is still true in other countries. Nothing produced in the present is considered by these peoples to possess as great value as the products of the past. They look backward rather than forward, so they train their children on ancient rather than on modern knowledge. They do not like the term "modern", and they look with suspicion upon individuals who advise them to become modern. However, the World War lessened the confidence of some of the Old World peoples in the superior value of things ancient, and just now there is talk in certain of these countries of modernizing the course of study. These are the same peoples that have condemned the schools of America because they have given a larger place to modern than to ancient studies. They have believed that America was making a mistake in giving such prominence in all schools to studies that aim to interpret present-day life and train pupils to adjust themselves thereto.

It was said in Chapter XVII that American educators are seeking to develop courses of study for all our schools which will assist the young directly to understand the world in which they live and to adjust themselves effectively thereto—not simply the physical world but also the intellectual, social, and aesthetic world. The slogan of American teachers during the last few years has been—"The school must prepare for the needs of actual life." Thousands of men and women are devoting themselves to a study of the question,—What is meant by "actual life" to-day in our country, and what education does an individual need in order to meet the requirements of actual life? There is one phase of this investigation which has been carried forward in America farther and faster than in any other country, and it has played and is now playing the dominant rôle in modifying courses of study in all our schools. This investigation

The Slogan of American Teachers: "The School Must Prepare for The Needs of Actual Life."

is seeking to determine to what extent, if at all, any particular study can train mental faculties so that power will be developed which can be applied in all the situations of actual life. It was said in preceding paragraphs that the course of study in European and Oriental schools is based largely upon the doctrine that the proper function of the school is to discipline the faculties of the mind, and any subject that is well adapted to this purpose will be valuable, even though it has no direct reference to any need which will arise in daily life.

We Are Abandoning the Doctrine of Formal Mental Discipline in Our Schools

People who rely upon "common sense" for their knowledge of human nature generally hold the view that the mind is so constructed that if it is exercised in any way it will acquire a power or strength or ability which can be used in any way whatsoever, just as if a muscle is exercised in any specific way the strength developed can be utilized in a general way. Thus if a person goes into a gymnasium and by pulling weights develops his arm and back muscles, he can use the strength he has thus gained in any way he wishes—in pitching hay, in chopping wood, in boxing, in rowing, in milking cows, or in any other activity. Is this proposition true? It has been shown time and again that it is not true as stated. People are specialists in muscular activities. In the high schools, colleges, and universities an adult is not likely to be good in all branches of athletics. One who is excellent in rowing may be no good at all in boxing, wrestling, vaulting, sprinting, or in baseball, football, or gymnastics. People who have endurance in walking on level ground may lack endurance in climbing mountains. Men who can walk all day long in a furrow behind a plow usually tire quickly when they walk on a sidewalk in the city.

Illustrations might be multiplied *ad libitum* to show that muscular skill gained in a special activity is confined almost wholly to that special activity. One who has tremendous strength and endurance in a special activity may have to begin *de novo* to build up strength and endurance if he engages in a different activity. There is probably some slight general training derived from any vigorous muscular activity in the way of developing breathing power and stimulating vital organs so that they can respond to vigorous demands. So far as any special kind of muscular activity will increase breathing capacity and strengthen digestive, assimilative, and eliminative organs, it will have general value, because when the individual takes up a different kind of muscular activity he will make use of the breathing, digestive, assimilative, and eliminative functions.

The principle that specific exercise develops specific and not general skill, ability, and endurance, has occupied the attention of our educational psychologists and teachers for the last twenty or twenty-five years more than any other single question in psychology or education. Innumerable persons have discussed the problem, in addresses and in articles, and many investigators have studied it experimentally. For a quarter of a century, men and women have fought and bled over this doctrine of formal mental discipline. While European and Oriental psychologists and educators have, for the most part, endorsed the doctrine that mental exercise in any specific field develops general mental power, American psychologists and teachers maintain that it has been demonstrated experimentally that the doctrine is untrue, at least as it has been utilized in determining the relative values of studies in the schools. Twenty-five years ago, it was generally maintained, alike by teachers and by laymen, that the studies of greatest value for all pupils were arithmetic and grammar, because these subjects more than any others developed the reasoning powers. Spelling was considered valuable partly because it developed memory. Of course, every teacher and probably every layman believed that the rudiments of reading, writing, spelling, and numbers had to be mastered by all children in order that they might get on in daily life; but a considerable part of each of these "tools of knowledge" was taught because it was deemed to be valuable for mental discipline, even if it were not of practical service in actual life. But the educational psychologists, and the teachers of an analytical and inquisitive turn of mind, who have been observing and investigating this matter for the last two decades, have reached the conclusion that it is wasteful and unjustifiable to teach any subject merely because of its theoretical value in disciplining the faculties of the mind. If a subject or topic will not function in any of the situations in which one will be placed in actual life, it will have slight value in his education, and it ought to give way to some other subject or topic that will be related directly to his physical, intellectual, social, or aesthetic needs.

The Doctrine of Formal Discipline is Still Believed by Some

It would require many volumes the size of this one to present a résumé of the discussions and investigations of the doctrine of formal discipline; and the debate is not yet concluded. Some persons, laymen particularly, though a few college presidents and professors should be included, still believe in the doctrine and try to base our courses of study on it. Speaking generally, but allowing for exceptions, the teachers of the classics and, to a lesser extent, the teachers of mathematics hold that a study is valuable just in the measure that it disciplines mental faculties, and not in the measure that it can be utilized directly in any of the experiences of daily life. Some of the teachers of English grammar hold the same view. The present writer has recently heard teachers of arithmetic complain because of the way in which the subject is being curtailed by the elimination of tables and measures and processes that are believed by those who have rejected the doctrine of formal discipline to be of slight value in actual life to-day. Some teachers maintain that even if the tables of stone or lumber measure, or cube root, or partial payments will not be used by one out of a thousand children who are now in the schools, nevertheless these matters should be studied because of the mental power which they develop.

The educational psychologists and the more "radical" teachers maintain that this is an illusion, and they demand that these topics, and others like them, should be deleted from the arithmetic required of all pupils. They point to experiments which have been made which show that pupils who have learned to reason in arithmetic may not be able on this account alone to reason much, if any better in grammar, logic, ethics, psychology, or in any of the practical situations of daily life. Further, they call attention to the fact that persons who have devoted many years to reasoning in mathematics or in languages or in mechanics, or in any other special field, may be quite incapable of sound reasoning in any department but the special one in which they have had special training. A grammarian, for instance, if he has had no training in economics, may reason very feebly and inaccurately in this latter field. The ability to reason is a specific and not a general ability. Indeed, persons who have been put through elaborate formal training in the elementary and high school and in college are often entirely incapable of dealing with the complicated problems that arise in connection with the work of a board of education, a board of health, a common council, a governor's office, a kitchen, or a nursery. It has frequently been noted by observers that some of the most conspicuous failures in the training of children are persons who have completed long courses of study based on the doctrine of formal discipline.

So in respect to the practice of attempting to train memory through the spelling of long lists of words that

But it Has Been Shown to be Fallacious

are not used in actual life,—it has been shown by investigators that the kind of memory trained by learning to spell words orally is of little or no service in the situations in which people are placed in daily life. It is not even of much service in spelling, because people who can spell a bookful of words orally often make blunders when they write these words in a letter or in an article. Memory is specific in its functioning. It may work well in the special way in which it has been trained but not in other ways. An experienced ticket agent may be able to remember details about fares and time-tables to a phenomenal extent, but he may not be able to remember people's names, or any facts of history, literature, or economics any better than, and often not as well as, a person who cannot remember very much about fares or time-tables.

The writer has colleagues whose memory for historical facts, or botanical facts, or mathematical facts, or psychological facts, is extraordinary, but outside their special fields their memory is very ordinary. One man has a marvelous memory for legal facts, including details of cases and decisions of courts and judges, but he often forgets the names of his friends, and he hardly ever remembers to go to his meals on time. He says he has forgotten all the mathematics he ever learned, even some parts of the multiplication tables. He has a wonderful memory for all details that belong to his profession, but he has a treacherous memory for other things. Every normal mind operates on this plan. This is why people who are in touch with the results of investigations say that it is wasteful to teach pupils ten thousand words, most of which they will never use in daily life, merely to discipline their memory.

So, while the problem of the extent to which mental activity in any specific field will develop power that can be utilized in different fields is still under investigation, nevertheless the question is practically settled so far as it affects educational procedure in most of our schools. During the past decade, educational psychologists, superintendents, principals, and teachers throughout the country have been examining all the studies in the elementary and high school with a view to selecting subjects and topics that relate quite directly to the needs of actual life and disregarding others. Topics and subjects that have been retained in courses of study merely for the purpose of training mental faculties have been marked for deletion. There is greater activity at the present moment in this than in any other phase of educational investigation and discussion in America. Already there is general agreement regarding many of the subjects and topics that should be taught in the schools, and agreement also regarding certain subjects and topics that have been taught heretofore but that have ceased to be of value and so they ought to be eliminated. It is impossible now to stop the movement in American schools to reconstruct courses of study on the basis of direct usefulness in actual life, although there are voices raised against this desecration of curricula, as they regard the matter.

Reconstructing Traditional Studies

The abandonment of the doctrine of formal discipline and the whole-hearted adoption by most educational psychologists and educators of the principle that the schools of whatever grade should teach pupils knowledge and skill that will be of service to them in daily life will explain what is happening to our courses of study, which so perplexes European and Oriental visitors to our country, and which is mystifying even to some of our own people. New subjects and topics relating to health, economics, citizenship, thrift, science, household arts, industry, agriculture, relations of capital and labor, music, art, etc., are being incorporated into the courses of study of the elementary and high schools, as well as the

Some Illustrations of What is Happening to Traditional Studies

colleges and universities. Traditional subjects, such as spelling, are being severely pruned. Twenty-five years ago pupils learned to spell from ten to fifteen thousand words; but as a result of investigations carried on during the past two decades, it has been found that the typical graduate of a high school does not need in his school work, and will not need in later life, to spell more than three thousand words at the outside, unless he engages in some technical pursuit, when it may be necessary for him to master a special and technical vocabulary. The typical American in his correspondence and in his writing for the newspapers rarely employs more than fifteen hundred different words; many of us never use more than half this number. In view of these facts, the course in spelling in the schools to-day is being constructed on the principle that the words that will be actually used in daily life should be mastered so that they can be spelled automatically, and the technical and unusual words that were formerly taught but that will probably never be used are being eliminated. Not a single word is being retained in present-day spelling courses on the theory that it will be valuable in the training of memory.

A quarter of a century ago, in the elementary school several years were devoted to the study of technical English grammar. But recent investigations have shown that many of the constructions which have been taught are never employed in daily life by the typical American. At the same time, some of the most frequently used grammatical constructions are most frequently violated. The appreciation of these facts is leading to a complete reconstruction of the course in grammar. Pupils are being taught to use correctly the constructions which they employ in ordinary speech and writing. These are presented in a great variety of linguistic situations so that by continued use in all the ways in which they will be employed later on, the pupil acquires the ability to use them correctly in an automatic manner. Before he leaves the elementary school he learns the parts of speech so that he knows their names and can recognize them, and he learns also the principles governing their proper use in sentences, and especially the kinds of sentences that he is likely to use in daily life. Farther than this he does not go in the study of English grammar. The time a pupil saves in curtailing this subject is devoted to the more thorough mastery of language as it is used in daily life, and also to gaining knowledge and skill in other fields which will help him to understand the world in which he lives and to reconstruct it so as to promote his well-being.

The elimination of topics in arithmetic has already been referred to. The only additional word needing to be said here is that no subject in the curriculum is being analyzed and overhauled more thoroughly than this one, which for generations has occupied the place of prestige in the course of study in the elementary school. Our educational psychologists and teachers see nothing about arithmetic that should entitle it to exceptional favors in the course of study. The reasoning power developed by arithmetic can be utilized in arithmetical situations only; but to-day these situations do not constitute a very large or the most important part of the life of the typical American. There are other kinds of situations concerned with political, social, ethical, moral, hygienic, domestic, artistic, and other relations and activities that play a more vital rôle than arithmetical situations do. The latter cannot be neglected, but they ought not to be over-emphasized in a course of study, and the appreciation of these facts is at the bottom of the thorough pruning which the subject is now undergoing and will continue to undergo during the next few years.

Space will not permit us to go through with every subject taught in schools for the purpose of showing what is happening to it, either by way of extending it because it is thought to be of increasing importance, or pruning it because it is believed to be of decreasing importance in actual life. It is enough to say that all curricula are being scrutinized with a view to deleting what has persisted in them on the supposition that it is valuable for the discipline of mental faculties; and also with a view to emphasizing topics that have been gaining in importance because of changes in American life or because of the development of new knowledge in various fields.

It should be added that no topic is likely to be retained in any subject merely because it is ancient. If it is of service in present-day life it will continue to enjoy a place in the curriculum; but age alone will not insure its retention. In this respect our American schools are distinguished from European and Oriental schools, in which age is one factor in determining the value of any topic or study. In these latter schools a person is not regarded as educated, or at least not cultured, unless he has amassed a considerable body of knowledge of ancient flavor. But in our country we are rapidly coming to the view that culture does not depend upon the mere possession of facts, whether ancient or modern. The cultured individual is one who has acquired knowledge and skill which make him of service to society, and habits of conduct which make him agreeable in association with his fellows. Knowledge which does not function in the life of the individual in his relations with others, to-day is not regarded by American teachers as of value for culture any more than for disciplinary purposes. The knowledge that will confer the greatest amount of culture upon the child is that which will enable him to interpret the nature and needs of the people among whom he lives, and to adjust himself to them in harmonious relations.

It should be acknowledged that there is at the present

moment a good deal of debate and even conflict between the friends of vocational education on the one hand, and cultural education on the other. It is recognized that vocational education is going forward throughout the country with great momentum. There is no stopping it, even if any individual or any group of individuals should wish to do so. Those who are directing the movement know quite definitely what they want, and they are proving that they understand how to secure it. This does not mean that every question concerning the character of vocational education is settled to the satisfaction of all its votaries; as a matter of fact, there is still difference of opinion expressed in vocational conferences respecting the balance which should be preserved between cultural training on the one side, and specific preparation for a particular vocation on the other. There are those, both within and without vocational education circles, who maintain that in the public schools boys and girls should pursue cultural subjects and master the *principles* underlying a vocation rather than to acquire the mechanical skill necessary to practice any vocation. Others hold the contrary view.

In some States vocational education is administered by boards created for the special purpose in various communities, while in other States all education, cultural and vocational, is put in charge of one and the same board—the board of education. In these latter States it is maintained that vocational training should be regarded simply as a phase of general education, while in other States it is believed by the votaries of vocational education that it can receive proper recognition and emphasis only when it is detached from cultural education and administered by boards that have a high respect for it, and that will see to it that the training is definite and specific. As a consequence of this distinction between vocational and cultural education, the former is more clearly defined,

Vocational vs. Cultural Education

387

is more definite and specific in States like Wisconsin, where it is in charge of special boards, than it is in some States which the writer has visited.

Courses of Study for Girls Should girls study the same subjects as boys throughout the elementary and high school? Many persons in our country are asking this question now. For the purpose of bringing the question before us, a portion of a letter written recently may be quoted here. The writer says that much of the strain and stress in our day arises from the fact that girls are educated away from the life they ought to live. He continues:

"I can cite my own household as an illustration. Mrs. M. completed a high school course and two years in a college. She never studied one thing that related to keeping a house. I am able to pay for a servant, but we seem to be unable to keep help very long. Whenever we are without help Mrs. M. prepares a meal or two and we take the rest out. But a half hour in the kitchen will put her into a frame of mind from which she does not recover during the rest of the day. But when the woman's club has some kind of doings she will work there all day and not be exhausted at all. The fact is, anything in the house gets on her nerves and she makes life a little disagreeable for all the family, but she can do anything outside with pleasure and without exhaustion. All her education really separated her from household duties, and now she detests the work. So, as a matter of fact, while I can pay the bills for a decent and comfortable home, we do not have such a one. There are other homes in this city just like mine."

One can hear many educational people saying about the same things now about the education of girls that Mr. M. says. Everywhere there is growing dissatisfaction with the "old-fashioned," conventional method of educating girls, and already important modifications are under way. In many places to-day, a girl in school has better opportunities for a useful education than Mrs. M. had when she was a pupil. Most up-to-date towns and cities have well-arranged courses relating to the making of a home, and all girl pupils are required to complete some of this work. In many high schools, girls may elect various studies in home making in the place of mathematics, physics, etc.

It is true that there are still sections of our country in which it is thought that girls should pursue only so-called cultural and disciplinary subjects. The present writer has heard it said a great many times that a girl has the same mind as a boy, and she should have it trained in the same manner. Some women's colleges still base their courses on this doctrine more than do the high schools or the elementary schools. The women's colleges, speaking generally but allowing for a few exceptions, have lagged behind other educational institutions in adapting their work to the requirements of present-day life. They have operated in the past— and some of them are still operating—on the belief that education means acquiring learning which cannot be applied in any way to the situations of actual life.

A suggestive illustration may be drawn from the educational aspirations of the negro. Those who are directing negro education, in the South particularly, have to fight constantly against the desire of the negro to study Latin, algebra, and other subjects which are regarded as "cultural" and "disciplinary" but not practical. The negro has reasoned thus: "In order to be a real aristocrat, I must study the things which the aristocrats study. Their studies have no practical application. If I should study agriculture, engineering, or household arts, I would have to work with my muscles, and so I would not be admitted to real society. Quality folks never work with their hands. They do not do any work at all. They are just polished, and Latin and

"Cultural," Not Practical Studies

algebra will put on a polish better than anything else."
Men like Booker T. Washington have had to spend
much of their energy in combating this naïve, absurd
educational philosophy. Somewhat of the same philosophy in principle has been and is now being followed
by some of the girls' schools and colleges.

Household
Arts On a
Scientific
Basis There is a vigorous movement in the public schools to
put all the work of home making on a scientific and
dignified basis. There are junior and senior high schools
throughout the country that are beginning to train girls
so that they will gain as much pleasure from home work
as they will gain from getting up a church supper or
attending a club meeting. The girl who looks upon the
kitchen as a laboratory; who understand the chemical,
bacteriological, and physiological principles which are
involved in all that takes place there, and who regards
cookery and whatever goes with it as a fine art, will not
be "all done up" when she spends an hour or two in
the kitchen, and she will not feel that she is doing menial
things then she gives attention to the sanitation,
decoration, etc., of her home.

It is the woman who has been brought up to regard
everything in the home as commonplace drudgery, fit
only for servants, who chafes when she is called upon to
perform any of the work herself. She is the one who fills
the house with complaining and who says, "I am not
going to be the servant of this family. I am nothing but
a drudge for the rest of you." At the same time, every
member of the family may be doing his or her work;
but women like Mrs. M. consider that any work connected
with the house is drudgery, and anything outside of it is
recreation.

The
Testimony
of Women
Regarding
the
Education
of Girls With a view to obtaining information regarding the
benefits which women believe they have derived from
different educational programs, the present writer, with
the coöperation of the United States Bureau of Education

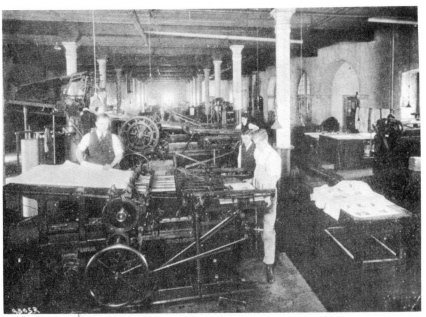

In some places pupils set up and print the publications and circulars issued by the Schools and the Board of Education.

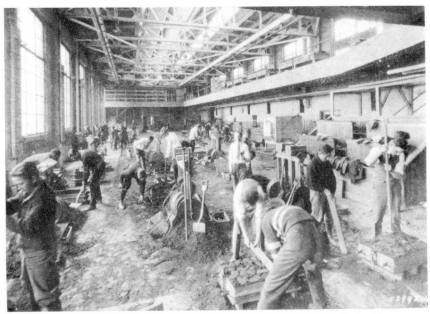

In an earlier day work like this would have been out of place in a school. Now it is regarded as a necessary part of a program.

and fourteen important colleges and universities, has secured testimonies from a large number of women who have had time and occasion to put their secondary and higher education to the test. There was prepared a list of five thousand college and university graduates of at least five years' standing, (there were representatives in every class from 1898 to 1915), so that they had had an opportunity to determine to what extent their education had proved to be of service in meeting the needs of actual life. In making up this list it was decided to secure an equal number from co-educational and from non-co-educational colleges, as follows: Northwestern, Bryn Mawr, Minnesota, Radcliffe, Illinois, Wellesly, Wisconsin, Goucher, Ohio, Smith, Colby, Chicago, Simmons, and Iowa.

A letter was sent to each of these five thousand graduates asking for information regarding the studies pursued in high school and college and for an expression of opinion, supported by concrete data, respecting the value of each study as tested by the needs of life. Each graduate was asked whether if she were now beginning her high school or college course, she would, in the light of her present knowledge, and if she were granted freedom of choice, elect the same subjects that she pursued originally. She was asked, further, whether she would advise a daughter to complete the same course of study that she completed in high school and college, and if not, what modifications she would suggest, and why.

Value of Each Study as Tested by Needs of Life

The women were asked to state their occupations. The occupations that were most numerously represented were, first, *teacher;* next, *home maker;* next, *mother.* Then in order—librarian, social worker, secretary, accountant, dean of women, business woman, writer, editor, clinician, pharmacist, Red Cross worker, artist, principal of schools, deaconess, lawyer, nurse, farmer, Y. W. C. A. worker.

The teachers, taken as a whole, are quite well satisfied

with the education they received in high school and college, although there is an occasional note of dissatisfaction because certain subjects were not taught so that they could be used in the practical situations of daily life. The home makers, mothers, and social workers are, with very few exceptions, discontented with their education. Only four of the home makers and mothers would elect the same course of study that they originally pursued if they had an opportunity to go over their high-school and college course again, because they failed to receive much help in solving the particular problems with which they have had to deal every day since they became home makers and mothers. The severest condemnation of the educational program was made by those who signed themselves as *mothers*. Very few of them had an opportunity to study subjects in either high school or college that pertained to the nature or training of children, and now they have to care for children and train them. They do not want their daughters to go through the same régime that they were compelled to pursue. They do not wish to have their daughters pursue studies that relate only to the care and training of children or to home making, but they would like to have them devote some time to these matters while they are in high school and college.

Lack of Courses in Home Making and Motherhood   It is worthy of special mention that graduates of colleges for women complain more generally of the lack of opportunities to pursue courses relating to home making and motherhood than do the graduates of co-educational universities. As a matter of fact, some of the women's colleges make only slight provision for studies which relate to home making in any of its aspects. The larger co-educational universities have departments or colleges of household arts in which there are courses that relate to every phase of home making, including the nature and training of children, and the girl students in these universities are electing such courses in constantly increasing numbers.

The greatest dissatisfaction with the training in high school and college is expressed by the oldest graduates, as is reflected in the following typical letters written by women who graduated fifteen or twenty years ago:

"I had no training that related specifically to home **Typical** making which I think I should have had. I graduated **Cases** before home economics was taught at........ Since two out of three women marry, I think home making as a profession should have consideration in the education of all girls."

"I regret that in neither high school nor college did I have an opportunity to take domestic science. I think all girls need training in the lines that the majority of women will either follow or direct. They need training in the consideration of community problems and oh, how I do wish that they would get some training that would teach them suitable dress. Our small high schools need more work in physical training for all, not just basketball for the one who likes it."

"My college education did not sufficiently equip me to become what I now am—the manager of a house and the mother of children. Having a trained mind has perhaps helped me to do my work and train my children more intelligently than some could have done these things, but I have always deeply felt the lack of practical knowledge of things pertaining to my special problems."

The curricula in our schools have changed greatly **Summary** during the past two decades. There has been such a rapid change that visitors from foreign countries think we are educationally unstable and are drifting with the tide. Changes in courses of studies are much more rapid and profound in our country than in any European or Oriental country.

The chief reason why our courses of study change more

rapidly than they do in other countries is because our educational system is plastic and mobile as compared with systems in foreign countries. In our social and political ideals and practices and in our manner of life we change very rapidly and profoundly as compared with people in foreign countries. The changes in education are not more rapid than they are in other aspects of our life.

A forward-looking people require constant changes in their social, political, and educational régime. It is inevitable that our courses of study should be modified so long as our people are going forward in all aspects and all phases of social, political, and industrial life.

A slogan of our teachers for the past two decades has been: "The School Must Prepare for the Needs of Life." Thousands of men and women are devoting themselves to a study of the question of what is covered by "the needs of life."

Chief Reason for Modification One of the chief reasons for the modification of our courses of study has been our abandonment of the doctrine of formal discipline. According to this doctrine, those studies are of greatest value that strengthen or sharpen the faculties of the mind even though the subjects themselves have no relation to any of the needs of life. When our curriculum was planned originally, it was believed that specific studies developed general mental ability, but our educational psychologists have shown that this is an erroneous doctrine and we no longer have faith in it, speaking generally.

Originally, certain studies were given a place of distinction in our courses of study in all our schools and colleges because it was thought that they developed reasoning power; other studies were given a prominent place because they trained memory; still others because they developed imagination. A movement is going forward now to eliminate from all courses of study all subjects and topics that have retained a place in the curriculum simply because they were supposed to be valuable for the training of perception, reason, memory, or imagination.

Traditional studies are being modified greatly with a view to retaining only the topics that appear to relate directly to the needs of contemporary life. Arithmetic, grammar, spelling, geography, Latin, and so on, are undergoing profound modification from this standpoint.

There is vigorous debate taking place between the advocates of cultural and the advocates of vocational education. The former maintain that the latter are seeking to abolish cultural training from the schools, but the latter maintain that all subjects can be taught so as to confer culture, and that no subject which is taught specifically for cultural purposes can yield culture in the highest degree. *Cultural vs Vocational Education*

During the past two decades the education of girls has received particular attention. Originally girls were trained in the same way as boys, but there has recently been vigorous protest against this program. It is now being maintained that girls should have opportunity to study household arts instead of, or at least as well as, subjects like algebra, geometry, Latin, etc. In many places all girls are now required to pursue subjects in the elementary and in the high school relating to home making. The testimony of women who have graduated from college regarding the education of girls shows that they believe that all girls should have training relating to homemaking as well as general training which will fit them for life outside of the home.

XIX

CHANGING METHODS OF TEACHING AND MANAGEMENT

What the
Critics of
Our Schools
Think of the
Newer
Methods

IT IS safe to say that there are readers who are in doubt concerning the wisdom of the changes they see taking place in the schools in the methods of teaching and of managing pupils. Quite often one reads articles in magazines and newspapers sharply criticizing the schools for their laxity and softness in the methods of teaching and of managing children. The present writer hears laymen say frequently, and teachers occasionally, that we are losing control of our pupils and that they are not learning to apply themselves diligently and continuously to their mental tasks. Laymen visit the schools and see pupils constantly in action. When they were in school themselves they sat in their seats and learned their lessons; but now pupils are out of their seats as much as they are in them while they are in the classroom. They are on their feet and are using their muscles in the performance of their tasks, and visitors frequently ask: "How is it possible for pupils to develop their minds properly unless they use their brains instead of their hands?" The writer recently received a letter from one critic of the newer methods who had been visiting the school attended by his two children, and the complaint he makes is often made by parents and laymen. He says:

"The children in the rooms I visited did not seem as quiet or did not apply themselves as thoroughly to their lessons as we children were required to do when I was in school, and I cannot see the reason for the way in which the pupils do some of their work. They seem to spend their time handling things instead of learning about them. It looks to me as though they are wasting their time. Certainly it would be better for them to learn the tables and then use them in solving problems instead of taking so much time to fool with the things themselves. I spent two hours in this school in order to see what sort of work my children are doing, and during the whole of those two hours the pupils moved about the room without asking the teacher, and I saw some instances in which a child went and sat with another one and they worked together. In their recitations the pupils sometimes talked directly to one another as though there were no teacher present. Now I don't believe that this is the best way to carry on school work. It is certainly very different from the way in which I had my schooling."

Visitors from European countries cannot understand why there is so much activity all the time in the typical American classroom. Compared with a European or Oriental school, an American school is unorganized, noisy, and even disorderly. In a classroom in a foreign country, speaking generally, pupils sit in their seats while they are preparing their lessons; they are forbidden to have any communication with their classmates; they cannot leave their seats without first securing the permission of the teacher. Their work largely consists in memorizing the lessons assigned them. For the most part, their plan of study consists in going over and over a lesson until they have fixed it so that they can reproduce it without error. They learn rules and formulæ by heart and then apply them to imaginary problems in their text books. In due course they are summoned to the teacher to recite on what they have learned and they make an effort to reproduce everything they have memorized.

What Foreigners Think of Our Methods

In brief, methods of teaching in most foreign countries consist principally in requiring pupils to learn verbatim certain facts, rules, and formulæ, and then apply them to problems found in the textbook. They must show to the teacher that they have memorized thoroughly what was assigned to be learned, and have applied the rules and formulæ accurately. Methods of management consist almost entirely in compelling pupils to be quiet and not to have any communication with classmates, so that everyone in the classroom may devote himself without distraction to the work in hand.

The American Slogan— Learn to Do by Doing American teachers, taken as a whole, have for the past few years been trying to base their methods of teaching upon the psychological principle that a child learns by doing rather than by memorizing exclusively. This principle was not discovered by American psychologists and teachers; the classic educational writers from Aristotle down to Herbert Spencer have emphasized the importance of *doing* for effective learning, and have condemned the practice of appealing to memory chiefly in teaching the young. Aristotle, in discussing the teaching of music, contended that in order to understand and appreciate it, the learner must actually *execute* it; without the latter, the former will be impossible.

Says Comenius: "The objects themselves, or, where this is not possible, such representations of them as can be conveyed by copies, models, and pictures, must be studied. In the case of the languages, arts, morality, and piety, impression must be insured by expression. 'What has to be done, must be learned by doing.' Reading, writing, and singing are to be acquired by practice. The use of foreign languages affords a better means of learning them than do the rules of grammar. Practice, good example, and sympathetic guidance teach us virtue better than do precepts."

Pestalozzi protested against the practice in his day of requiring pupils to learn the contents of books. He says: "I believe that the first development of thought in the child is very much disturbed by a wordy system of teaching, which is not adapted either to his faculties or the circumstances of his life. According to my experience, success depends upon whether what is taught to children commends itself to them as true through being closely connected with their own observation. As a general rule, I attached little importance to the study of words, even when explanations of the ideas they represented were given."

Milton, though a linguist himself, advised against the emphasis that was placed upon linguistic study in the schools of his time. Among other criticisms of the methods of the schools, he says that, "Though a linguist should pride himself to have all the tongues that Babel cleft the world into, yet if he have not studied the solid things in them as well as the words and lexicons, he were nothing so much to be esteemed as any yeoman or tradesman competently wise in his mother dialect only."

But even in the face of the severe condemnation of mere verbal learning which was uttered by Comenius, Locke, Rousseau, Bacon, Pestalozzi, Herbart, Herbert Spencer, and many others, memorization has continued to play the chief rôle in the schoolrooms of most foreign countries, and of our own country until very recently. In such schools the pupil as a learner means the pupil as a *memorizer;* and the teacher is a hearer of recitations for the purpose of ascertaining whether pupils have fixed their lessons in memory so that they can recall them without error, and have correctly applied rules and formulæ to imaginary situations presented in the textbooks. Laymen who visit such schoolrooms are likely to approve them because of the quiet which prevails in them and also because of the apparent diligence of pupils who are busy conning over their tasks so that they can be recited exactly as they are given in the text books.

But during the past few years, educational psychologists in America have been presenting the results

The Persistence of Mere Memory Work

of experimental studies showing that a pupil may be able to recite a rule correctly and apply it accurately to a textbook problem, but that at the same time he may not be able to apply it to an actual problem as he has to deal with it in daily life. Special investigation, as well as observation and experience, have shown that mere word knowledge may not, and for that matter usually does not, give understanding of actual, concrete situations unless a pupil has translated his rules and formulæ into concrete terms and used them in solving actual problems. A pupil may learn all the rules in the textbook regarding banking (as an instance), so that he can recite them accurately; but if he has not employed his rules in actual banking procedure by performing the processes described by the rules, he may be about as ignorant of banking as he was before he learned his rules. And what is true in respect to banking is true of every other process in arithmetic or of any other subject for that matter.

Readers of this volume can easily make observations that illustrate this psychological and educational principle. If any reader's children attend a school in which the work is of the verbal type,—the learning of facts, rules, and formulæ in text books and reciting them for the purpose of revealing whether they have been memorized accurately,—he can test his children when they come home to see in how far they can apply in actual, concrete situations what they have learned in school. Parents often complain that their children do not make any use in the home or outside of what they are learning in school; and yet these same parents sometimes approve methods of teaching which require pupils to memorize verbal knowledge without actually performing the actions to which the knowledge relates.

During the past few years, a new term has been introduced into educational literature in our country, and it suggests what we are striving to attain in our methods of teaching. This is the term *dynamic*, which is contrasted with the term *static;* the former refers to the kind of teaching which requires pupils actually to *do* what they are learning. If, for instance, they are learning linear measurement, they must use the units—inches, feet, yards, rods—in actual measurements, and in this way they will learn the value of each unit and the relations between the several units. In concluding their study of the units of linear measurement they construct a table and memorize it, but this is the last and not the first step in the mastery of the subject. And so with every table in arithmetic; it is constructed only after pupils have had experience in actually *using* the units of the table. They cannot understand the relations of the various units in any measurement until they discover by actual trial how many of one unit are required to make each of the other units. This is the type of work that the father, whose letter was quoted in the second paragraph of this chapter, complains about because the pupils seem to be "fooling" with the measures when they ought to be memorizing the tables and applying them to imaginary problems in the textbook. This parent would approve the *static* method of teaching whereby pupils would never handle any object or perform any process they were studying.

American Education is Becoming Dynamic

Any adult ought to know that he cannot master a new object or process merely by learning rules concerning it; one always wants to handle new objects or try out new actions before he is satisfied that he understands them. While most adults appreciate this principle so far as their own need is concerned, still they frequently fail to interpret a child's need as of the same character and urgency as their own. Whenever a normal adult comes in contact with a wholly new situation he tries to experiment with it or test it in some way so that he can gain an understanding of it in terms of what he can do with it, or how it is composed, or what it can do to him; but when a child does the same with a new object or situation which he encounters, he is thought by some to be wasting his time or merely "fooling" with things that he ought to learn about in his textbook.

How Words Gain Meaning or Content Words are merely *symbols;* they have no meaning for a learner unless they are embodied in concrete experience. Our early ancestors who developed words had the experiences first which they denoted; the words came after vital, concrete contact with the objects, situations, and phenomena to which they referred. But in teaching children according to the static method, which was universal in our own schools in an earlier day and which is still almost universal in foreign schools, words are learned ahead of the experiences which they denote on the theory that a novice can appreciate the experiences of those who developed words merely by memorizing the words. This is the great illusion in education which educational psychologists and teachers in America are trying to dispel from the schoolroom. All of the changes that are taking place in the methods of teaching in our schools are based on the principle that children can gain real knowledge that will be of service to them only by concrete experience in manipulating the objects and performing the processes they are learning. To comprehend adequately the characteristics of any occupation or activity, one must actually reproduce the movements and adjustments of that activity or occupation. Merely to read about the work of the blacksmith or carpenter or farmer, or even to look at them while they are busy in their several ways, or to listen to them describe their daily round of duties, will yield at best only vague and blurred outlines of their functions; but when a pupil cultivates a garden or makes a hand sled or fashions into desired shape a piece of iron—these and other like tasks that the young take delight in performing will serve best to give real and accurate knowledge of these activities. In our country, in all our teaching, we are going over completely onto this dynamic principle. The present writer has discussed this matter in his book *Mental Development and Education*, and a few paragraphs from that book are here reproduced: "In the modern kindergarten, for example, the pupil devotes much of his time to constructive activities that are planned to meet his every-day needs. A well-conducted kindergarten is a place of testing, of experimenting, of constructing, of practicing in play the serious enterprises of later life. The pupil does not spend his time simply memorizing the names of things; he works with the things themselves. He may not be able to read or write the words *clay, hammer, knife, flower,* and so on, but it is planned that he should come to *know* these things by *working with them* directly. Again, the cordial welcome which our people have given the Montessori methods indicates that we appreciate a system of teaching and training based on the dynamic nature and needs of the young.

"In the *'Houses of Childhood'* the children are always *doing;* they are not required to sit in seats and memorize words. They are engaged in buttoning and lacing frames, performing such acts as they need to perform in buttoning and unbuttoning their own clothes, and in lacing and unlacing their shoes. They build towers with blocks of varying sizes. They match colored spools. They use their fingers to trace letters or geometrical figures, or to measure distances. They employ their muscles to estimate the relative weight of different objects. They are blindfolded and then fit geometrical inserts into their proper forms; in this way they must discover through feeling the characteristics and relations of different forms. They learn to read in part by constructing words from letters cut out of cardboard. They learn to write by tracing words on the sand, the floor, or on the blackboard.

The Dynamic Principle Illustrated in the Montessori Schools

"The Montessori system is based on the principle that the child can learn only through sense activity and motor action. Dr. Montessori did not discover this fundamental principle of learning. Every serious student of childhood and education from Locke to the students of our own day has emphasized it. Dr. Montessori has applied the principle skilfully in devising apparatus which exercises the senses and stimulates constructive activities. She is not a 'discoverer' or a 'wonder-worker'; she is simply a clever and resourceful teacher who is familiar with what many investigators have done and many teachers have accomplished; and she has made some advance upon what others have achieved in the practical training of young children.

"The Montessori apparatus has been regarded by some as possessing mystic value. But it is not necessary to have this apparatus in order to apply the Montessori principles. Any ordinary home or school could afford children much of the sensory and motor experience that can be gained from the Montessori apparatus. This apparatus is designed to give children training in doing some of the important things they will need to do in daily life and to stimulate them to observe and discriminate carefully through all the senses. A child from three to six years of age who is allowed considerable freedom in the use of objects in the home, and who can be with his mother in the kitchen and elsewhere and participate in her activities will gain the sort of experience that he is expected to derive from the use of the Montessori apparatus. Further, if he has a sand pile and a collie dog, and tools such as a hammer and saw and the like, and a few pieces of gymnastic apparatus,—a rope ladder, and a swing and trapeze, for instance,—he will gain more varied experience than he could acquire if he should be confined to the Montessori apparatus alone.

"The dynamic principle is being applied in the

elementary, grammar, and high schools, as well as in the kindergarten and the Montessori schools, though, as we shall see later, the higher the pupil ascends in school, the more his work must consist in organizing and interpreting his experiences. But the fundamental aim of progressive schools of every grade to-day is to have pupils master *things* and *actions* as well as *words* and *rules*. We are hearing much about the Gary schools, the Fairhope school, and others of similar character; but they are merely conspicuous illustrations of tendencies to be seen everywhere throughout the country. He is regarded as the most skilful teacher who is most resourceful in leading his pupils actually to experiment with the objects or to perform the actions which he is teaching them. On the other hand, he who is regarded as the most ineffective teacher, the one who is farthest behind the times, is he who simply has his pupils sit in their seats and memorize rules and apply them to imaginary rather than real, every-day problems. There are certain sections of the country in which teaching is still largely of the latter sort, and these sections are regarded by educational people everywhere as retarded in their educational development.

"It is encouraging to note the change which is taking place in the textbooks in arithmetic. Those now coming from the press are requiring the pupil to react upon his environment in ways which will compel him to use the arithmetic he is trying to learn. The mere memorizing of definitions or fundamental operations and applying them in the solution of problems entirely remote from the pupil's daily life is passing, though it has not disappeared altogether by any means. The boys who take part in the annual corn-raising contests in the country schools of Winnebago County, Illinois, for instance, thoroughly master a large part of the essentials of arithmetic, for they must make careful measurements of the land on

The Dynamic Principle Applied to All School Work

which the corn is raised, careful computation of the amount of seed needed, of the yield from each hill of the value of the crop, and the percentage of profit.

Even Formal Studies Can Be Taught Dynamically "The principle in question is universal in its application to the work of the schoolroom. One cannot make a mistake in saying that a pupil will gain effective command of reading and spelling only by *using* these arts in some vital way. They must not be set apart from his active life, but must be made the means of acquiring useful knowledge, recording it, and communicating with his friends. As early as the tenth year children will strive with all their might to write well when they wish to send a letter to some friend. Then they will give attention to chirography and spelling. They will work out the meaning of words, securing help from every available source when they wish to decipher the story in some interesting book. In the same way the college student will attack with zest and enthusiasm the difficulties of a foreign language when he is looking forward to a trip abroad. The chief function of both teacher and textbook should be to create situations appealing so strongly to the learner's interests and impulses that he will largely disregard the drudgery of mastering the technique of a subject, as he fixes his attention upon the end to be reached and eagerly presses toward it.

"The subject which has offered the greatest resistance of any in the elementary school curriculum to the application of dynamic methods is grammar. It has been more than any other study the despair of teachers and the bugbear of pupils. Yet it is possible to combine the use of language and the technique of grammar and to relate both to the pupil's actual experience in such a way that he will come to appreciate the help that he will receive from the study of grammar. The sentence, as the pupil himself uses it, especially in written expression, should be made the basis of grammatical study. His own

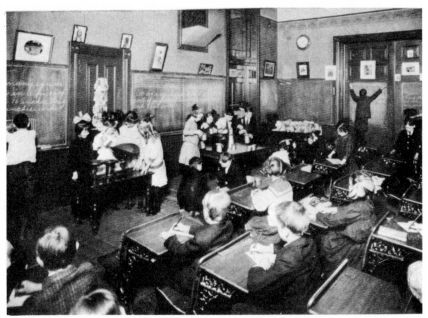

Pupils construct tables by actually working with the various units of measurements.

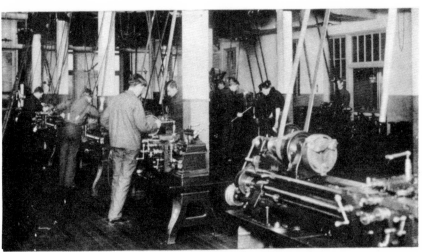

In the mechanical department of a High School.

compositions upon subjects in which he is vitally interested will furnish all the materials necessary for gaining a mastery of the essentials of grammar. From his own essays he may be led to see what the nature of a sentence is; what various functions words perform; the changes that occur in words as they are used in varied relations; the necessity for different kinds of sentences, and the characteristics of each. In short, he may be so taught that he will come to regard grammar as a useful tool, which, like the ability to read and to write, he sees to be necessary as a rule for the adequate interchange of thought."

A further illustration of the dynamic principle, as it is being applied in our schools, is found in the teaching of history. Doubtless some of our readers can remember the time when the learning of history consisted of memorizing dates and names of important persons, mainly warriors, and the wars in which they participated, with the outcome thereof. History learned in this way never functioned actively in the daily life of the learner. The facts he memorized by great effort remained static in his associations with people, either individually or in groups. Let any reader ask himself this question: "How much of the history I studied in the schools fifteen or twenty years ago has played any rôle in my life, either by way of helping me to interpret the trend of human affairs about me, or by way of enlightening me in respect to my duties as a citizen?" The answer to that question probably would be convincing to most of those who should ask it, that history has not played a prominent part in the intellectual, moral, or civic life of most persons trained in schools twenty or twenty-five years ago.

How does the dynamic principle apply to the teaching of history? If you have not recently observed the work of a class in history in a progressive school, you are

The Dynamic Principle and the Teaching of History

urged to visit such a class and note the ways and means by which history is made vital and illuminating in the lives of pupils. The past is reconstructed as fully as possible. Every sort of concrete evidence that can be obtained is used to help children to visualize and appreciate the epochs which they are studying. They dramatize the people, situations, and events which are described in the authorities which they consult. They are shown motion pictures made by students of history of dramatizations of important historical epochs. They make models of the homes and assembly places occupied by the people during the epoch which they are studying. In other ways the men and women who have lived in earlier times are made to pass in review before present-day pupils so that their habits of life—personal, social, political, industrial, and so on,—can actually be observed.

It is probably no exaggeration to say that every teacher in our country, who has felt the spirit of American education, is endeavoring to devise new and better ways of applying the dynamic principle in all his teaching. The educational magazines—there are literally hundreds of them in our country—are filled with accounts of experiments conducted for the purpose of showing how a particular topic in the various subjects of study in the elementary and high schools can be taught in a more dynamic way than it has been taught before. Departments of education in the universities and normal schools are publishing bulletins by the hundreds giving results of investigations relating to problems of dynamic teaching. At every educational meeting, teachers describe the results of their experiences in teaching subjects so as to give pupils actual experience in doing the things they are learning. This will explain why the atmosphere in a typical schoolroom in our country is very different from what it was twenty-five years ago. It will explain why pupils are on their feet much of the time and using their hands while they are studying. It will explain why there appears to be so much more going on in a typical schoolroom to-day than in almost any schoolroom a quarter of a century ago.

There is one subject which is rapidly coming to occupy first place in the work of teaching the young, not only in the elementary and high school but also in the home; and it is of supreme importance that it should be taught in a dynamic way, so that special mention may be made of it in this place. By way of introducing the problem with which we have to deal it may be asked: "Is there any good reason why one who lives in America should love his country?" Let one ask this question of the first ten adults one meets on the street or elsewhere and note the answers he receives. The majority of them will probably not be very clear or emphatic in their responses. Ask them what the country does to promote their welfare and most of them will be hazy and uncertain in their answers, because they have never thought in concrete terms regarding the service which our country renders to all its citizens. The present writer sometimes talks with adults who do not feel that the country is a real thing with a heart; it is to them a sort of abstract and remote thing which does not come close to the life of anyone. *(Methods of Teaching Children to Become Good Americans)*

Will the persons who are reading these lines please ask their children at the first opportunity whether they really love their country? They will probably all be demonstrative in their assertions of affection and loyalty; but then ask them to explain why they love their country, and the responses will certainly be a revelation to many who have taken it for granted that young people really feel an attachment for our country and understand why they should have love for it.

The writer has visited many classes in different sections of the country in which pupils have been reciting

in "civil government." He has heard lessons on Ameri-
canization. He has listened to recitations on the duties
and responsibilities of each individual to the government.
Further, he has heard pupils reproduce what they had
learned about the way States, counties, cities, and districts are governed, but he has not often heard pupils say
a word which would show that they were actually con-
ceiving of the country, the State, the city, the town, and
the district as playing an important rôle in determining
their comfort, happiness, and feeling of security. He has
frequently asked pupils during recitations in civil government to mention one thing the national government
had done for them that day or week which had promoted
their welfare, and the responses have rarely been satisfactory. As a rule, the pupils who have been questioned
never connected the government directly with their own
daily experiences. They did not think that the country
had made it possible for them to have an education, or to
earn their living, or to enjoy any other advantage.
Pupils have said to the writer time and again that the
clothing they wore, the food they ate, the houses they
lived in, the automobiles they rode in, and so on, were
earned as a result of their own industry or that of their
parents; and they did not appreciate that the country
had anything to do with the advantages which they
enjoyed.

Every reader will undoubtedly agree that one cannot
love any person or any thing unless that person or thing
has some vital connection with his own life—is essential
to his intellectual, physical, emotional, moral, or
aesthetic well-being. We cannot have affection for a
mere abstraction, or for anything that does not in any way
affect our happiness or prosperity; so the chief requisite
in developing love of country in young people is to lead
them to feel that the country is very real and that without
its constant assistance, watchfulness, protection, and

guidance we would not have the comforts, the safety, and the freedom which we now enjoy.

We must begin with very concrete experiences to awaken in our pupils a consciousness of the benefits which they receive from the government. Let us start with the school. "Who built this school building and equipped it with all that is needed to carry on our work? Who pays for the teachers and for the heat? Suppose that every pupil had to pay his share of the cost of these things, how many of them would have any schooling? There are children in some countries who cannot go to school, because there is no school for them to attend; and children in other countries who can attend school but for a short time because they cannot afford it, since they have to pay all the cost of their schooling. Most of the people in these countries go through life ignorant, and the only thing they know how to do is to work at hard manual labor. They do not have time or the means for enjoyment. They can earn scarcely enough food and clothing to keep body and soul together. But in most of the States in our country, everyone who wishes to do so and who is industrious and capable may go to a free school for at least sixteen years—eight years in the elementary school, four years in the high school, and four years in the state university. Who is it that pays the expenses of all this education? The district, city, town, county, State, the United States, all help to pay it, so that every individual may make the most of his life. Every day a child is in school he is indebted to his country for the advantages he enjoys."

Again, the parent or teacher must lead the child to see that without the care and assistance received from his country he would constantly be exposed to dangers and hardships. Take his health, for instance. How could he protect himself in times of epidemic of scarlet fever, typhoid fever, yellow fever, cholera, or other

The Country Helps the Individual in a Very Real Way

411

diseases unless the town, city, county, State, and nation came to his aid? In other countries these diseases often kill a large part of the people because their countries do not give them the right kind of help in time of need. There is not a child of any age who cannot be impressed with this story. And when the impression is made, let the parent or teacher ask: "Here we are receiving help all the time, so that we may keep well and enjoy life, and what should we do for the country that helps and protects us?"

Even a young child can be led to appreciate that the country is a very real thing, that it is constantly helping every person to solve his problems, and that without its aid we would all be helpless. This is why we should love our country and be loyal to it. It cannot go on helping everyone unless everyone will coöperate with it. Anyone who stands in its way is an enemy of everyone. Any person who accepts the benefits which our country offers him—and everyone does accept them—and who is then unappreciative and disloyal is greedy and mean, and he does not deserve to receive any assistance.

How the Country Assists Rural People Young people, and older ones as well, who live on farms, are often unable to see how they are assisted or protected by the country. They usually find fault with it, and they see nothing about it to admire or respect. They have to work hard, and they think that whatever they possess they have earned by the sweat of their brow without aid from any source. Here is a good opportunity for a parent in a rural home or a teacher in a rural school to lead young people to see that farmers as well as those who work in banks, in stores, in factories, or in offices of any kind are helped and protected by the county, State, and nation. How could farmers combat diseases that attack their crops and their animals unless the nation had studied these diseases and had devised ways and means of controlling them? In foreign nations, where the tiller of the soil works without much, if any, help from his country, these diseases often completely destroy his crops and his livestock, and millions of people may starve because there is not enough food. Children should be led to understand that great progress has been made in farming during the last fifty years, and this has been made possible almost entirely because of the watchfulness, assistance, and protection of the country. Our country supports stations where every problem which the farmer encounters is scientifically investigated, and as soon as information which will be of help to him is secured it is conveyed to him in books, in institutes, and in other ways.

A hundred years ago farmers traded their wheat, corn, and cattle directly for clothes, flour, etc. They had to carry their grain to the man with whom they wanted to make a trade; but our country has developed a system of transportation, so that now practically every farmer, no matter where his farm is located, can send his grain to Chicago, to Seattle, to New Orleans, or to New York City and get money for it with which he can buy what he wishes. He is no longer obliged to trade his products with somebody in the neighborhood.

Young people admire and respect a person or a thing that is strong, powerful, and capable of meeting any emergency. Pupils ought to be impressed with the fact that America is a great, powerful, and courageous country. Sometimes parents think it is not desirable to speak of our nation as a great and powerful country, and so they miss one opportunity to arouse the admiration, affection, and loyalty of children. Young people cannot be made to admire a weak or flabby person or thing, and there cannot be any harm in indulging their love for strength and magnitude. The more a parent can impress upon his children the vast power and resources of our country the warmer attachment they will have for it.

Of course, our nation's vast power must be used in an

Young People Admire Courage and Strength

413

honorable way. Young people do not like a bully. They admire a strong person if he is fair, if he will not pick on those who are smaller and weaker than he is himself; so the teacher must not fail to impress her pupils with the fact, for fact it is, that our country is using its strength for the betterment of all people and not for the enslavement of any of them. Just now, a teacher can impress this idea more strongly than it would have been possible to do four years ago. Our country has taken the lead in offering to abandon our great ships and to cease building any more for a considerable period. America could build ships more easily than any other country and yet our country is willing to give weaker nations a chance. We are not using our power to take advantage of any weak people. Throughout the World War, and since then, we have stood for freedom for all peoples, weak or strong. We will not exploit weaker nations than our own, and we do not want any other strong nation to take advantage of those who are not so strong.

The American ideal is freedom for all people so long as they live in accord with rules and regulations which are essential to the welfare of all. While we have might, still we stand strongly against the idea that might makes right. No nation in the world's history has ever emphasized this principle so strongly as America has done both by precept and by example during the last decade. A parent ought to put this idea before his children very concretely on every suitable occasion. Nothing will strengthen the admiration, affection, and loyalty of children as they grow older more than this idea of great strength held in check in order that those who are not so strong may have a chance to live their lives unhampered and unterrified.

Teaching Children Health Habits Next to the teaching of citizenship in our schools, the teaching of health is coming to occupy the place of chief importance, and we are making extraordinary progress in applying the dynamic principle to the method of teaching this subject. There is a peculiar situation to deal with since children do not naturally feel any concern about health, and it is difficult to make them careful in respect to health matters. It takes a skilful parent or teacher to convince a five or six-year-old child that if he puts dirty fingers in his mouth he may suffer from internal pains, or become sick so that he will have to stay in bed. Nature seems to say to a young child: "Put your fingers in your mouth whenever you want to. Then when you take them out of your mouth, and they are covered with saliva, pick up dirty objects if you wish to, and then put your fingers in your mouth again. Don't pay any attention to dirt." In the same way, nature encourages a child to run out in the rain, to lie down in the grass or sand when he is overheated, to gulp down his food, to eat anything he likes at any time he can get it and especially to eat an excess of sweets, to give no attention to the care of his teeth, eyes, or skin; in short, nature apparently says to children: "Go ahead and do anything you want to, enjoy yourself in any way you wish, and don't take any thought about your health."

In teaching any health habit, it must be connected directly with the child's wish to run faster, to climb higher, to throw straighter than rivals, and to be always able to take part in the games that are going on. If he throws himself down on the ground, for instance, when he is overheated, he will not be able to do any of these things as well as if he would stand up and keep moving when he is perspiring. As a matter of fact, this is one of the health habits that it is difficult to lead young children to observe; it is difficult to induce children in the teens even to observe it.

How to Impress the Value of Health

Further, pains and aches must be connected directly with unhygienic habits. It is of no use to say to a child that he will have a pain if he violates a health rule; but when the pain comes, the parent can lead him to see the cause of it; and when this is done systematically the child will make the connection in due course. Then when he is tempted to crack a nut with his teeth, say, the thought of the pain that is likely to follow may restrain him. Of course, one cannot expect that one or two warnings will hold impulses in check. Only by constant and unvarying repetition for many months can a child establish the connection between unhygienic habits and pain, sickness, and lessened ability to do what he wishes to do.

How the Dynamic Principle is Being Observed in the Teaching of Formal Studies

It will not be possible to show in detail how dynamic methods are coming to be used in all the subjects of study, but space may be taken to point out briefly how the dynamic principle is being observed in the teaching of the so-called formal or mechanical studies. Take spelling, for instance. Formerly pupils stood up in a row and spelled orally the words pronounced by the teacher. To-day in any progressive school the pupils write the words, as well as spell them orally, and they use them in sentences as they are likely to use them in writing letters, reports, or essays. It has been shown experimentally that one may be able to write isolated words in a list accurately and readily, but he may not be able to write them so accurately or so readily when they occur in sentences, for the reason that spelling habits, like all other habits, are very specific. When one has learned to spell a word in a certain situation, he can spell it in that situation but not so readily, if at all, in a different situation; that is to say, when the circumstances in which a word has been learned are altered even slightly, an individual may not show a secure mastery of it. Spelling of familiar words ought to be largely *automatic*, which requires that they should be learned in school as they will be used in daily life; that is, they should be written in the types of sentences in which they most frequently occur.

Again, the dynamic method is being observed in the teaching of handwriting. According to the static method, the pupil learns to write by reproducing copies in a special copy book. He first practices the elements of the letters, and later he combines these as they occur in letters; and finally he combines the letters into short words first and then into longer words. As a result of this system of training, the pupil may be able to write æsthetically in his copy book, but he may write altogether differently when he needs to use handwriting in the expression of his thoughts. A pupil taught in this way thinks of handwriting as an accomplishment for a special handwriting period. He has not used it as a medium for the expression of thought, so that it is regarded as a sort of thing in itself, possessing characteristics of inherent value. In learning to write he gave his attention mainly to the mechanical processes involved, so that when he writes now he has to continue to give conscious attention to the mechanical processes.

When handwriting has thus been practiced in a special period during eight years, with attention focused upon the *mechanics* of the process, it cannot then be used automatically merely as a medium of expression. One may see in the schools of foreign countries, and he may still see in some of our own schools, pupils who cannot use writing automatically in conveying their ideas to others. When they take their pens in hand to express themselves, their thinking ceases. One may observe children who have practiced handwriting as a special exercise for ten or fifteen minutes a day all through the elementary school, whose mental processes are slowed down by the pen. When they are asked to express themselves on any topic on which they could talk freely and at great length or to write a letter to a friend, they do not know what to say and they ask for assistance. With such children the pen has become a barrier to the expression of thought.

But when pupils are taught according to the dynamic principle, they acquire their handwriting in connection with the expression of their ideas in the different subjects of study in the school and in communication with their friends outside of school. *They learn to write by writing.* Of course, they must devote some attention at the outset to the mere mechanics of constructing letters and words, but they are required at the earliest possible moment to express their thoughts through the medium of handwriting. As they pass through the grades they have an increasing amount of experience in readily employing handwriting in the expression of ideas, so that by the time they reach the eighth grade handwriting becomes largely an automatic medium of expression for most of them. The pen can be used then in graphic expression much as the tongue is used in oral expression. If a pupil had been required to spend fifteen minutes a day all through the grades in the study of the mechanics of speech, and if he had not had training in the use of oral language in conveying his experience and his views to others, he would not be able to use oral language any more freely in the eighth grade in expressing thought than he can use handwriting when he has learned it as a thing in itself and not as medium of expression. This psychological fact is accountable for the change which is taking place in our country in the teaching of handwriting in the schools. The old copy books are going, and in many places have gone completely.

The Dynamic Principle in the Teaching of Reading

Take another illustration—the teaching of reading. In our schools a few years ago, pupils prepared each reading lesson by studying the new and difficult words so they could pronounce them. When they came to recite, their effort was centered chiefly upon pronouncing the words accurately. Classmates kept watch of each reader in order to note whether he miscalled any of the words. This method of teaching has been or is being abandoned in every progressive school system. Instead of emphasis being placed upon the correct pronunciation of words, it is now placed upon the gaining of thought readily and accurately and expressing it easily and pleasingly. It has been shown experimentally that a pupil may be able to read a page without error in pronunciation and still he may have only a hazy notion of the meaning of what he reads. Also, he may read slowly and painfully. But in actual life his chief concern will be to get the content of his reading rapidly and accurately, for otherwise he will be handicapped, since the amount which one must read in order to keep in touch with the life about him is already enormous and is constantly increasing. Furthermore, the need for oral reading is constantly declining. A large proportion of persons in present-day American life are hardly ever called upon to read orally; but they are constantly called upon to read *rapidly* in order to gain an understanding of, and to keep in touch with, the life about them. Practically all of the reading of most persons to-day is "silent." It is not necessary that they should pronounce the words they read; on the contrary, it is better that they should not pronounce them, actually or internally, for the reason that the pronunciation of words slows down the process of gaining thought. Any reader of these lines may test himself; if he mentally pronounces all the words he reads, he is a slow and ineffective reader. On the other hand, if he can grasp the meaning of phrases or clauses without mentally pronouncing the words, he is more likely to be a rapid and effective reader. The larger the units he can interpret without being conscious of the words—or at least without pronouncing them—the better reader he will be, so far as the needs of contemporary American life are concerned.

Now, if in teaching a child to read, emphasis is constantly placed upon correct oral pronunciation of words, he will acquire mental habits which will make it difficult if at all possible for him to read as rapidly and effectively, so far as grasping the content of his reading is concerned.

as if he had had much experience at the outset in reading solely for the purpose of gaining meaning accurately and rapidly. For this reason, we are striving in our schools to have children from the first grade on throughout all the grades read silently for a large part of each reading period and then state in their own words or to act out the thought of what they have read. They are trained to read as rapidly as possible so that they will not be halted in the gaining of meaning by giving attention to separate words, since explicit awareness of separate words in one's reading delays and often confuses the process of interpreting the thought contained in the reading.

The Dynamic Principle Applied in the Teaching of Foreign Language We may mention one further illustration of the application of the dynamic principle in the method of presenting studies in American schools to-day. Probably most of the readers of these lines have studied French, German, Spanish, or Italian in school. If they studied any of these languages twenty or twenty-five years ago, they know that chief emphasis was then placed upon grammar. They learned the vocabulary of the languages by connecting each word with its English equivalent. They did not *use* the foreign language in the classroom; they always recited in the native tongue. Their reading in the foreign tongue was designed principally for the purpose of illustrating the grammatical rules which they had memorized. Consequently pupils did not gain the ability to speak the language, to read it readily, to understand it when spoken, or to write it easily. Investigations recently made have shown that pupils in the high school who have spent four years in studying a foreign language have often found themselves utterly unable to use the language when in need of it while visiting the country in which it is the native tongue. Anyone who has seen much of Americans in France, Germany, or Italy knows that only very rarely can they use the native language of any of those countries though they may have studied it for a number of years. They were taught the language in a static way and consequently it is not of service to them now.

The static method still prevails in the teaching of foreign languages in our schools more largely than it does in the teaching of any other subject probably, but still it is being abandoned in many places in favor of the dynamic method. One may visit progressive schools in which pupils are actually *using* the foreign language which they are studying. Emphasis is placed upon speaking, reading, and understanding a language, rather than upon a mastery of its technique. The pupils are required to interpret the teacher's communications in the foreign language; they exchange ideas with one another in the language; they write it as well as speak it, and they read it without waiting to get a complete knowledge of its grammatical construction. That is to say, they learn the foreign language in the way in which they will need to employ it. They do not neglect grammatical study, but it plays a decidedly subordinate rôle; it is resorted to principally in order to help the learner to interpret correctly what he reads or hears. So long as he can interpret accurately without grammatical study, he is permitted and encouraged to go forward with the *use* of the language.

During the past two decades the methods of teaching **Summary** in our schools have changed rapidly and profoundly. The critics of our schools think that our newer methods give children too much freedom, and especially that they substitute too largely the use of the hand for the exercise of the brain. Visitors from foreign countries are always forcibly impressed by the *activity* which they observe in our schoolrooms. In practically all foreign countries the methods of teaching consist mainly in requiring pupils to memorize contents of books and to recite them without verbal error.

A slogan of our American teachers for the past two

decades has been, "Learn to Do by Doing." The great writers on education from John Locke to Herbert Spencer have endorsed and emphasized this principle.

During the past few years our educational psychologists have shown that a pupil may be able to recite a rule correctly and apply it accurately to a textbook problem, but that at the same time he may not be able to apply it to an actual problem such as he has to deal with in daily life. So our teachers say, "Have the pupil learn things in the school in the way in which he will have to use them outside of school."

The term, *dynamic*, is becoming common in our educational literature. It is used in contrast to the term, *static*. It means that in our methods of teaching we aim to have pupils learn by actually performing the processes they are studying, rather than by sitting in their seats and memorizing words about the processes.

We are coming to believe that words are merely *symbols* and that they gain meaning only as they are learned in connection with concrete, dynamic experience. The changes that are taking place in our methods of teaching are based upon this principle. The aim of all progressive schools to-day is to have pupils master *things* and *actions* as well as words and rules.

Each subject in the curriculum, even so formal a subject as spelling, can be taught in a dynamic as contrasted with a static way. The most resourceful teachers are the most successful in devising dynamic methods in presenting all subjects. The more completely a pupil can *do* what he has learned, the more completely he attains the ideal we are striving for in the methods of teaching in our schools. This principle applies to spelling, handwriting, reading, and other formal subjects, as well as to content studies.

In no subject is the dynamic principle being applied more thoroughly or with greater success than in the

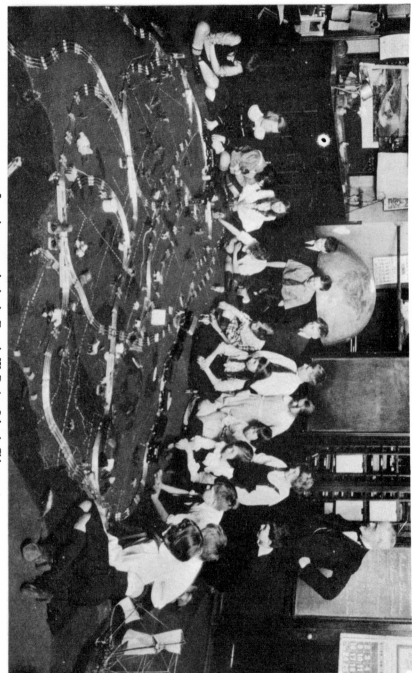

Learning geography in the Francis W. Parker School, Chicago.

teaching of children to become good citizens. Formerly pupils studied civil government by memorizing the contents of a textbook; now they organize their school into a community and administer it as a miniature society. They also study concretely how the government of the town or city in which they live is actually carried on and with what results. Pupils come to appreciate their country and gain a love for it because they are led to understand how it cares for them, protects their well-being, and safeguards them at home and abroad.

The teaching of health in our schools is being profoundly affected by the dynamic principle. Formerly pupils learned definitions of the organs of the body and their functions. To-day they become familiar with the requirements for maintaining health and vigor so that they may accomplish the objectives in which they are interested and avoid losing time and suffering pain because they violate the laws of nature.

XX

PROMOTING THE HEALTH AND PHYSICAL DEVELOPMENT
OF SCHOOL CHILDREN

Revelations
Concerning
the Physical
Development
and the
Health of
Our People

THE medical examination of young men during the World War revealed a surprising situation in respect to the health and physical development of our people, as Dr. Winslow has shown in Chapter XI of this volume. We had been assuming that we were a strong, vigorous, healthy nation. We had been going ahead in our work, our amusements, and all our undertakings at such a rapid pace that we had taken it for granted that our people were in good health or they would have had to slow down in their activities. But the results of the medical examination of soldiers put an end to our assumptions regarding our superior physical condition. A large proportion of young men in the prime of life were found to be physically defective in one way or another and to be below par in general health. Most surprising of all, it was found that a larger proportion of young men born and reared in the country than in the city were suffering from maldevelopment of various sorts and were not up to the standard in physical vigor. They bore the effects of early diseases that left weaknesses and deformities sufficiently serious to unfit them for military service. They showed lack of normal development of the different members of the body which, even if they were not marked enough to prevent them from entering the war, would nevertheless prove a handicap in the enterprises of daily life.

Even the Federal health authorities were impressed by the evidence of the inferior physical condition of young men at a time in life when bodily and mental vigor should be at the maximum and maldevelopment should be least conspicuous. The newspapers as well as the medical, and to some extent the general, magazines have been devoting much space to a discussion of the reasons why so many of our young men are not better developed physically and are below a reasonable standard of health so that they cannot meet the requirements of the sort of life they would have to undergo in the army. The chief conclusion which must be drawn from this discussion is that we have not undertaken to solve the problem of the sound physical development and the promotion of the health of the young in as thorough-going a way as we have undertaken to solve most of our other problems. We have been so busy developing our natural resources that we have overlooked to a harmful extent the development of our human resources; and we have been so impressed by our material successes and prosperity that we have not as a people been much impressed by the prevalence among us of physical defects and deficiencies and ill-health. Professor Fisher and others, especially persons connected with the Life Extension Institute, have been saying for some time that a large proportion of our people are losing from ten to thirty or forty per cent of their time and energy because of preventable diseases, and that this constitutes a very serious economic loss, to say nothing about the distress which is caused thereby. We have had such unequalled success in the development of machines to take the place of human hands that most of us have not noted the fact that workers in factories are laid off and our pupils in school are absent frequently, caused by diseases that could quite easily be avoided.

Our people are becoming thoroughly aroused in regard to this matter and are determined that the physical development and the health of our school children shall be improved. A large number of national, state, and local organizations have been and are being formed for the purpose of investigating the health conditions of the young, and are taking proper steps to improve these conditions. As these lines are being written, the organization of the Child Health Association of America is being completed, and Herbert Hoover, Secretary of Commerce, is taking the leadership of the Association. This is a significant fact because it indicates how seriously our people are taking hold of the task of promoting the health and physical development of the young. The Federal Children's Bureau has been devoting some attention for years to the subject of the health of school children, and it is proposed to devote much more attention to it in the future. State and city boards of health throughout the country are awakening to the necessity of getting at the causes which made it impossible for so large a proportion of our young men to meet the requirements of service in the army, and then to modify or eliminate those causes.

The first point of attack in the promotion of the health and normal physical development of school children is the hygiene of school buildings. There can be no doubt that a considerable part of the preventable disease and maldevelopment among the young is due to the fact that most of our children are in school buildings from three to five hours a day for an average of five days a week, forty weeks in the year, from the age of six to the age of fourteen—the period when physical development is most rapid and when defects and deformities can become established most easily. Nature undoubtedly intended that the young should live an active muscular life out in the open during the developmental period. When the human body was being constructed, man lived out of doors and he had to engage in an active muscular life for subsistence. Almost over night, as such things should be measured, we have changed our mode of living so that instead of being out in the open, hunting and fishing, etc., for a living, we now spend our time indoors, usually in a sitting posture, and we exercise the brain principally instead of the muscles. This change in our habits of living has an unfavorable effect upon the young particularly. Nature is more insistent that the young should live a motor life than that adults should do so; but we put our children in a school building at the age of five or six and keep them there a considerable part of their waking life for from eight to twelve years. And to add to the injurious effect of such a life for the young, the educational methods which have been in vogue heretofore have required that children should sit in seats learning lessons or reciting them during practically all of their time in school buildings. The wonder is that a larger proportion of them have not been defective or deformed or their vitality weakened so that they could not resist disease.

Serious attention is now being given to the improvement of the hygiene of school buildings and their equipment. First of all, an effort is being made to provide air within school buildings which shall be, as near as possible, like the air out of doors. It has been shown that a large proportion of the diseases from which school children suffer are due to the unhygienic atmospheric conditions in school buildings. Numerous investigations have impressed the fact that the air has been too dry and too hot and that it has contained dust which carried disease germs. Too often it has been "dead," which is chiefly responsible for the prevalence of respiratory diseases among school children. These facts are now quite generally understood by educational people and, to some extent, by laymen; and in the new school buildings that are being erected, special appliances are being installed so that the atmospheric conditions will be more healthful

The Problem of Hygienic Ventilation in School Rooms

than has been the case heretofore, speaking generally. Older school buildings are being reconstructed with a view to improving the ventilation so that the air in the schoolroom will closely approximate the air out of doors in every quality except temperature. Some States have enacted laws requiring that plans for every new school building shall be submitted to expert authorities who are charged with the responsibility of securing proper ventilating and heating arrangements so as to conserve the health of school children.

The problem of the one-room rural school is the most difficult to solve, but even here conditions are being rapidly improved through the installation of better heating, ventilating, and humidifying devices. A number of States have passed laws requiring that all stoves in school rooms shall be provided with jackets so that the heat may be distributed with some degree of uniformity throughout the schoolroom. There is a movement also in the direction of requiring that every schoolroom heated by a stove shall be provided with an inlet for fresh air to be heated and distributed about the room. However, the writer has very recently inspected rural schools in certain States in which no intelligent attention has yet been given to problems of heating, ventilating, or humidifying the air. In such schoolrooms a large proportion of pupils are afflicted throughout the fall and winter months with respiratory troubles.

Defects Due to Bad Posture in the Schoolroom The medical examination of soldiers showed that defects due to unhygienic posture during the developmental period—spinal curvature, for instance—were found among young men. And the discussion of the matter by physicians, teachers, and laymen has emphasized a fact already understood by many persons, that school seats improperly adjusted to the children who sit in them are responsible for certain defects in physical development. During the past two or three decades,

superintendents, principals, and teachers have been calling the attention of boards of education and patrons of
the schools to the necessity of providing seats for school
children properly adjusted to their physical measurements. If a short child and a tall child are required to use
a seat and desk of the same height, one or the other will
have to assume an unhygienic posture, and if this is
continued for several hours each day for a number of
years, it is practically certain that there will be maldevelopment in some respect. Even before the prevalence
of physical defects among young people was revealed by
medical examiners during the World War, school buildings
were beginning to be equipped with seats which were
adaptable to the physical measurements of pupils. One
may safely predict that it will not be long before school
children throughout the country will not have to use
while they are in the schoolroom furniture which will
habitually require them to assume unhygienic postures.

And not only are school buildings and furnishings
being determined in view of the requirements for the
promotion of the health and physical development of the
young, but the program of school work is also being
scrutinized from the same standpoint. The school day
of children in the various grades and in the high school
is being studied in order to ascertain how the various
tasks can be arranged and performed so as to avoid
unnecessary fatigue. It has been shown by investigations
that studies which require substantially the same mental
or motor processes, if they follow one another directly
in the day's program, will be more likely to cause fatigue
in pupils than if studies that do not use the same mental
or motor processes are alternated. Further, the hygiene
of each branch of instruction is being studied in order to
determine how it can be pursued with the least nervous
wear and tear. In short, every phase of the problem of
schoolroom fatigue has recently been or is now being

*The Hygiene
of the
School
Program*

investigated, and it may be predicted that, in due time teachers will be able to arrange the daily, weekly, and monthly programs of work and present each branch of instruction so that the energies of pupils will not be wastefully dissipated.

Relieving Young Pupils of Fine, Highly Coördinated Tasks As a result of investigations already concluded, one reform has been achieved in our schools. Formerly very young children were required to perform tasks requiring a high degree of muscular control and coördination. Thus pupils in the first grade were expected to write with pens having sharp points, to do fine work in sewing, and to thread needles having small eyes. They were provided with small blocks for building purposes. In fact, all their school activities were based on the false principle, that the smaller the child the more delicate his fingers and muscles and the finer and more highly coördinated tasks he should be required to perform. But this program has been completely changed in the progressive schools of our country. Instead of requiring the youngest children to do the finest work, while permitting older children large freedom in this respect, the order is reversed. The youngest children now do not generally write with pens or if they do it is with those that have coarse points. The pencils they use have soft lead. The youngest children are not required to write in small spaces demanding precise muscular control; they write a large, coarse hand. They have large blocks for building purposes. If they engage in sewing at all, they do coarse work and use large needles with large eyes.

The youngest children are not required to toe a line and maintain a controlled attitude in their recitations for a very considerable period, but this may be required of the older children whose nervous development makes it possible for them to perform such tasks without overstrain. Each year as they develop they are required to work with smaller implements and to perform tasks

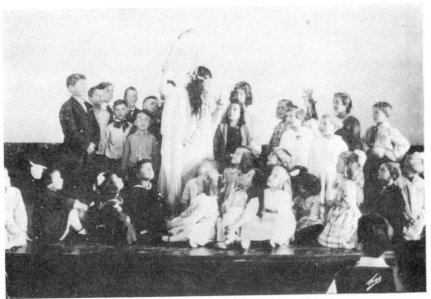

Health habits are being impressed through dramatization.

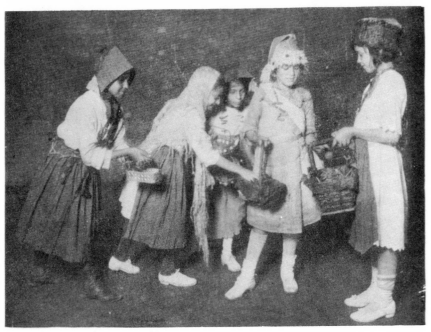

Learning the food values of vegetables.

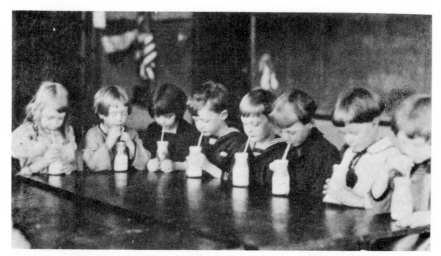

A nutritious lunch in the middle of the forenoon.   A small bottle of milk and a straw.

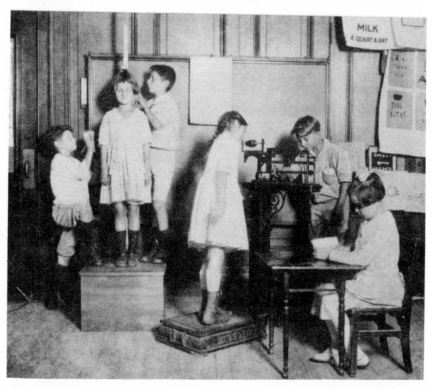

Pupils keep a record of their height and weight and compare their score with the standards for their age.

demanding increasingly fine coördinations, on the principle that in the development of the nervous system the centers that govern large muscles and coarse, nonprecise movements should be exercised earlier than the centers that control highly coördinate movements. When young children attempt to execute highly coördinated activities for which their nervous development has not adequately prepared them, they become fatigued easily. Much of the schoolroom fatigue of the era now passing has been due to the excessive demands made on pupils in the performance of precise and complicated motor tasks.

It is not intended to convey the impression that school children do not show any overstrain in our schools to-day; quite the contrary is true, in fact. It is claimed by medical inspectors in the various cities of our country that a sufficiently large proportion of school children are overstrained to invite the serious attention of parents, teachers, and boards of education. It is believed that one cause of this overstrain is malnourishment. The children are not sufficiently nourished to provide energy for all the demands that are made upon them. In the attempt to solve this problem, schools everywhere are instituting a program of school feeding for children who show under-nourishment or overstrain. Milk is furnished to such children in the middle of the forenoon session, by school authorities and sometimes in the middle of the afternoon. It is becoming the practice to furnish school lunches at noon to children who reveal deficiencies in their nutrition. Of course, malnourishment is not always due to an inadequate amount of food; it is due as frequently to improper food or to the environments in which a child lives, which keep him in a highly tense or irritated condition so that he cannot properly assimilate the food which he consumes. In New York, Chicago, Boston, and other cities, the whole subject is under investigation by

Dealing With the Problem of Malnourishment

civic or private welfare organizations. The general phases of the problem have been discussed in Chapter IX, and it will not be necessary to go into the matter in further detail here.

Overstrain
Among
School
Children
Due to Over-
Stimulating
Environ-
ments
It is beginning to be appreciated that the overstrain so often seen in school children is not due principally or even largely to the excessive demands of the school curriculum upon nervous energy but rather to the conditions surrounding children, especially in towns and cities. The present writer has called attention in another connection to the over-stimulating effect upon the young of contemporary life in our country and a few paragraphs may be quoted because they bear directly upon the problem of fatigue among school children.

"From one point of view we would not expect either children or adults to be overtaxed in these times. We do not work as hard now as our forefathers did fifty years ago. In former days, the young and the old alike arose with the sun and were often busy at hard labor until the sun went down. This program was carried out day after day, week after week, and month after month. Nowadays, there are fewer hours of labor, and work is not so heavy as it was formerly, for we have learned how to make machines perform the heaviest parts of our tasks.

"And yet we learn from many sources that there is overstrain among the young as well as among adults. This is undoubtedly due to the fact that the majority of young persons, as well as adults, to-day do more work that overtaxes brain and nerves than they did thirty years ago. There is a difference between being muscularly tired and being nervously tense and strained. Modern urban life tends to put children's nerves on edge. Even if a child does not have to do any hard work, mental or physical, he can still hardly escape from being intensely stimulated much of the time. To-day he must adapt himself to many more people than would have been required of him twenty-five years ago, and this is likely to develop nervous tension. Following a plow all day long is easy on nerves compared with meeting different people throughout the day and adjusting oneself to them. In addition, a large proportion of young persons must be on crowded streets a considerable part of each day, dodging vehicles, getting out of the way of pedestrians, being angered because of the apparent meanness or selfishness of adults, or being intensely stimulated in rivalry with competitors, or in anticipation of approaching exciting events.

"One who is using his muscles mainly is working along lines of least resistance, as compared with one who is using his brain constantly, whether in study, in social adaptation, or in dealing with complicated and constantly shifting situations such as city life presents. In following a plow the work soon becomes largely automatic, and the mind moves along unobstructedly in a sort of day dream. The plowman is not constantly wrestling with difficult problems. His energies are being expended mostly through his muscles, thus relieving his nervous system. When he has finished his day's work he can lie down and he may be asleep as soon as his head touches the pillow.

"But it is quite the reverse with one who has been chiefly using his brain all day, who has been trying to solve involved problems of one kind or another, and who has not used his muscles very actively. When night comes the brain and nervous system of such a person are likely to be unduly stimulated and he cannot relax immediately. Often he will lie awake for hours after he retires. He may talk in his sleep and be partially aroused during the night. His nervous system does not become entirely relaxed at any time. But the plowboy probably can secure profound sleep during the entire night.

"Take a young person who is in contact with many people of different dispositions, who is in a large, complex school for several hours each day, who has parties to give and to attend, whose home constantly, is in a more or less excited state because of the complicated life which is streaming through it,—such a child is very likely to become overstrained. He may have 'colds' or indigestion or a fever, but the fundamental cause is nervous overstrain.

The Chief Cause of Overstrain
"In remedying this condition, the first point to appreciate is that overstrain results from the effort to adapt oneself to too many and too complex situations. Every reader of these lines has probably at some time had the experience of having half a dozen problems pressing upon him for solution at the same time. His attention was drawn first here and now there and again in another direction, and he could not go forward in any direction because he was in the hands, so to speak, of conflicting and competing ideas and desires. He was literally torn by mental conflict. So long as competing or conflicting ideas prevent one from working through first one problem and then another, he will be tense and he will feel strain and stress. Some persons, children as well as adults, are able to deal with complicated situations much more easily than other persons, because they have the power of shutting out every problem but the one they are working on at the moment. When the one in hand is solved they take up the next one, and so they go on; and they get through a relatively large amount of difficult mental work without overstrain.

"In preventing overstrain in a child, then, we must limit the number of problems that press upon him at any moment. This is always an individual matter. The parent or the teacher who knows the child alone can determine how complicated a life he can live—whether he can do all the work of his grade in school, whether he can participate in competitions and contests, whether he can endure all the examinations that are ordinarily given in the school, and whether he can take part in outside activities—practice music, for instance, and attend parties. Some children can do all these things and not show overstrain, while other children would be broken in trying to carry through so complicated a program.

"The home and school should make an attempt to counteract the exciting influences of the street. At certain periods, every pupil in school and every member of a family should be quiet. Young and old alike should learn to sit still. Merely to tell children to keep quiet will not accomplish much, of course; this is more likely to accentuate restlessness than to subdue it. But if someone will tell or read a captivating story every day, or describe an interesting event or object or natural law, so that all who hear it will listen and be still, it will prove an excellent discipline and a restorative for the nervous system.

"It is peculiarly unfortunate that the voices of American parents and teachers often increase the tension and excitability of the young. A high-pitched, rasping, loud, restless voice will overstimulate the majority of children within its reach. Even adults cannot listen quietly to such a voice. On the other hand, a well-placed, well-controlled, modulated voice is soothing to an overwrought nervous system. One who will make observations can see persons who are tense and restless becoming calm under the influence of such a voice. Parents and teachers should keep this fact in mind, for one can control the quality of his voice to some extent. If he allows himself to become tense the evil effect will be apparent in his voice, which is delicately responsive to one's mental and nervous condition.

"Something could be done in the school, too, to offset the lack of poise in the life outside. In the Montessori schools there are brief periods of quiet each day. A signal is sounded on the piano, the room is darkened, and children become relaxed and quiet. They remain so for a little time; then another signal is sounded, the room is made light again, and the work progresses. Every schoolroom should have several brief periods during the day when the pupils should relax. There is no danger of overdoing relaxation in American life. The danger is on the other side,—that there will not be enough of it, no matter what program we may follow in the effort to secure it."

Medical Inspection in Schools Reference has been made to the investigations being conducted by medical inspectors throughout the country. It should be added here that there are very few communities of ten thousand or more inhabitants in which there is not at least one physician or trained nurse who is employed to make physical examinations of school children and recommend proper treatment of defects, deficiencies, or diseases. In some of the largest cities— Chicago, Philadelphia, New York, San Francisco, and the like—there is a large staff of well-trained physicians and nurses who devote their entire time to promoting the health and physical development of school children. They examine every pupil at least once, and often twice, a year. They make reports to parents or guardians respecting the condition of the health and physical development of each child. When they find defects of posture and development, they outline a remedial program. If they discover that a child is suffering from adenoids, infected tonsils, carious teeth, or defective vision or hearing, they advise parents respecting the procedure which should be followed in order to correct the difficulties. Nurses visit the home to see if the recommendations of the medical inspectors are carried out. Some States have laws requiring that medical inspectors or nurses be provided for rural as well as for town and city schools, and it is probable that all the States soon will enact legislation of this character.

Not only do the medical inspectors and nurses make examinations in order to discover defects or diseases already contracted, but they are on the alert to prevent the spread of disease among school children and the contracting of diseases due to improper posture or misuse of the senses or members of the body, particularly the eyes. In consequence of very active investigation and discussion of these matters during the past two decades, there is to-day less strain put upon the eyes in an up-to-date American school than there was formerly. The print in text books has been improved and this has helped to correct bad posture of pupils in school work.

With a view to promoting sound physical development among our children, schools everywhere are adopting a program of physical education, which includes gymnastics and games and plays of all sorts. States like Wisconsin require that there shall be a certain amount of physical training in all the schools of the State. New school buildings are being equipped with gymnasiums and sometimes with swimming pools, and teachers are engaged who have had special training in physical education with a view to teaching the young. Normal schools and universities are establishing courses in physical education for teachers in the public schools so that they may direct the physical training of the young, and the enrollment in these courses is increasing with extraordinary rapidity. There can be little doubt that we have entered upon a program which if carried through to completion will secure better physical development and better health among school children than has been the case in the past. *Physical Education as a Regular Part of School Work*

There is one movement which promises to accomplish a good deal in promoting the physical development and the health of our young people, and this is the establishment of playgrounds in towns and cities, and even in rural sections, and arranging the work of children of all ages so that every day they will have opportunity for plays *The Establishment of Playgrounds for all Children* and games. There is apparently complete agreement among those who have charge of the care and culture of the young that health and physical development can be promoted more effectually by plays and games than by formal gymnastics, though the latter have a place in the child's physical education. Everywhere there is an insistent demand that a playground be established within the reach of pupils in every school, and that it be properly equipped and be under the supervision of a trained play leader. A slogan frequently heard throughout our country to-day is,—"Playground facilities for every child in elementary and high schools!" High schools and universities are endeavoring to secure adequate playground space so that every student may have an opportunity to participate in games. Some high schools and colleges are requiring all students to play one or more games as a regular feature of their program. Swimming is being made a requirement for graduation in some places.

Country Children are Least Well Provided for

One often hears it said that the children in the city are greatly handicapped because they have no place for games and plays except the street, but that the children in the towns and in the country are more fortunate, since they have plenty of open space in which to play. But, as a matter of fact, most towns and country districts have inadequate facilities for play. In some such communities recently visited by the writer, little effort has been made to provide opportunities for games and plays. The children are often limited to a vacant lot; but even if vacant lots could be used for play, they are usually not suitable therefor, since it is rare that one can find such a lot which is adapted to baseball, football, or any of the tag games, and certainly not for any gymnastic activities.

The country school building is often located on a small plot of ground which does not afford sufficient space for the games and plays which children like and in which they should indulge. The farmers protest if the pupils make

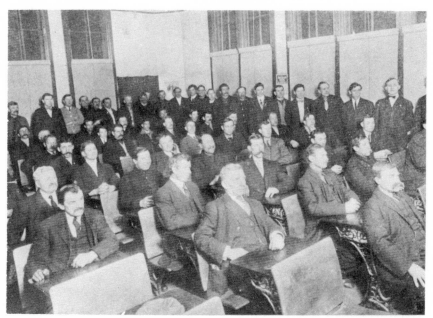

Many nationalities gather at the public schools to gain knowledge and inspiration.

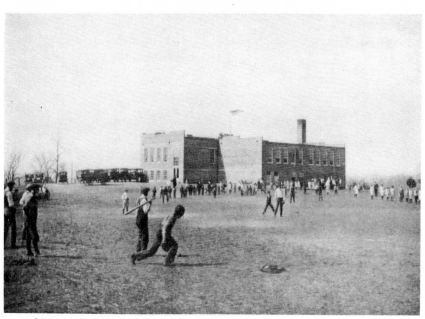

Memorial Consolidated School, Hart County, Kentucky, provides for athletics and games.

use of the fields adjoining the school grounds for any of their games. In some rural districts the teacher is under constant criticism because her pupils over-run the property adjoining the school, when they do not have room to play their games on the school grounds. Some important surveys of country life recently have been completed and they show that, except in rare instances, no one has devoted time or thought to providing facilities for plays and games for children in the country.

Fortunately, the country roads as well as the untilled fields and the woods afford opportunities for the young to play some of the games in which they take delight; but they do not provide for all their needs. The children in the typical country school have no place where they can play baseball, for instance, or football or basketball or any of the ball games of which they are passionately fond. Country children, contrary to popular belief, do not play as great a variety of games as children in towns or cities where there are playgrounds. They are handicapped particularly in respect to facilities for gymnastic activities, so that the city child who is within reach of a well-conducted playground is better off, even with all the disadvantages of city life, than the country child for whom no provision has been made.

The rapid drift of population to the cities makes the problem of promoting the health and physical development of the young largely an urban problem. In an earlier day, cities were planned as though children were not to live in them, or at least were not to enjoy any special rights in them. We have been hearing a good deal in the last few years about the rights of different groups of persons—women's rights, employers' rights, workers' rights, and so on. We have rarely heard anything said, until quite recently, though, about children's rights. Do they have any special rights? This is being very actively discussed now in a city which the writer

The Health and Physical Development of City Children

is studying. Many of the children have roller skates. Nearly every one of them has an express wagon or a coaster or a racer of some kind. They indulge in roller skating and operate their wagons on the sidewalks at all hours during the day. It need hardly be said that they make a lot of noise. Roller skating is a noisy pastime, and riding in a cart which does not have rubber tires is even noisier. A number of citizens in the city under observation have written to the newspapers complaining about the "frightful racket" which the children make. They say it has become so annoying that it is impossible to secure an hour's quiet anywhere in the city. Nervous people say they are made ill by these incessant, irritating noises. The police have been asked to put an end to the nuisance, but they are unwilling to proceed against the children, because they say there are no laws which make it an offense for children to skate or run carts on the sidewalks.

This is a typical problem which has to be solved sooner or later by every city of any size. Children who play on the streets of a crowded city are always a disturbing factor. They not only make noise but they get in the way of pedestrians and commerce. In some cities rigorous laws are put on the statute books compelling children to keep off the streets. If there are no public playgrounds, then they are required to play in their own homes. Of course, they often take a chance and try to play on the streets, but they are always being chased by the police and frequently penalties are inflicted upon them or their parents for violating the laws.

We are coming to see that no city can solve this problem satisfactorily which does not proceed on the principle that children as well as adults have rights which must be respected. Does this mean that children should be allowed to roller skate in a city whenever and wherever they choose, and also to operate their express cars, throw snowballs, roll hoops, and run over lawns? It means nothing of the kind. When a large proportion of the adults claim that they are irritated by the noise which the children make, the latter must be restrained to some extent. Either they must indulge in their noise-making activities in certain streets set aside for them or, if this is not feasible, then they must play their noisy games at certain times during the day and not at other times. Adults who are frightened by roller skates, carts, and the like might be able to work out a program so that for two hours each day, say, the children could engage in these pastimes, if during the rest of the day the adults could be sure that they would not be disturbed; but the latter should not be expected to submit to a regimen which will make it impossible for them to have any hour during the day when they can be free from irritation and annoyance.

Finally, something should be said regarding the movement to have all pupils in our schools pursue physiology and hygiene as a regular subject of study. It has been taken for granted that knowledge pertaining to the structure and function of the human body will lead a child to observe the laws of health. An interesting illustration of this general belief is found in the fact that in most States there are laws requiring that all pupils be given instruction regarding infectious diseases and the effects of alcohol and narcotics upon the human body; and many States are now considering the establishment of laws requiring instruction relating to sex hygiene, patent medicines, and other matters concerning health.

The Study of Physiology and Hygiene for the Promotion of Health and Physical Development

In all times, the majority of people have believed that knowledge will not only give power, but that it will influence conduct. At the same time the conviction has been deepening among educational people in our country that *knowing* and *doing* are two different and sometimes antagonistic things. One hears it said everywhere now

Will Knowledge Influence Conduct?

that a person may acquire learning without gaining wisdom. Since the days of John Locke, educational reformers have called attention to the failure of much of the learning of the schools to influence the behavior of the learners. The classic writers all seem to agree upon the principle that a child may learn rules pertaining to good behavior, but he may habitually act directly contrary to these rules.

Testimonies Regarding the Value of Physiology With a view to securing some first-hand information relating to the outcome of the study of physiology in the schools upon the health habits of pupils, the writer has had a large number of university students write out a detailed account of their own experience in regard to the matter; and people in various walks of life have contributed to the investigation. These persons have all had the ordinary instruction in physiology. Most of the students could give the names of many of the bones of the body and accurately locate them. They could give the names of the more important vital organs, locate them, and describe their structure and principal functions. They could also state a number of rules relating to the character and quantity of food required, the methods of preparing it for assimilation in the organism, the hygiene of breathing, exercise, bathing, of abstinence from alcohol and tobacco, and the like.

But the testimonies of these persons regarding the influence of this learning upon their health habits were negative in the majority of cases. All of the subjects stated that they had memorized statements to the effect that drinking ice water was harmful to health, but two-thirds of them indulged in it without restraint. They had memorized rules regarding the thorough mastication of food, but practically all of them testified that they had given no attention to the matter until the recent popular agitation about "Fletcherizing" had attracted their attention. The men had all learned that tobacco is injurious to health and efficiency; but the majority of them used it in one form or another. These students had memorized rules to the effect that health could be preserved only when one retired early and rose early, but hardly a student had observed this rule. They all declared that what they had been put through in physiology had exerted little or no influence upon their habits in regard to sleep or work. Again, most of the students had learned in their books that candy is injurious to the digestive organs and the teeth; but not one student in ten refrained from eating sweets because of this instruction. The list of instances showing how instruction had failed to influence conduct might be extended *ad libitum*.

Among those who gave testimony in this inquiry were a number of students of medicine. Of course, medical students have a more extensive knowledge of the structure of the human body than have students of arts and letters; and one might expect that the former would practice rules of hygiene more fully than the latter, or than laymen in general. But the medical students said that in no respect did they live more hygienically than do people who have little or no knowledge of the construction of the body. They testified that they, as do most physicians, used tobacco freely; that they did not abstain totally from alcoholic drinks; that they were not more temperate and restrained in their dietetic habits than are other people. According to the observation of the writer, no more regard is paid to securing fresh air in a classroom or convention hall of physicians than of lawyers or ministers or farmers. Medical students are apparently less restrained in regard to the use of tobacco and alcohol than are those studying for the ministry or for teaching; but it is not the study of physiology which has developed hygienic habits among ministers and teachers; it is the traditions of their professions.

Why has so much of the instruction in physiology and

Testimony of Medical Students

443

Why Has the Study of Physiology Been so Fruitless? hygiene in the past failed to take effect in conduct? The reason seems clear; the instruction has been too technical, too anatomical, too cold, and too remote from the everyday life of pupils. Memorizing technical terms about bodily structure or rules about general hygiene will not influence conduct greatly so far as health matters are concerned. Again, the aim of preserving health merely as a formal or moral idea does not appeal strongly to the typical boy or girl. We have to reckon first with the indifference which children manifest toward health. Primitive man, whose heir the child of to-day is, had to bolt his food and to pay little attention to its quality. He probably never thought of having a balanced ration, but ate what he could get and had his fill of it. In various other ways primitive man was indifferent to conditions which if ignored to-day would seriously lessen the individual's vitality or eliminate him altogether. As the arts of civilizations have increased, and man has been freed from his subjection to nature, he has at the same time lost some of his original resistance to discomfort and disease. It is this difference between primitive and civilized life, with the child tending to live on a primitive program under conditions of civilization, that makes instruction in hygiene at once imperative and unusually difficult.

The First Aim in Hygiene Teaching As suggested in Chapter XIX, the first thing to aim at in instruction in hygiene is to lead the child to appreciate that certain health habits will make him more efficient than he otherwise could be in attaining the ends which he wishes to achieve. If it can be made apparent to him in a very concrete, dramatic way that preserving his teeth, chewing his food thoroughly, restraining himself in the use of candy, taking his food at regular times, breathing through his nostrils, having fresh air in his sleeping room, avoiding extreme fatigue, bathing at regular intervals, changing his clothing if it becomes wet—that in these ways he can gain more strength, be more alert, have greater endurance, and so on, he will be in a frame of mind to profit by his instruction. This will be particularly true if the teacher can show that the boys and men in the community who excel in dynamic activities owe their superiority to their hygienic life.

We are beginning to appreciate further, that it holds in physiology and in hygiene as in other studies, that instruction in order to be effective must be adapted to the particular interests and needs of the individuals for whom it is designed. This means that what is taught in the eighth grade may not be well suited for the fifth grade and *vice versa*. Knowledge which might prove of great practical advantage in the life of the adolescent may be wholly without value for a child nine or ten years of age. It is a fundamental principle of development that knowledge will take effect in the life of the individual only when it is related to his needs and interests. Human nature is not so constituted that an immature individual can store up knowledge in anticipation of some future time of need. Knowledge so acquired will either remain dormant or it will be eliminated altogether. That knowledge alone will persist which plays some rôle in determining the individual's welfare in his everyday efforts at adaptation to the environment around him. *(Instruction Must Be Adapted to Age and Special Needs)*

The World War revealed a surprising situation in respect to the health and physical development of our people. Even Federal health authorities were impressed by the evidence of the inferior physical condition of young men at a time in life when bodily and mental vigor should be at the maximum. *(Summary)*

Our people are becoming thoroughly aroused to the necessity of providing for better physical development of our young people than we have had heretofore. Many national, state, and local organizations have been and are being formed for the purpose of investigating the health conditions of the young and using effective means to improve these conditions. The first step in promoting the health and physical development of school children is improvement in the hygiene of school buildings. It has been shown that a considerable part of the mal-development and ill-health of children is due to the fact that we compel all our young people to spend several hours a day for about forty weeks a year and for at least eight years in school buildings that are often not hygienic in respect to ventilation, seating, or lighting.

The hygiene of the school program is being investi-gated. Already we are relieving young children of fine, highly coördinated tasks. We are constructing the daily program so that pupils will not be kept seated for long periods at a time. Opportunities are being provided for a variety of games and plays every day.

The problem of malnourishment is being studied, and effective remedies are being applied. The conviction is becoming widespread that in towns and cities, our children are being injured by overstimulation and many persons are working on the problem of securing less stimulating environments for children both in the home and in the school. We are endeavoring to work out a program which will make it possible for pupils to secure periods of quiet and relaxation every day.

In order to promote the physical well-being of our children, we are providing medical inspection of school pupils not only in the cities but also in the rural schools. Certain States have enacted laws requiring health inspec-tion of pupils in all schools, rural as well as urban.

Physical education is becoming a regular part of school work. In some States, teachers must have training in physical education and must conduct this work in their schools. Playgrounds are being established in connection with public schools. There is a movement now starting

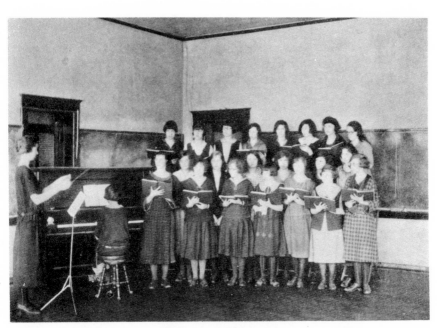

Girls' Glee Club, Spartanburg School, Randolph County, Indiana.

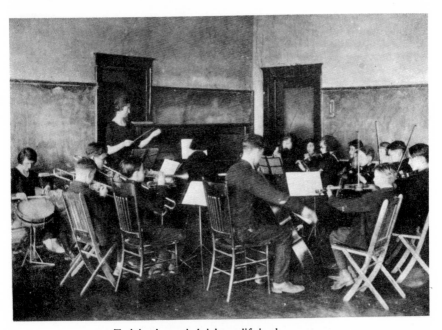

Training in music brightens life in the country.

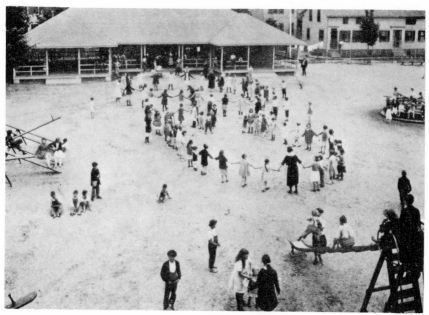

Children learn valuable social lessons in coöperating in their play.

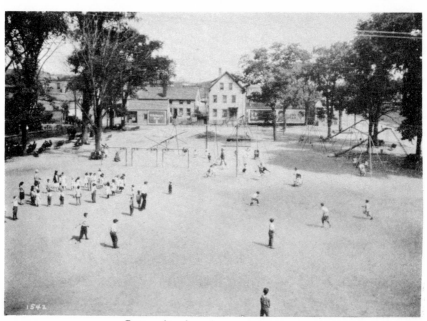

Coöperation through competitive games.

to provide playgrounds and playdays for country children, who have been largely overlooked heretofore.

Our chief problem to-day is to promote the health and physical development of urban children, since a majority of children now live under urban conditions. It is beginning to be appreciated that children in the cities have a right to use the streets for play, if there is not adequate provision in playgrounds; and cities are recognizing this right by setting aside certain streets for certain kinds of play, such as coasting.

The study of physiology and hygiene is to-day being required of all pupils in every progressive community. This study aims to develop health habits in respect to diet, posture, sleep, exercise, the care of the teeth, of the skin, etc., etc. It is the aim to have instruction in hygiene properly adapted to the age and special needs of the children for whom it is designed.

XXI

EXTENDING EDUCATIONAL FACILITIES, OPPORTUNITIES, AND REQUIREMENTS

In America the School is the Most Conspicuous and Imposing Social Institution

THE maxim of American teachers, boards of education, and a large majority of laymen at the present time seems to be,—"The more education the better for the individual, the community, the State, and the nation." As evidence that our people are devoted to the increase of educational facilities, opportunities, and requirements in every direction, one has but to make an inspection trip throughout the country and observe what is taking place in the way of providing new school buildings and elaborate equipment, and extending the school year and the period of compulsory education. The most prominent and imposing buildings in all sections of the country are those devoted to education. They always make a deep impression upon visitors from foreign countries, and many of our own people speak in complimentary terms of our magnificent educational plants. In the Old World, the buildings that attract attention are mainly the cathedrals, mosques, parliaments, and military establishments. But in our country the school buildings dominate the landscape. The different wards in cities vie with one another in erecting structures that compel admiration on account of their architectural beauty and their massiveness.

Whether or not our people have consciously accepted the principle that the well-being of a people depends chiefly upon thoroughgoing education of the young, they are at least putting the principle into practice. It would not, of course, be quite true to the facts to say that all our people approve the expansion of the educational program, involving the expenditure of vast sums of money for buildings, equipment, and teachers, and involving also increasing demands upon the time and attention of the young. It should be added, though, that those who are hostile to the extension of our educational work have not been able thus far to retard educational expansion in an important degree.

Those who are leading in the enlargement of our program are proceeding on the principle that as a nation develops, its educational opportunities, facilities, and requirements must be increased. They hold that when the expansion of the educational program is arrested, the development of a people will be arrested at the same time. They point to certain countries of the Old World as an illustration of the apparent law that a nation goes forward in its material, intellectual, political, social, and moral development just in the measure that its educational program is enlarged to provide for the increasing complexity of life in the community, State, and nation. The progress of a people means increasing knowledge in respect to every phase of human life, regarded individually or politically. When a people cease to add to knowledge affecting human welfare, they cease to make advance in the arts of civilization, and apparently they begin to return in their course. There have not been many nations that have remained static for a long period; when they have not gone forward, they have gone backward. One can go around the Mediterranean Sea and observe numerous illustrations of this apparent law. Nature seems to say to a people: "Keep going forward or your days will be numbered."

As a Nation Develops, Its Educational Program Must be Increased

As society grows more complex, and knowledge essential to the maintenance of its stability and the promotion of its welfare is increased, it is imperative, of course, that the young should be put into possession of this knowledge so that it will not be necessary for them to begin where their ancestors began, and re-discover the arts of living. This is why schools are maintained,—so that the young may take advantage of the experiences of their forbears in solving the problems of individual and social life. Primitive people, whose society is extremely simple, do not need schools because there is not much knowledge to transmit to the oncoming generations; but a highly developed people need highly developed schools in order to maintain the position which they have reached in their development. If the schools cannot transmit to the young the knowledge which their predecessors have accumulated, then a people begin to return in their course. One can see just this thing happening to-day in some of the countries of the Old World. They are not as strong, stable, and prosperous as they were several centuries ago. Certain of these countries had attained to a high degree of culture, but their schools were not developed so that they could pass on this culture to future generations and it is passing out of the life of the people. Remains of earlier culture may be seen in the churches, art galleries, museums, and other institutions but the people have not assimilated the culture, so that they are dropping backward instead of going forward in civilization. And once a people begin to go downward, it seems that nothing can stop them. They lose their enthusiasm for knowledge and return inevitably to a point where practically their sole interest consists in securing indulgence of their appetites.

The More Education the Better So the slogan of our people—"The more education the better for individual and social well-being"—is unquestionably based upon true and profound principles of human nature. And how are we putting our slogan into effect? First of all, we are increasing the number of days each year that the young may and *must* attend school. Probably some readers can remember when children attended the rural school for not more than one hundred days, at the most, in any one year; and in some States the majority of rural pupils did not attend more than seventy-five days in any year until quite recently. But at the present time many States require a yearly attendance of at least one hundred fifty days, and we are apparently moving in the direction of a program which will require that every rural school pupil must attend school between the ages of six and fourteen for at least two hundred days every year. In town and city schools in most sections of the country, pupils are now required to be in school from one hundred eighty to two hundred days each year from the age of six to fourteen.

Our people are not yet satisfied with the length of the school year. Everywhere throughout our country voices are being raised in favor of all-year schools. During the last decade, boards of education in various places have taken action looking toward the curtailment of the long vacation. Many of the superintendents who have recently reported upon the desirability of having school the year 'round have said that the only barrier to continuous sessions in their several communities is the financial one. If they could obtain the necessary funds to meet expenses, they would immediately go onto the all-year program.

Not every one who has expressed himself on the subject favors an all-year school. Some say that both children and teachers need substantially three months in the summer to recuperate from nine months intellectual work. Still others maintain that the summer time is not suitable for school activities. Most parents who have offered their opinions upon this topic have expressed themselves in favor of a longer session than we now have, because they appreciate that it is a difficult matter to keep children happily and wholesomely occupied for three months at a stretch; but there are some parents

The Pros and Cons on an All-Year School

who have said that they do not want to keep their children in school during the summer because they prefer to have them spend the time in travelling or in the study of nature out of doors. Farming people—some of them, not all of them—think their children ought to help in the fields during the summer after they have reached the age of ten. Our present plan of part-year schools was instituted long ago largely in deference to the wish of farming people who needed their children to work in the fields several months each year. Only a very small fraction of our young people are now required to work in the fields or have an opportunity to do so, but in most places we still continue to shut up our schools during the summer months.

It has been shown that pupils who are out of school for ten or twelve weeks during the summer lose much that they have gained during the nine months while they are in school, and it takes some time at the opening of school in the fall to recover lost ground. Pupils not only forget what they learn but they slip back into habits which make it difficult for them to apply themselves to intellectual pursuits. This latter consequence of the long vacation is probably the most serious of all. It is difficult at best in present-day American life to develop habits of concentrated application among pupils; there is so much that is distracting going on outside of the schoolroom and the home that pupils are continually lured away from their studies. The motion picture theatre, the pool hall, the dance hall, the automobile, the playground, the call of the street,—all make a tremendous appeal to young persons of both sexes. Intellectual work seems dull and uninteresting in comparison with these exciting emotional activities in the world outside the school. Even rural school pupils feel the lure of the town and the city, because many of them now have automobiles so that the motion picture theatre, the dance hall, and other seductions are practically as near to them as if they actually lived in the city.

The records of juvenile courts show, and the testimony of parents reinforce the court records, that young people engage in disorderly conduct more frequently during the long vacations than at any other season of the year. A boy or girl who frequently attends motion pictures, the pool rooms, or dance halls, and who does not have regular occupation during the day, will be very likely to think up mischief. Systematic intellectual application is the best antidote to the unwholesome influence of places of amusement in contemporary life. In fact, the only safeguard of young persons who indulge in the dissipations of these times is mental application for a number of hours every day for at least five days in the week. When boys and girls are left without occupation for two or three months at a stretch, the chances are that some of them will commit offenses against the customs and conventions and possibly against the laws of the communities in which they live.

There is another important reason why our people are beginning to think that we should conduct schools on an all-year program. The countries in Europe which are our rivals in competition for commercial supremacy are quickening the pace in their educational work. They are considering the establishment of all-year school programs, and they are even developing an extensive night-school régime. They know that the nations that will lead in the future are those that can accomplish the most in their schools. The wars hereafter will probably be fought more largely in the schoolrooms than on the battle fields of the world. We have thus far had an advantage over most nations, probably all of them, in our educational work, but unless we enlarge our present program, we may drop behind in the procession of the nations.

The Educational Race Among the Nations

Should We Extend the School Day? We must in the future accomplish more during the school life of our children than we have been able to do heretofore, and so we must have them under school influences for a larger portion of their time than we have had them in the past. There is no escape from this requirement if we are to meet the new conditions in the world. There is widespread belief that we ought not to make the school day longer than it now is in most places; but in any community which is provided with playgrounds, it might prove of advantage if they could be placed under the direction of school authorities so that pupils could be subjected to school influences during the entire day. Also, if our schools could all be provided with well equipped manual arts and household arts laboratories, pupils might with advantage to their intellectual development and without prejudice to their health or recreation, spend an hour or two in manual and household activities beyond the regular school day. But we must gain more time for school work mainly by utilizing the long vacation. In some cities it would be of advantage to pupils if they could be in school Saturday forenoon instead of being left with nothing to do except to run the streets. School buildings are the most sanitary and healthful places in many communities, and most children are better off in them than they are in their own homes or on the streets. This is not true in all communities, but it is true in a great many of them.

A Hygienic Program of School Work It has been urged in the past that pupils would become mentally and nervously fatigued unless they could have two days' vacation each week and three months' vacation in the summer. Modern studies have shown that the best way to avoid fatigue from intellectual work is to have frequent relaxation periods. From the standpoint of conserving energy and avoiding overstrain in school work, it would be better to follow an all-year program in which there would be five or six one-week vacations scattered

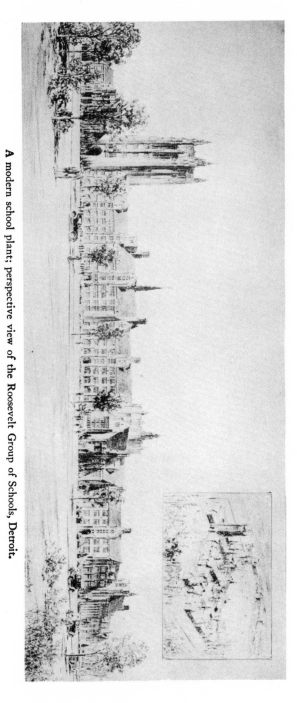

A modern school plant; perspective view of the Roosevelt Group of Schools, Detroit.

throughout the year, with one-day vacations each week, and several relaxation periods during each school day. It is a wasteful plan to crowd children until they become fatigued and then have a very long break for recuperation. When one actually becomes fatigued nervously, it is a slow process for him to regain his accustomed vigor, whereas if he could have a relaxation period before he becomes fatigued, his energies would be more readily restored.

Of course, an all-year session presents difficult problems from the teacher's standpoint, but these problems have been solved in normal schools and colleges that have practically continuous sessions. A few years ago, all higher educational institutions had a three-months' vacation in the summer, and now practically none of them follow this program. It can be arranged in the public schools, as it is in colleges and normal schools, so that teachers can have long vacations when they need them for study or rest. This plan is already in operation in many places. There are barriers to be surmounted, but our people are becoming disposed to work out a program to surmount them.

Many cities are attempting to solve the practical problems of an all-year school, and various plans are being tried out; they differ in details but agree in the fundamental aim of providing facilities and opportunities for school work during the summer months. Some cities have established an extra term and have called it a summer school. A few have instituted summer work especially to help backward children. As an instance of the tendency of the times in respect to the establishment of an all-year school, the action of Mason City, Iowa, may be mentioned. The year is divided into four quarters of twelve weeks each. During the summer months, the forenoon session begins at eight o'clock and continues until twelve o'clock. It is devoted to regular work with

Various Plans for an All-Year School

a liberal amount of supervised play. The afternoon session is devoted to supervised play, field sports, and folk games.

Seattle established an all-year school in 1923. The attendance the first summer was very large; many more pupils attended than were expected. It was planned to make the summer work of value especially to those who were able to push ahead of their grade, and also those who were behind in their work and needed assistance in order to be promoted.

Extending the Compulsory School Age

Not only are we striving to work out feasible plans for an all-year session of public schools in order to economize time in education and save the waste due to a long summer vacation; we are also working out programs for extending the compulsory school age. It has been thought heretofore that pupils ought not to be required to remain in school after they had reached their fourteenth birthday; but in all the more progressive States in our country now, a child is not permitted to detach himself completely from school at the age of fourteen. He must at least attend a vocational or continuation school for part of his time until he is sixteen, and in Wisconsin, for instance, until he is eighteen years of age. If after the age of fourteen he takes a position in a store, a factory, a shop, or a bank, his employer must allow him enough time off each week to meet the requirements of the compulsory education law.

In some sections of the country the educational system is being reconstructed in certain particulars so as to encourage pupils to continue in school full time until they are eighteen. Formerly the elementary school comprised eight years and the last year was conducted as though it were a finishing year. When the length of the elementary school period was settled upon originally, it was the belief of those who decided it that only a very few children in a community would continue their schooling beyond the eighth grade. So the elementary school became an educational unit sharply marked off from the secondary school unit. The program of the former was worked out on the theory that it must provide all the education which at least ninety-five per cent of the children in a community would receive. The secondary school program was constituted on the theory that its proper function should be to prepare pupils for college; the studies and the methods of presenting them universally adopted in the secondary schools had reference solely to the requirements of entrance upon college studies. No attention was paid to the so-called practical needs of secondary school pupils.

But the courses of study in the public high schools to-day are administered largely without reference to special requirements for entrance upon college work. It is true that in every high school in a community of five thousand or more inhabitants there is a course of study offered which is designed principally as a preparation for college, but this course does not absorb a large part of the time and energy of teachers and of the resources of the high school. The college preparatory course is subordinate to other courses in the typical American high school to-day; the organization and administration of the high school is conducted mainly, though not entirely, with a view to meeting the needs of pupils even if they do not go any farther in their schooling. The high school to-day is really a continuation of the elementary school, not a separate unit detached from the first unit and administered for an altogether different purpose.

During the past decade an institution has been developing the purpose of which is to facilitate transition from the elementary to the high school, and this is the junior high school. It is often spoken of as the connecting link, and those who originated it and who are responsible now for its development have really had in view the

The Junior High School

457

establishment of a school which would bridge the chasm between the elementary and the high school so that there would be one continuous school from the kindergarten to the senior year of the high school. The rapidity with which the junior high school is being adopted in small as well as in large communities is evidence that we are moving onto a program wherein a large proportion of pupils will continue in school full time for twelve years. It may be predicted that the compulsory full-time period will soon be extended to the eighteenth year, or to the completion of twelve years of standard educational work, even if some pupils must take thirteen or fourteen years to complete it.

Enforcing Compulsory Education Laws

A few years ago, the Russell Sage Foundation conducted an investigation to determine the success which the various States were having in enforcing compulsory education laws. The investigation revealed the fact that the total number of days spent in school by children in certain States was only one-half or one-third of the number of days spent in school by children in other States. It was found that some of the States were so lax in enforcing the compulsory education laws that many children of school age did not attend school at all after nine or ten. Even in such a progressive State as Ohio, it was discovered that parents frequently kept their young children out of school to work and nobody said anything about it. A number of southern States practically ignored compulsory education laws, and they were shown up when it was revealed during the World War that a surprisingly large proportion of drafted men could not read or write. A small percentage of them were foreign born; but most of them were born and bred in the United States. The results of these investigations have impressed our people with the fact that while we have provided a complete and exceedingly expensive educational system, some of our children have not enjoyed the advantages thereof.

The State of Ohio has already been referred to; it has just enacted a law which will make it possible for school officers to keep every child of school age in school every day during the school year, provided he is physically and mentally capable, and making exceptions only for extraordinary circumstances such as a death in a family. The problem of regular school attendance in States like Ohio is in the way of being solved. Every teacher in the State becomes an assistant to attendance officers in locating children of school age in her district or ward and seeing to it that every such child is in school continuously unless he is incapacitated.

Heretofore the attendance problem has been most serious in rural schools. Farmers in some sections of the country have thought nothing of keeping children out of school who could work any time when there was work to be done. During the last two or three years, when the attendance problem has been receiving special attention at educational meetings, the writer has heard teachers in rural schools in almost every State say that when there was any work that children could do on the farm, it was impossible to keep them in school. This is one reason why children reared in the country are at a disadvantage as compared with city children in respect to the breadth and thoroughness of their education. If the schooling of boys and girls reared in the country can be broken into whenever there are any chores to be done at home, it is certain that they will be handicapped in maturity. Educational men as well as laymen everywhere are aroused to the seriousness of this problem, and there is a determination sweeping over our country to *compel* country children to go to school and to remain in school as regularly and for as long a period each year as do the children in towns or cities.

It must be acknowledged that regular attendance at school is not considered to be necessary in sections of the

Parents from Foreign Countries Often Resist Compulsory Laws

country where there are parents who have come from countries where no effort has been made to get pupils int school and keep them there for eight or ten years. In some of these countries, the favored classes have encouraged parents in the less favored classes to keep their children out of school and make them work. These parents have brought such notions to our country, and they do not now understand why it is necessary that their children should go to school, and they are sometimes in a rebellious and defiant attitude. The writer knows from experience that it is not easy to convince some of these parents that they have no right whatsoever to handicap a child by keeping him out of school to work. A resourceful teacher can frequently win over an obstinate parent so that he will willingly keep his children in school during at least the compulsory school period; but if he cannot be won over, we are coming to believe that he must be *compelled* to keep his children in school.

The Truancy Problem

Of course, there are children who play truant whose parents do not keep them out of school to work. There is scarcely a district or town or city in our country which does not have to deal with the truant problem. Nature has endowed some boys and girls with such strong nomadic impulses that she seems to say to them: "You must keep out in the open. You cannot stand it if you sit in school three or four hours a day. It will be better for you to run away from school and even from home and hunt in the woods, or fish or swim or hide in straw stacks and steal your food from farmers, or join a gang and make raids on fruit shops, candy stores, and the like."

Fortunately, we are reducing truancy in some measure by making school life less irksome for boys and girls who feel an irresistible longing to be constantly doing something adventurous. The writer knows of schools which are being conducted so that there is but slight temptation for boys or girls to play truant. They are given a good deal of manual work and have opportunity for games and plays; and they even like their reading, number, geography, and history lessons because they are made concrete and interesting. It is not impossible that the time may come when we shall be able to teach children so that even the most restless of them will about as soon be in the school as to be climbing trees, throwing stones, roaming about the country, or forming gangs and fighting other gangs.

But the schools in most places are not yet able to prevent truancy, and so there must be officers who will keep track of truants and see that they conform to the law and remain in school full time every day when it is in session until they are at least fourteen years of age. These truant or probation officers have a very important and at the same time a very delicate task to perform. Rough, unsympathetic men can do and have done great harm both to the children who are truants and even to their parents, who are sometimes in sympathy with them. As suggested above, there are families in many communities, usually fresh from the Old World, in which there is a lack of appreciation of the need of keeping children in school until they are fourteen years of age or older. Most—fortunately not all—foreigners think their children should begin to work so as to increase the income of the family when they reach the age of nine or ten. Truant or probation officers have a difficult task to make such persons understand the American ideal in educating all children, whether or not the parents wish to have them educated.

The Problem of the Truant or Probation Officer

We are coming to accept the view that truant officers should be connected with the office of the county or city superintendent of schools in every community and not with the courts. They certainly should not be agents of the courts. A truant should not be regarded as a criminal and he should not be dealt with by any one who acts for the courts. Parents who do not keep their children in school should not in the first instance be regarded as criminals and should not be dealt with by court officers.

Heretofore, truant and probation officers have as a rule had no training whatsoever for their special work. They have often been selected because of their rough-shod ways with people. This has been due to the fact that a truant has been regarded as a criminal who needed chastisement. An officer who regards truants from this standpoint is likely to do them more harm than good.

It is being emphasized by educational people to-day that a truant officer should have made special preparation for his work. He should be a student of child nature and of the sociological conditions which lead to truancy. He should know how to handle people diplomatically, and he should have sympathy with young persons who cannot restrain their impulses so that they can submit to the restrictions of the school. From one standpoint, it is not to the discredit of a boy that he feels a longing to be out in the open, living an adventurous life; and he should not be treated as though he were guilty of some heinous crime when he runs away from school. The task of the truant officer is to make the school seem attractive to the truant rather than to drive him into the school with the rod.

The Problem of the One-room Ungraded Rural School It may appear to some readers that while we are extending educational facilities, opportunities, and requirements for children in towns and cities we are not following the same program for children in rural sections. It must be acknowledged that in our educational progress the rural school has, speaking generally, lagged behind urban schools. But our people are aware of this fact and a considerable part of educational investigation to-day has reference to the devising of ways and means of improving rural education. The isolated, one-room school, which is still the dominant type of school found in rural sections throughout the country, is out of date in American life, and children living in the country who must attend such a school are seriously handicapped when compared with children who live in towns and cities. It is still regarded in some States as a matter of course that a child in a district or village school cannot have the educational advantages enjoyed by any child who can attend a town or city graded school. But the times are changing rapidly in respect to this matter. One may hear it said freely to-day in all sections of our country that a child reared in the country should receive as good schooling in every way as if he were reared in the city. This means that the one-room, isolated country school must be greatly improved, or it must be abandoned and in its place must be provided a community school as well equipped with capable teachers and with apparatus as are city graded schools.

The writer recently, spent some time in Colorado observing developments there in rural education. It is impressive and encouraging to observe the progress made in various sections of that State in developing consolidated community schools offering all the advantages of well-organized and well-conducted city graded schools. These schools are found scattered throughout the mountains, the valleys, and the plains of the State. The physical barriers to consolidation of schools in all parts of Colorado are as great as they are in most other States. The population is sparser than it is in many sections of our country. The weather in winter is more rigorous and the snow is deeper in the mountains and valleys than is the case in most other places. And yet, consolidation is going forward with rapidity and enthusiasm in every part of Colorado. Some of the consolidated school buildings are as attractive and as healthful, well-lighted, and well-equipped, as are the school buildings in the cities of any State. In a number of the counties, attractive homes adjoining the community

The Establishment of Consolidated or Community Rural Schools school buildings have been provided for the teachers. The pupils are brought to the schools and returned to their homes in auto busses that are warmed in winter, so that the trip to and from school is comfortable. These busses are operated by the teachers, at least in a number of the consolidated districts, who apparently enjoy this phase of their work as fully as they do their teaching.

There is slight chance that rural education can be greatly improved unless rural people will coöperate so that they can secure educational advantages equivalent to those of the city, in some such way as they are doing in the rural districts of Colorado, Indiana, Iowa, and other States. And a farmer who has the welfare of his children at heart will think better of a first-rate school located five miles away than of a tenth-rate school located at the turn of the road. Any good school that his children attend every day will be close enough in space and in spirit so that he will feel a personal interest in it. And when he sees what superior intellectual, social, and hygienic advantages he and his children gain from a well-equipped, well-conducted graded school, as compared with a poorly-equipped, ungraded, isolated school, he will not fail to give it his support. Such a school will be of direct service to him in his business as a farmer, whereas the one-room school can hardly ever be of any material assistance to him.

How Can Impoverished Communities Support an Enlarged Program? And we come now to a vital question: How can this great program of extension of educational facilities, opportunities, and requirements be supported by communities that are not well situated financially? The program which is being worked out in the more progressive and prosperous States is a very expensive one, and it would manifestly overtax the resources of less financially fortunate communities. A recent publication of the Bureau of Economic Research gives an estimate of the income of the people of a number of States. From this report we find that the per capita incomes in the States showing the lowest income are as follows: Alabama, $345; Mississippi, $352; Tennessee, $365; Arkansas, $379; North Carolina, $383; Kentucky, $392. Contrasted with these figures are those for the States in which the people enjoy a large income. These States show the following incomes per capita: Massachusetts, $788; Ohio, $789; Delaware, $792: New York, $874; California, $820; Nevada, $850.

Is there any way out of the difficulty of providing for an expanding educational program in communities and States that are not as well situated financially as are other communities and States? Our people are beginning to take the view that equal educational facilities and opportunities should be available for all our children, no matter where they may be born or reared. Because a child happens to be born and to be reared in an impoverished State or in a rural section of a wealthy State, is no reason, we are coming to see, why he should be handicapped in respect to his education at maturity as compared with a child born and reared in a prosperous State. A child brought up on a farm may not remain on the farm when he becomes mature. American life is so mobile that the country child is as likely to spend his mature years in a city as in the country; it should not be assumed that because he is born in a certain place he will remain there throughout his life. We are coming to see the educational bearings of the fact that society is so fluid in America that probably the majority of persons do not live out their lives in the place or under the social or economic conditions of their birth.

We are committed in America to the principle that education is essential to the welfare of every person, whether regarded as an individual or as a member of society. It has already been said that we are establishing rigid compulsory laws based upon this principle. We are constantly saying that a child who is trained by a capable

Equal Educational Opportunities for all the Young

teacher and in a well-equipped and hygienic school building will have an advantage over one taught by an inferior
teacher and in a poorly ventilated, poorly lighted, and
poorly equipped school. There is only one conclusion
to be drawn from these elementary principles,—we must
earnestly strive to equalize educational opportunities for
all our children, whether they live in a wealthy or in an
impoverished section, or in the country or in the village
or in the city. In order to accomplish this, the more
fortunate sections of a State in respect to financial
resources must assist the less fortunate sections. The
cities must help the rural districts to provide educational facilities equal to those enjoyed by city children.
The educational work of a State must be paid for mainly
or wholly from state funds, since education is properly
a state or national and not a local function. The nation
must equalize opportunities as between the wealthier
and the poorer States, so that children born and reared
in impoverished localities will be helped by contributions
from more prosperous sections. A child born and edu-
cited in Vermont or New Hampshire is about as likely
to become a resident of California, or Wisconsin, or
Massachusetts when he is mature as he is to live out his
life in Vermont or New Hampshire. When we really
appreciate this fact we will see the necessity, looking at
the matter from the standpoint of national well-being,
of providing as good educational opportunities for the
children in Vermont or New Hampshire as for the children
in California, Wisconsin, or Massachusetts. Doubtless
this will seem idealistic to some readers; but let all
doubters take note of the fact that we have already
entered upon this equalizing program, and it is being
carried forward successfully in some parts of the country.

Summary   The maxim of all our people seems to be: "The more
education the better for the individual, the community,
the State, and the nation." Anyone will be impressed

with the rôle which the school is playing in American life if he will take a trip through the country and observe our school buildings and facilities for carrying on school work; and we are constantly increasing our facilities and extending our opportunities and requirements.

We are appreciating that as a nation develops its educational program must be constantly enlarged. Nations that remain stationary educationally for a long period tend to go backward and ultimately to disappear altogether.

We are becoming convinced that we must require our pupils to spend more time each year in school than has been the practice heretofore; so we have gradually extended the school year until now plans are being formed in some places for the establishment of an all-year school. Already a few cities have adopted this program. The arguments in favor of an all-year school apparently outweigh the arguments against it.

There is a race among the nations for supremacy in respect to matters that depend upon education. Our people are awakening to this fact, and many of them already appreciate that we cannot hold our own unless our young people have more schooling than they have had in the past.

There is a tendency to enforce compulsory laws more rigorously than has been done in the past. Some States have recently enacted laws which will make it practically impossible for any boy or girl of school age to be absent from school except for sickness. Our people are becoming convinced that an uneducated individual is a menace to the community. The World War showed that a considerable proportion of our young men were illiterate. This revelation has strengthened our people in their conviction that no child in America should be permitted to escape at least an elementary school education.

The compulsory school age is being extended quite

generally throughout our country. In many sections a boy or girl must be in school for full time until fourteen years of age, and part time from fourteen to sixteen, seventeen, or even eighteen years of age.

Constant pressure is being put upon pupils to continue in school for full time after completing the elementary school curriculum. With a view to facilitating the transition from the elementary to the high school, the junior high school is being widely established. This is designed to bridge the gap between the elementary and the high school.

Our people are confronting a difficult problem in extending the compulsory school period or even enforcing attendance of all pupils for the length of the present compulsory period. Parents from foreign countries sometimes resist enforcement of compulsory laws; but there is an increasing determination on the part of our people to compel all parents to keep their children in school during the compulsory school age. Truant or probation officers are being appointed each year for the purpose of enforcing the compulsory laws.

The one-room rural school constitutes the most serious problem in present-day American education. The solution of the problem seems to be in the direction of consolidating one or two-room rural schools into graded community schools, properly equipped to do as efficient work as is done in the typical graded city school. The establishment of such consolidated schools has the effect universally to promote better attendance among rural school pupils.

BIBLIOGRAPHIES

I

BRIDGING THE GAP BETWEEN OUR KNOWLEDGE OF
CHILD NATURE AND THE TRAINING OF CHILDREN

1. Bagley, W. C. The Educative Process. New York, Macmillan Co., 1905.
2. Baldwin, B. T. Educational Research. U. S. Bureau of Education Bulletin 42, 1923.
3. Baldwin, B. T. An Introduction to Physical Measurements and Tests. Yonkers, N. Y., World Book Co. (In preparation.)
4. Baldwin, B. T., and Stecher, L. I. Mental Growth Curves of Normal and Superior Children. The Iowa Child Welfare Research Station Studies. Vol. II, No. 1, 1921.
5. Baldwin, J. M. Mental Development in the Child and the Race. New York, Macmillan Co., 1895.
6. Binet, A. and Simon, T. The Development of Intelligence in Children. Baltimore, Williams, & Wilkins, 1916.
7. Claparéde, E. Experimental Pedagogy and the Psychology of the Child. (Tr. by M. Loud and H. Hohman.) New York, Longmans, Green & Co., 1911.
8. Colvin, S. S., and Bagley, W. C. Human Behavior, a First Book in Psychology for Teachers. New York, Macmillan Co., 1918.
9. Dewey, J. The School and Society. Chicago, Univ. of Chicago Press, 1900.
10. Freeman, F. N. How Children Learn. Boston, Houghton Mifflin Co., 1917.
11. Froebel's Pedagogics of the Kindergarten. (Tr. by Josephine Janis.) New York, D. Appleton & Co., 1917.

12. Gates, A. Psychology for Students of Education. New York, Macmillan Co., 1923.

13. Hall, G. S. Youth, Its Education, Regimen and Hygiene. New York, D. Appleton & Co., 1906.

14. James, W. Talks to Teachers on Psychology and to Students on Life's Ideals. New York, H. Holt & Co., 1899.

15. Judd, C. H. Psychology for Teachers. New York, D. Appleton & Co., 1903.

16. Kirkpatrick, E. A. Fundamentals of Child Study. New York, Macmillan Co., 1917.

17. McCall, W. A. How to Measure in Education. New York, Macmillan Co., 1922.

18. Montessori, M. Montessori Method. (Tr. by A. S. George.) New York, F. A. Stokes Co., 1912.

19. Norsworthy, N., and Whitley, M. T. Psychology of Childhood. New York, Macmillan Co., 1918.

20. O'Shea, M. V. Dynamic Factors in Education. New York, Macmillan Co., 1907.

21. Pintner, R. Intelligence Testing. New York, H. Holt & Co., 1923.

22. Pyle, W. H. Psychology of Learning. An Advanced Text in Educational Psychology. Baltimore, Warwick & York, 1921.

23. Rousseau, J. J. Émile. Abridged. (Tr. and annotated by W. H. Payne.) New York, D. Appleton & Co., 1917.

24. Rugg, H. O. Statistical Methods Applied to Education. Boston, Houghton Mifflin Co., 1917.

25. Stern, W. The Psychological Method of Testing Intelligence. (Tr. by Whipple.) Baltimore, Warwick & York, 1914.

26. Terman, L. M. The Measurement of Intelligence. Boston, Houghton Mifflin Co., 1916.

27. Thorndike, E. L. The Principles of Teaching Based on Psychology. New York, A. G. Seiler, 1906.

28. Whipple, G. M. Manual of Mental and Physical Tests. Baltimore, Warwick & York, 1910.

II

THE CHILD'S INSTINCTS AND IMPULSES

1. Abbott, E. H.   On the Training of Parents.   Boston, Houghton Mifflin Co., 1908.
2. Anonymous.   A Young Girl's Diary.   New York, Thomas Selzer, 1921.
3. Birney, Mrs. T.   Childhood.   Chapter III.   New York, Stokes Co., 1905.
4. Hall, G. S., and others.   Aspects of Child Life and Education.   Chapters 6 and 7.   Boston, Ginn & Co., 1907.
5. Howard, W. L.   Start Your Child Right.   Chicago, F. H. Revell & Co., 1910.
6. Major, D. R.   First Steps in Mental Growth.   Chapter IV.   New York, Macmillan Co., 1906.
7. Moll, A.   The Sexual Life of the Child.   New York, Macmillan Co., 1912.
8. Norsworthy, N., and Whitley, M. T.   The Psychology of Childhood.   Chapters III, IV.   New York, Macmillan Co., 1918.
9. O'Shea, M. V.   First Steps in Child Training.   Valparaiso, Indiana, Lewis E. Myers & Co., 1920.
10. O'Shea, M. V.   Social Development and Education.   Boston, Houghton Mifflin Co., 1909.
11. Pyle, W. H.   Outlines of Educational Psychology.   Chapters III, IV, V.   Baltimore, Warwick & York, 1912.
12. Saleeby, C. W.   Parenthood and Race Culture.   New York, Moffatt, Yard & Co., 1909.
13. St. John, E. P.   Child Nature and Child Nurture.   Chapter IV.   Boston, Pilgrim Press, 1911
14. Thorndike, E. L.   Briefer Course in Educational Psychology.   New York, Teachers College, Columbia University, 1919.
15. Watson, J. B.   Psychology from the Standpoint of a Behaviorist.   pp. 198-206.   Philadelphia, J. B. Lippincott Co., 1918.
16. Wile, I. S.   Sex Education.   New York, Duffield & Co., 1912.

III

THE ACTIVE NATURE AND NEEDS OF CHILDHOOD

1. Campbell, Y. Practical Motherhood. New York, Longmans, Green & Co., 1910.
2. Curtis, Henry S. Education through Play. New York, Macmillan Co., 1915.
3. Dearborn, George V. Motor-Sensory Development. Baltimore, Warwick & York, 1910.
4. Fisher, Dorothy Canfield. Mothers and Children. New York, Holt & Co., 1915.
5. Fisher, Dorothy Canfield. A Montessori Mother. New York, Henry Holt & Co., 1912.
6. Johnson, G. E. Education by Plays and Games. Boston, Ginn & Co., 1907.
7. Lee, J. Play in Education. New York, Macmillan Co., 1921.
8. Major. First Steps in Mental Growth. New York, Macmillan Co., 1906.
9. O'Shea, M. V. Dynamic Factors in Education. New York, Macmillan Co., 1909.
10. Sies, A. C. Spontaneous and Supervised Play in Childhood. New York, Macmillan Co., 1922.
11. Smith, C. F. Games and Recreational Methods for Scouts, Camps, Clubs. New York, Dodd, Mead & Co., 1924.
12. Tyler, J. M. Growth and Education. Boston, Houghton Mifflin Co., 1907.

IV

THE DEVELOPMENT OF THE INTELLECT IN CHILDHOOD AND YOUTH

1. Book, W. F. Psychology of High School Seniors. Philadelphia, J. B. Lippincott & Co., 1922.
2. Dearborn, W. F., Shaw, E. A., Lincoln, E. A. A Series of Form Board and Performance Tests of Intelligence. Harvard Monographs in Education, Series I, No. 4. Harvard Graduate School of Education.
3. Jennings, H. S., and others. Suggestions of Modern Science Concerning Education. New York, Macmillan Co., 1917.

4. Kuhlmann, F. A. Handbook of Mental Tests. Baltimore, Warwick & York, 1922.
5. Norsworthy, N., and Whitley, M. T. The Psychology of Childhood. New York, Macmillan Co., 1918.
6. O'Shea, M. V. Mental Development and Education. New York, Macmillan Co., 1921.
7. Pintner, R. Intelligence Testing. New York, H. Holt & Co., 1923.
8. Pintner, R., and Patterson, D. G. A Scale of Performance Tests. New York, D. Appleton & Co., 1921.
9. Preyer, W. The Development of the Intellect. New York, D. Appleton & Co., 1895.
10. Terman, L. M. The Intelligence of School Children. Boston, Houghton Mifflin Co., 1919.
11. Terman, L. M. The Measurement of Intelligence. Boston, Houghton Mifflin Co., 1916.
12. Tracy, F. Psychology of Childhood. Boston, D. C. Heath & Co., 1909.

V

The Child's Moral Equipment and Development

1. Adler, F. Moral Instruction of Children. New York, D. Appleton & Co., 1892.
2. Coe, G. A. Law and Freedom in the School. Chicago, University of Chicago Press, 1924.
3. Dewey, John. Schools of To-Morrow. New York, E. P. Dutton & Co., 1915.
4. Dewey, E. New Schools for Old. New York, E. P. Dutton & Co., 1919.
5. Fisher, D. C. Self-Reliance. Indianapolis, Bobbs-Merrill Co., 1916.
6. Gould, F. J. Moral Instruction; Its Theory and Practice. New York, Longmans, Green & Co., 1913.
7. Griggs, E. H. Moral Education. New York, B. W. Huebsch, 1916.
8. Iowa Plan Character Education Methods. National Institution for Moral Instruction. Washington, D. C., 1923.

9. MacCunn, J. The Making of Character. New York, Macmillan Co., 1913.
10. Neumann, H. Education for Moral Growth. New York, D. Appleton & Co., 1923.
11. O'Shea, M. V. Social Development and Education. Boston, Houghton Mifflin Co., 1909.
12. Sharp, F. C. Education for Character. Indianapolis, Bobbs-Merrill Co., 1917.
13. Sneath, E. H., and Hodges, G. Moral Training in the School and Home. New York, Macmillan Co., 1913.

VI

The Social Traits of Childhood and Youth

1. Bolton, F. E. Everyday Psychology for Teachers. New York, Chas. Scribner's Sons, 1923.
2. Clark, T. A. The High School Boy and His Problems. New York, Macmillan Co., 1920.
3. Dewey, John. School and Society. Chicago, University of Chicago Press, 1907.
4. Dewey, John. Schools of To-Morrow. New York, E. P. Dutton & Co., 1915.
5. Hall, G. S. Aspects of Child Life and Education. Boston, Ginn & Co., 1907.
6. Howells, W. D. A Boy's Town. New York, Harper & Bros., 1890.
7. King, I. The High School Age. Indianapolis, Bobbs-Merrill Co., 1914.
8. Norsworthy, N., and Whitley, M. T. The Psychology of Childhood. New York, Macmillan Co., 1918.
9. O'Shea, M. V. Faults of Childhood and Youth. Valparaiso, Lewis E. Myers & Co., 1920.
10. O'Shea, M. V. First Steps in Child Training. Valparaiso, Lewis E. Myers & Co., 1920.
11. O'Shea, M. V. Social Development and Education. Boston, Houghton Mifflin Co., 1909.
12. O'Shea, M. V. The Trend of the Teens. Valparaiso, Lewis E. Myers & Co., 1920.
13. Puffer, J. A. The Boy and His Gang. Boston, Houghton Mifflin Co., 1912.

14. Romanes, G. J. Mental Evolution in Man. New York, D. Appleton & Co., 1889.
15. Sharp, F. C. Education for Character. Indianapolis, Bobbs-Merrill Co., 1917.
16. Swift, E. J. Youth and the Race. New York, Chas. Scribner's Sons, 1912.

VII

THE CHILD'S MASTERY OF THE ARTS OF EXPRESSION—
LANGUAGE, DRAWING, AND MUSIC

1. Clark, A. W. Public School Penmanship. Boston, Ginn & Co., 1909.
2. Colby, L. E. Talks on Drawing, Painting, Decorating for Primary Teachers. Chicago, Scott, Foresman & Co., 1909.
3. Freeman, F. N., and Dougherty, M. L. How to Teach Handwriting. Boston, Houghton Mifflin Co., 1923.
4. Freeman, F. N. Psychology of the Common Branches. Boston, Houghton Mifflin Co., 1916.
5. Kendall, C. N. and Mirick, G. A. How to Teach the Special Subjects. Boston, Houghton Mifflin Co., 1918.
6. Lemos, P. J. Applied Art, Drawing, Painting, Design, and Handicraft. Mountain View, Cal., Pacific Press Pub. Assn., 1920.
7. O'Shea, M. V. Linguistic Development and Education. New York, Macmillan Co., 1907.
8. O'Shea, M. V. Mental Development and Education. Chapter VI. New York, Macmillan Co., 1921.
9. Parker, S. C. Types of Elementary Teaching and Learning. Boston, Ginn & Co., 1923.
10. Patterson, A. How to Speak. Boston, Houghton Mifflin Co., 1922.
11. Row, R. K. The Educational Training of the Manual Arts and Industries. Chicago, Row, Peterson & Co., 1909.
12. Sargent, W. Fine and Industrial Arts in Elementary Schools. Boston, Ginn & Co., 1912.

VIII

BRIDGING THE GAP BETWEEN OUR KNOWLEDGE OF CHILD WELL-BEING AND OUR CARE OF THE YOUNG

1. Gesell, A. The Pre-School Child. Boston, Houghton Mifflin Co., 1923.
2. Goddard, H. H. Human Efficiency and Levels of Intelligence. Princeton, N. J., Princeton Univ. Press, 1922.
3. Goddard, H. H. Juvenile Delinquency. New York, Dodd, Mead & Co., 1921.
4. Hall, G. S. Adolescence. New York, D. Appleton & Co., 1904.
5. Lucas, W. P. The Health of the Runabout Child. New York, Macmillan Co., 1923.
6. Mateer, F. The Unstable Child. New York, D. Appleton & Co., 1924.
7. Miller, H. C. The New Psychology and the Teacher. New York, Thomas Selzer, 1922.

IX

RELATION OF NUTRITION TO MENTAL DEVELOPMENT

1. Baldwin, Bird T. The Physical Growth of Children from Birth to Maturity. University of Iowa, Studies in Child Welfare, Vol. I, No. 1, 1921.
2. Barker, L. F. How to Avoid Spoiling the Child. Mental Hygiene, Vol. III, No. 2, April 1919.
3. Burnham, W. H. Success and Failure. Boston, Massachusetts Society for Mental Hygiene, 1919.
4. Emerson, W. R. P. Nutrition and Growth in Children. New York, D. Appleton & Co., 1922.
5. Holt, L. E. Food, Health, and Growth. New York, Macmillan Co., 1922.
6. McCollum, E. V. The Newer Knowledge of Nutrition. New York, Macmillan Co., 1922.
7. Robinson, J. H. Mind in the Making. New York, Harper & Bros., Physical 1921.
8. Rude, A. E. Physical Status of Pre-School Children, Gary, Indiana. Government Printing Office, 1922.

X

Nervous and Mental Hygiene Among Children in Present-Day Life

1. Emerson, L. E. Nervousness, Its Causes, Treatment, and Prevention. Boston, Little, Brown & Co., 1918.
2. Flügel, J. C. The Psycho-Analytic Study of the Family. London, The International Psycho-Analytical Press, 1921.
3. Hinkle, B. M. The Re-Creating of the Individual. Chapter II. New York, Harcourt, Brace & Co., 1923.
4. International Conference of Women Physicians, Proceedings. The Health of the Child. New York, The Woman's Press, 1920.
5. Jones, Ernest. Papers on Psycho-Analysis. (3d edition.) Chapters XXXIV, XXXV, XXXVI, and XXXVII, particularly the last two. New York, W. Wood & Co., 1913.
6. Miller, H. C. The New Psychology and the Parent. New York, Thomas Selzer, 1922.
7. Miller, H. C. The New Psychology and the Teacher. New York, Thomas Selzer, 1922.
8. Patri, A. D. Child Training. New York, D. Appleton & Co., 1922.
9. Payne, G. H. The Child in Human Progress. New York, G. P. Putnam's Sons, 1916.
10. Positive Health Series. Pamphlet Four. Mental Health. New York, Women's Foundation for Health, Inc., 1922.
11. Wells, F. L. Mental Adjustments, New York, D. Appleton & Co., 1917.
12. White, W. A. The Mental Hygiene of Childhood. Boston, Little, Brown & Co., 1919.

XI

The Prevalence and Treatment of Sense Defects

1. Cornell, W. S. Health and Medical Inspection of School Children. Philadelphia, F. A. Davis Co., 1922.

2. Fisher, I., and Fisk, E. L.   How to Live.   New York, Funk and Wagnalls, 1922.
3. Hoag, E. B.   The Health Index of School Children. San Francisco, Whitaker & Ray-Wiggin Co., 1910.
4. Hough, T., and Sedgwick, W. T.   The Human Mechanism.   Boston, Ginn & Co., 1918.
5. Newmayer, S. W.   Medical and Sanitary Inspection of Schools.   Philadelphia, Lea & Febiger, 1913.
6. O'Shea, M. V., and Kellogg, J. H.   The Body in Health.   New York, Macmillan & Co., 1923.
7. O'Shea, M. V., and Kellogg, J. H.   Making the Most of Life.   New York, Macmillan & Co., 1923.
8. Winslow, C-E. A.   Healthy Living.   Book II. New York, C. E. Merrill Co., 1917.
9. Winslow, K.   The Prevention of Disease in the Individual.   Philadelphia, W. B. Saunders Co., 1923.

XII

THE TREATMENT AND PREVENTION OF DELINQUENCY

1. Bibliography for Parents.   Federation for Child Study, 2 West 64th St., New York.
2. Bigelow, M. A.   Sex Education.   New York, Macmillan Co., 1916.
3. Gruenberg, B. C.   Parents and Sex Education.   New York, American Social Hygiene Association, 1923.
4. Harrow, B.   Glands in Health and Disease.   New York, E. P. Dutton & Co., 1922.
5. Healy, W.   Honesty.   Indianapolis, Bobbs-Merrill Co., 1915.
6. Healy, W.   The Individual Delinquent, A Text Book of Diagnosis and Prognosis.   Boston, Little Brown & Co., 1915.
7. Healy, W.   Mental Conflicts and Misconduct.   Boston, Little, Brown & Co., 1917.
8. Healy, W.   The Practical Value of the Scientific Study of Juvenile Delinquents.   Washington, U. S. Children's Bureau Publication No. 96.
9. Miller, H. C.   The New Psychology and the Parent. New York, Thomas Selzer, 1922.
10. Thomas, W. I.   The Unadjusted Girl.   Boston, Little, Brown & Co., 1923.

XIII

THE CARE OF INTELLECTUALLY INFERIOR CHILDREN

1. Anderson, M. Education of Defectives in the Public Schools. Yonkers, N. Y., World Book Co., 1917.
2. The Boston Way. Special Class Teachers of Boston. Concord, N. H., The Rumford Press, 1917.
3. Gesell, A. Exceptional Children and Public School Policy. New Haven, Conn., Yale University Press, 1921.
4. Gesell, A. The Normal Child and Primary Education. Boston, Ginn & Co., 1912.
5. Gesell, A. The Pre-School Child from the Standpoint of Public Hygiene and Education. Boston, Houghton Mifflin Co., 1923.
6. Hollingworth, L. S. The Psychology of Subnormal Children. New York, Macmillan Co., 1920.
7. Holmes, A. Backward Children—Childhood and Youth Series. Indianapolis, Bobbs-Merrill Co., 1915.
8. Holmes, A. The Conservation of the Child. Philadelphia, J. B. Lippincott & Co., 1912.
9. Lepage, C. P. Feeble-Mindedness in Children of School Age. Manchester, Eng., University Press, 1911.
10. Plaisted, L. L. Handwork in Early Education. Oxford, Oxford University Press, 1913.

XIV

PROVISIONS FOR INTELLECTUALLY SUPERIOR CHILDREN

1. Baldwin, B. T., and Stecher, L. I. Additional Data from Consecutive Stanford-Binet Tests. Journal of Educational Psychology. Vol. 13, No. 9, pp. 556–560. 1922.
2. Baldwin, B. T. Measuring Scale for Physical Development. Iowa Child Welfare Research Station. 1919.
3. Burt, C. Experimental Tests of General Intelligence. British Journal of Psychology. Vol. 3, pt. 1–2, pp. 94–177. 1909.

4. Cobb, M. V., and others. The Special Opportunity Class for Gifted Children, Public School 165, Manhattan. Ungraded. 1923.

5. Coy, G. L. The Interests, Abilities, and Achievements of a Special Class for Gifted Children. New York, Teachers College, Columbia University, 1923.

6. Dickson, V. E. Treatment of Gifted Children in Oakland and in Berkeley. San Jose Teachers College Bulletin. 1923.

7. Freeman, F. N. Provision for Superior Children. Elementary School Journal. 1920.

8. Galton, F. Hereditary Genius. New York, Macmillan Co., 1914.

9. Gillingham, A. Superior Children—Their School Progress. Journal of Educational Psychology. Vol. XI, No. 6, pp. 327–346. 1920.

10. Hollingworth, L. S. Special Talents and Defects. New York, Macmillan Co., 1923.

11. National Society for the Study of Education. Year Book. 1924.

12. Peter, R., and Stern, W. Die Auslese befähigter Volksschüler in Hamburg. Zeitschrift für Angewandte Psychologie. 1922.

13. Race, H. V. A Study of a Class of Children of Superior Intelligence. Journal of Educational Psychology. Vol. IX, No. 2, pp. 91–97. 1918.

14. Seashore, C. E. The Psychology of Musical Talent. Boston, Silver, Burdett & Co., 1919.

15. Specht, L. F. A Terman Class in Public School No. 64, Manhattan. School and Society. Vol. IX, No. 222, pp. 393–398. 1919.

16. Terman, L. M. The Intelligence of School Children. Boston, Houghton Mifflin Co., 1919.

17. Terman, L. M. A New Approach to the Study of Genius. Psychological Review. Vol. 29, No. 4, pp. 310–318. 1922.

18. Thomson, G. H. The Northumberland Mental Tests. British Journal of Psychology. 1921.

19. Whipple, G. M. Classes for Gifted Children. Bloomington, Ill., Public School Publishing Co., 1919.

20. Woodrow, Herbert. Brightness and Dullness in Children. Philadelphia, J. P. Lippincott & Co., 1919.
21. Yoder, G. F. The Study of the Boyhood of Great Men. Pedagogical Seminary. Vol. III, pp. 134–156. 1894.

XV

THE ADOLESCENT PERIOD; ITS PROBLEMS, REGIMEN AND HYGIENE

1. Bigelow, M. A. Sex Instruction. New York, American Social Hygiene Association, 1912.
2. Bigelow, M. A. Sex Education. New York, Macmillan Co., 1916.
3. Galloway, T. W. The Boy and the Community. New York, Education Dept., American Social Hygiene Association, 1923.
4. Galloway, T. W. Father and His Boy; the Place of Sex in Manhood Making. New York, Association Press, 1921.
5. Hall, G. Stanley. Youth, Its Education, Regimen and Hygiene. New York, D. Appleton & Co., 1907.
6. Hall, W. S. From Youth into Manhood. New York, Association Press, 1919.
7. Hall, W. S. Girlhood and Its Problems. Philadelphia, J. C. Winston Co., 1919.
8. Hall, W. S. Youth and Its Problems. Philadelphia, J. C. Winston Co., 1919.
9. Hall, W. S. A set of Four Booklets: John's Vacation, Chums, The Doctor's Daughter, Life Problems. Chicago, American Medical Association, 1913.

XVI

BRIDGING THE GAP BETWEEN OUR KNOWLEDGE OF EDUCATION AND OUR EDUCATIONAL PRACTICE

1. Bizzell, W. B., and Duncan, M. H. Present-Day Tendencies of Education. Chicago, Rand McNally & Co., 1918.
2. The Elementary School Journal. Published by the University of Chicago Press, Chicago.

3. Finney, R. L. The American Public School. New York, Macmillan Co., 1921.
4. Fisher, S. G. American Education. Boston, Richard G. Badger, 1917.
5. Flexner, A. A Modern College and a Modern School. New York, Century Co., 1923.
6. Freeland, G. E. Modern Elementary School Practice. New York, Macmillan Co., 1919.
7. Horn, J. L. The American Elementary School. New York, Century Co., 1923.
8. McMurry, C. A. How to Organize the Curriculum. New York, Macmillan Co., 1923.
9. Meriam, J. L. Child Life and the Curriculum. New York, World Book Co., 1920.
10. Phillips, C. A. Modern Methods and the Elementary Curriculum. New York, Century Co., 1923.
11. U. S. Bureau of Education. Bulletin, No. 8, 1916.
12. U. S. Bureau of Education. Bulletin, No. 34, 1920.

XVII

Changing Objectives in American Schools

1. Adams, J. Modern Developments in Education Practice. (2d impression.) London, University of London Press, Ltd., 1922.
2. Andrews, B. R. The School of To-Morrow. New York, Doubleday, Page & Co., 1911.
3. Bourne, K. S. The Gary Schools. Boston, Houghton Mifflin Co., 1916.
4. Caldwell, O. W., and Courtis, S. A. Then and Now in Education, 1845:1923. Yonkers, World Book Co., 1924.
5. Cubberley, E. P. Public Education in the United States. Boston, Houghton Mifflin Co., 1919.
6. Cyclopedia of Education. Edited by Paul Monroe. New York, Macmillan Co. (Articles on education in the various States, especially in the Colonies, 1911-13.)
7. Dewey, John. The School and Society. Chicago, University of Chicago Press, 1916.
8. Dewey, John. Democracy and Education. New York, Dutton & Co., 1922.

9. Dopp, K. The Place of Industries in Elementary Education. Chicago, University of Chicago Press, 1903.
10. Gessell, A. The Normal Child and Primary Education. Boston, Ginn & Co., 1912.
11. Hollingworth, H. L. Vocational Psychology. New York, D. Appleton & Co., 1916.
12. Judd, C. H. Fundamental Educational Reforms. Elementary School Journal, Vol. 23, pp. 333-41, January, 1923.
13. Keith, J. A. H., and Bagley, W. C. Nation and the Schools. New York, Macmillan Co., 1920.
14. Miller, I. E. Education for the Needs of Life. New York, Macmillan Co., 1917.
15. Moore, E. C. What is Education? Boston, Ginn & Co., 1915.
16. Moore, E. C. What the War Teaches Us About Education. New York, Macmillan Co., 1919.
17. Reisner, E. H. Rationalism and Education since 1789, Chapters XV to XVIII. New York, Macmillan Co., 1922.
18. Roman, F. W. The New Education in Europe. New York, Dutton & Co., 1923.
19. Ruediger, W. C. The Principles of Education. Boston, Houghton Mifflin Co., 1910.
20. Snedden, D. S. Vocational Education. New York, Macmillan Co., 1920.
21. Weeks, A. D. The Education of To-Morrow. New York, Sturgis & Walton, 1916.

XVIII

CHANGING COURSES OF STUDY

1. Bagley, W. C. Educational Values. New York, Macmillan Co., 1911.
2. Blake, K. D. Revising the Elementary Curriculum. Journal of the National Education Association. Vol. 11, pp. 355-59, November, 1922.
3. Bourne, R. S. The Gary Schools. Boston, Houghton Mifflin Co., 1916.

4. Caldwell, O. W. Principles and Types of Curriculum Development. Journal of Education, Vol. 97, pp. 428–32, April 19, 1923.

5. Charters, W. W. Curriculum Construction. New York, Macmillan Co., 1923.

6. Davis, C. O. High School Courses of Study. Yonkers, N. Y., World Book Co., 1914.

7. Dewey, E. New Schools for Old. New York, E. P. Dutton & Co., 1919.

8. Dewey, John. Schools of To-Morrow. New York, E. P. Dutton & Co., 1915.

9. Hill, D. S. Introduction to Vocational Education. New York, Macmillan Co., 1920.

10. Judd, C. H., and others. Measuring the Work of the Public Schools. Cleveland, The Survey Committee of the Cleveland Foundation. 1916.

11. Lapp, J. A., and Mote, C. H. Learning to Earn. Indianapolis, Bobbs-Merrill Co., 1915.

12. McMurry, F. M. Elementary School Standards. Yonkers, N. Y., World Book Co., 1913.

13. McMurry, O. L., and others. Teaching of Industrial Arts in the Elementary School. New York, Macmillan Co., 1923.

14. Merian, J. L. Child Life and the Curriculum. Yonkers, N. Y., World Book Co., 1920.

15. Miller, I. Education for the Needs of Life. New York, Macmillan Co., 1917.

16. Moore, E. C. What the War Teaches About Education. New York, Macmillan Co., 1919.

17. O'Shea, M. V. Education as Adjustment. New York, Longmans, Green & Co., 1903.

18. Sears, J. B. The Boise Survey. Yonkers, N. Y., World Book Co., 1920.

19. Thompson, F. V. Commercial Education in Public Secondary Schools. Yonkers, N. Y., World Book Co., 1915.

20. Weeks, R. M. The People's School. New York, Macmillan Co., 1912.

21. Wells, M. E. A Project Curriculum. Philadelphia, J. B. Lippincott & Co., 1921.

XIX

CHANGING METHODS OF TEACHING AND MANAGEMENT

1. Ayer, F. C. The Present Status of Promotional Plans in City Schools. American School Board Journal, Vol. 66, pp. 37–39, April, 1923.

2. Ayres, L. P. Laggards in Our Schools. New York, Survey Associates, Inc., 1909.

3. Bagley, W. C. School Discipline. New York, Macmillan Co., 1917.

4. Bankes, W. J. The Model Platoon School. Journal of Education, Vol. 97, pp. 63–65, January 18, 1923.

5. Book, W. F., and Norvell, L. An Experimental Study of Incentives in Learning. Pedagogical Seminary, Vol. 29, pp. 305–62, December, 1922.

6. Branson, E. R. An Experiment in Arranging High-School Sections on the Basis of General Ability. Journal of Educational Research, Vol. 3, pp. 53–55, January, 1921.

7. Clerk, F. E. The Arlington Plan of Grouping Pupils According to Ability in the Arlington High School, Arlington, Massachusetts. School Review, Vol. 35, pp. 26–47, January, 1917.

8. Cox, P. W. L. Providing for Individual Differences by Means of Grouping by Ability. Ninth Annual Schoolmen's Week Proceedings, University of Pennsylvania Bulletin, Vol. 23, No. 1, p. 233.

9. Fisher, D. C. Mothers and Children. New York, H. Holt & Co., 1915.

10. Fisher, D. C. Self-Reliance. Indianapolis, Bobbs-Merrill Co., 1916.

11. Freeland, G. E. Modern Elementary School Practice. New York, Macmillan Co., 1919.

12. Healy, William. The Individual Delinquent. Boston, Little, Brown & Co., 1922.

13. Holmes, Arthur. Backward Children. Indianapolis, Bobbs-Merrill Co., 1915.

14. Kennedy, E. V. Dayton's Achievement in Special Education. School Progress, Vol. 1, pp. 3–4, February 23, 1923.

15. Merriam, J. L. Child Life and the Curriculum. Yonkers, N. Y., The World Book Co., 1920.
16. Miller, H. L. Directing Study; Educating for Mastery Through Creative Thinking. New York, Chas. Scribner's Sons, 1922.
17. Morehouse, Frances. The Discipline of the School. Boston, D. C. Heath & Co., 1914.
18. O'Shea, M. V. Dynamic Factors in Education. New York, Macmillan Co., 1909.
19. O'Shea, M. V. Every-Day Problems in Teaching. Indianapolis, Bobbs-Merrill Co., 1912.
20. Parker, S. C. Types of Elementary Teaching and Learning, Including Practical Technique and Scientific Evidence. Boston, Ginn & Co., 1923.
21. Parkhurst, Helen. Education on the Dalton Plan. London, G. Bell & Sons, 1922.
22. Rousseau, J. J. Emile. Tr. by Payne, New York, D. Appleton & Co., 1908. Tr. by Worthington. Boston, D. C. Heath & Co., 1885. Tr. by Foxley. (Everyman's Library) New York, E. P. Dutton & Co., 1911.
23. Satchell, J. K. Student Participation in School Administration. School Review, Vol. 30, pp. 733-41, December, 1922.
24. Stoner, W. S. Natural Education. Indianapolis, Bobbs-Merrill Co., 1916.
25. Swift, E. J. Learning and Doing. Indianapolis, Bobbs-Merrill Co., 1914.
26. Taylor, J. S. Grading and Promotion. School and Society, Vol. 17, pp. 405-9, April 14, 1923.
27. Thorndike, E. A. Individuality. Boston, Houghton Mifflin Co., 1911.
28. Wells, Margaret. A Project Curriculum. Philadelphia, J. B. Lippincott Co., 1921.
29. Wilson, G. M. Teaching Levels, Teaching Technique, and the Project. Journal of Educational Method. Vol. 2, pp. 323-29, 385-93, April, May, 1923.
30. Wilson, H. B. The Motivation of School Work. Boston, Houghton Mifflin Co., 1916.

XX

Promoting the Health and Physical Development of School Children

1. Addams, J. The Spirit of Youth and the City Streets. New York, Macmillan Co., 1923.

2. Allen, W. H. Civics and Health. Boston, Ginn & Co., 1909.

3. Andress, J. M. Health Education in Rural Schools. Boston, Houghton Mifflin Co., 1919.

4. Ayres, L. P. Open-Air Schools. New York, Doubleday, Page & Co., 1910.

5. Burks, F. W. Health and the School. New York, D. Appleton & Co., 1913.

6. Curtis, C. H. Education Through Play. New York, Macmillan Co., 1915.

7. Evans, E. The Problem of the Nervous Child. New York, Dodd, Mead & Co., 1920.

8. Gulick, L. H. and Ayres, L. P. Medical Inspection of Schools. New York, Survey Associates, 1913.

9. Lee, J. Play in Education. New York, Macmillan Co., 1915.

10. New York (State) University. General Plan and Syllabus for Physical Training in the Elementary and Secondary Schools of New York State. Albany, published by the State of New York.

11. Physical Education, Courses in, for Washington, Michigan, Alabama, Kentucky, Missouri, New Jersey, West Virginia, Wisconsin, in bulletins published by the State Department of Education in each State.

12. Rapeer, L. W., ed. Educational Hygiene. New York, Chas. Scribner's Sons, 1915.

13. Terman, L. M. The Hygiene of the School Child. Boston, Houghton Mifflin Co., 1914.

14. Wells, W. L. Mental Adjustment. New York, D. Appleton & Co., 1917.

XXI

EXTENDING EDUCATIONAL FACILITIES, OPPORTUNITIES, AND REQUIREMENTS

1. Abel, J. F. Extending the Reach of the School. School and Society. Vol. IX, Nov., 1923.
2. Bourne, R. S. The Gary Point of View. *In his* The Gary Schools. pp. 76–77. Boston, Houghton Mifflin Co., 1916.
3. Brim, O. G. The Curriculum Problem in Rural Elementary Schools. Elementary School Journal, Vol. 23, pp. 586–600, April, 1923.
4. Butterfield, K. L. The Education of the Rural People. Journal of Rural Education, Vol. 3, pp. 166–74, December, 1922–January, 1923.
5. Carney, M. Country Life and the Country School. Chicago, Row, Peterson & Co., 1912.
6. Claxton, P. P. School and the Summer Vacation. Journal of Education, Vol. 79, pp. 726–27, June 25, 1914.
7. Corson, D. B. All-Year Schools. American City, Vol. 22, pp. 588–92, June, 1920.
8. Deffenbaugh, W. S. Summer Sessions of City. Schools. *In* U. S. Bureau of Education. Bulletin, 1917, No. 45, pp. 1–45.
9. Hall, O. E., and Betts, G. H. Better Rural Schools. Indianapolis, Bobbs-Merrill Co., 1914.
10. Judd, C. H., and others. Rural School Survey of New York State. Administration and Supervision. Ithaca, N. Y., 1923.
11. Kennedy, J. W. All-Year Schools. *In* National Education Association. Proceedings and Addresses, Vol. 55, pp. 795–801, 1917.
12. Kirkham, F. W. Utah's Year-Round Educational Program, authorized by the Legislature of 1919. Vocational Summary, Vol. 3, pp. 154–56, February, 1921.
13. Krause, C. A., and Hoffman, A. L. The Organization and Administration of a City Vacation High School. New York, Chas. Scribner's Sons, 1923.

APPENDIX

Biographical Data Regarding Contributors to "THE CHILD: HIS NATURE AND HIS NEEDS"

PROFESSOR BIRD THOMAS BALDWIN, Author of Chapter I

Professor Baldwin secured his first degree in science at Swarthmore College, and his master of arts and doctor of philosophy degrees at Harvard. He has studied at the University of Pennsylvania and the University of Leipzig, Germany. He was for a time supervisor and principal of Friends' Schools in Pennsylvania, and was for two years assistant in education and later in psychology and logic at Harvard. He was then appointed professor of psychology in the Pennsylvania State Normal School at West Chester. He was lecturer on psychology and education at Swathmore for four years, and at the University of Chicago for one year, and was professor of education and head of the School of Art of Teaching at the University of Texas for two years. He was professor of psychology and education at Swarthmore from 1912 to 1916, professor of educational psychology at John Hopkins for several summers, and was later lecturer in educational psychology at Johns Hopkins. In 1917 he was appointed research professor in educational psychology and director of the Iowa Child Welfare Research Station at the State University of Iowa. For a year and one-half he served as major in the Sanitary Corps of the U. S. Army, in the office of the Surgeon General of the Army, and chief psychologist and director of the rehabilitation of disabled soldiers in the Walter Reed General Hospital, Washington, D. C. He has written numerous important articles, bulletins, and reviews on educational and psychological topics, and is associate editor of psychological and educational journals. He is a Fellow of the American Association for the Advancement of Science, and is a member and officer of a number of psychological and educational associations. He is the author of the following works: *Physical Growth and School Progress; Physical Growth of*

Children from Birth to Maturity; Educational Research; The Rehabilitation of Disabled Soldiers; joint author of the *Mental Growth Curves of Normal and Superior Children,* and *The Psychology of the Pre-School Child.*

DEAN FREDERICK E. BOLTON, Author of Chapter VI

Dean Bolton was reared on a farm in Wisconsin. He has had experience in teaching in all kinds of schools, including rural schools, high schools, normal schools, and four universities. He has organized and headed two Schools of Education, one at the State University of Iowa, the other at the State University of Washington. While in Iowa he was chosen by Governor Albert B. Cummins to be chairman of a committee to revise the school laws of the State and suggest new legislation. He was President of the Iowa Child Study Association, and Secretary of the Wisconsin Child Study Association. He was secretary for six years of the National Association of College Teachers of Education. He is a Fellow of the American Association for the Advancement of Science. He studied Psychology under Wundt in Leipzig, President Hall at Clark, and Professor Jastrow at Wisconsin. He is author of *The Secondary School System of Germany; Principles of Education,* of which it has been said, "Bolton did for Education what James did for Psychology"; *Everyday Psychology for Teachers;* besides nearly one hundred magazine articles in educational, psychological, and literary magazines. He has lectured extensively at teachers' institutes, public school commencements, college and normal school commencements, and state teachers' associations. He is chairman of a committee of the American Council on Education in standardizing teacher-training institutions in the United States.

PROFESSOR WALTER FENNO DEARBORN, Author of Chapter IV

Professor Dearborn prepared for college at Phillips Exeter Academy and studied at Wesleyan, Columbia, Wisconsin, and Chicago Universities in this country, and the Universities of Göttingen, Heidelberg, and Munich in Germany. He has received the following academic degrees: A.B. and A.M. from Wesleyan University; Ph.D. from Columbia; and M.D. from the University of Munich. He has taught in the Departments of Education and Psychology at the University of Wisconsin, Chicago University, and Harvard University. He is now Professor of Education at Harvard University and in charge of the Psycho-Educational Clinic of the Graduate School of Education. He is a member of the American Psychological Association and of various educational and scientific associations and is a Trustee of the Massachusetts State Infirmary. He is the author of the following Monographs and of various articles in psychological and educational Journals: *The Psychology of Reading; The Relative Standing of Pupils in the High School and University; School and University Grades; Formen des Infantilismus mit Berüchsichtigung ihrer klinischen Unterscheidung.* He is joint author of *Standard Educational Tests in the Elementary Training Schools of Missouri;* and *A Series of Form Board and Performance Tests of Intelligence.*

PROFESSOR WILLIAM ROBIE PATTEN EMERSON, Author of Chapter IX

Dr. Emerson graduated from Dartmouth College in 1892 and from The Harvard Medical School in 1899. Among the positions he has held in which he has dealt with the problems concerned in this chapter have been Professor of Pediatrics at the Tufts College Medical School; President of Nutrition Clinics for Delicate Children, Incorporated; Major (retired) National Guard; President, Board of Military Examiners, State of Massachusetts, 1908-1913; Member of the Committee on Height and Weight Standards, National Child Health Council; Consultant of the Elizabeth McCormick Memorial Fund, Rochester Public Schools, Tuberculosis and Public Health Association, and International Grenfell Association. He is author of many articles in social, educational, and medical journals, and also of a series of twenty-eight articles which have appeared in the "Woman's Home Companion." He has recently published *Nutrition and Growth in Children.*

PROFESSOR ARNOLD GESELL, Author of Chapter XIII

Dr. Gesell received his first degree from the University of Wisconsin. The degree of doctor of philosophy was secured from Clark University, and the degree of doctor of medicine from Yale University. He held the position of professor of psychology in the Los Angeles State Normal School for two years and was assistant professor of education in Yale University from 1911 to 1915. He was then appointed professor of child hygiene in the Yale Graduate School, which position he now holds. He was associate for a number of years in the School for Special Training of Defective Children in New York University. He established the Yale Psycho-Clinic in 1911 and has been director of it since that time. He became school psychologist under the State Board of Education of Connecticut in 1917. In 1919 he was appointed to the Connecticut Commission on Child Welfare. He has been consulting psychologist of the New Haven Hospital since 1920. He is chairman of the Executive Committee of the Connecticut Society for Mental Hygiene, and is a member of various medical, psychological, and psychiatrical associations, and is a director of the American Child Health Association. He is a member of Phi Beta Kappa Fraternity. He is the author of the following works: *The Normal Child and Primary Education; Manual on Defective Children; School Provisions for Exceptional Children; Exceptional Children and Public School Policy; Hemihypertrophy and Mental Defect; Handicapped Children in School and Court; Mental and Physical Correspondence in Twins; The Pre-School Child, from the Standpoint of Public Hygiene and Education.*

PROFESSOR HENRY HERBERT GODDARD, Author of Chapter VIII

Professor Goddard secured his first and second degrees at Haverford College. He was Fellow in Psychology at Clark University for three years, and secured the doctor of philosophy degree there. He studied in German universities for one year. He served as academy and seminary principal for several years, and was Professor of Psychology in the Pennsylvania State Normal

School at West Chester for seven years. In 1906, he was appointed Director of the Department of Research in the Training School for Feeble-Minded Children, Vineland, New Jersey, which position he held for twelve years. In 1918 he was appointed Director of the State Bureau of Juvenile Research in Columbus, Ohio. Later he was appointed Professor of Abnormal and Clinical Psychology in the Ohio State University, which position he holds at the present time. He is a member of Phi Beta Kappa and numerous scientific, psychological, and kindred societies. He has written and lectured much on education, eugenics, treatment of feeble-mindedness, and related topics. He is the author of the following works: *The Kallikak Family; Feeble-Mindedness; The Criminal Imbecile; School Training of Defective Children; Psychology of the Normal and Subnormal.* He is a contributor to Jelliffe and White's *Modern Treatment of Nervous and Mental Diseases* and to *Reference Handbook of the Medical Sciences.*

PROFESSOR LETA S. HOLLINGWORTH, Author of Chapter XIV

Professor Hollingworth was born in Dawes County, Nebraska, in 1886. She was graduated from high school in the State of Nebraska, and took the degree of B.A. from the University of Nebraska, in 1906. From 1906 to 1909, she taught in Nebraska high schools. In 1913, she took the M.A. degree in education, at Columbia University. From 1913 to 1916, she served as mental examiner for the City of New York, first at The Post Graduate Hospital, and later at Bellevue Hospital. The duties of this office included particularly the examination of mental deviates among juvenile applicants for admission to institutions. In 1916, she received the Ph.D. degree in education, with special reference to educational psychology, at Columbia University, and later in the same year she was appointed instructor in educational psychology at Teachers College, Columbia University, where she is now associate professor of education. She is the author of *The Psychology of Special Disability in Spelling; The Psychology of Sub-Normal Children; Special Talents and Defects;* and of various articles dealing with exceptional children, published in educational periodicals. She is a member of various educational, psychological, and research associations.

DOCTOR WINFIELD SCOTT HALL, Author of Chapter XV

Dr. Hall secured his B.S. degree at Northwestern University in 1887 and his M.S. in 1889. He received the degree of doctor of medicine at the University of Leipzig, Germany, in 1894 and the degree of doctor of philosophy in 1895. He was professor of biology in Haverford College for four years and professor of physiology in Northwestern Medical School for twenty-four years. He was junior dean of the medical faculty for twelve years. He is now professor emeritus of Northwestern University Medical School. He is also medical director of the Board of Temperance and Moral Welfare of the Presbyterian Church of the U. S., and has been head of the work of social hygiene since 1919. He has been exchange professor with l'Université Internationale, Brussels, Belgium, since 1921. He is a member of Phi Beta Kappa and Sigma Xi fraternities. He is a member and officer of a great many medical and welfare organizations. He is the author of the following works: *Laboratory Guide in Physiology; Anatomy of the Central Nervous System in Man and in Vertebrates; Textbook of Physiology; Elementary Anatomy, Physiology and Hygiene; Intermediate Physiology and Hygiene; Manual of Experimental Physiology; Textbook of Normal and Pathologic Physiology; The Biology, Physiology, and Sociology of Reproduction; Sex Hygiene; Essentials of Physiology and Hygiene; From Youth into Manhood; Nutrition and Dietetics; The Strength of Ten; Instead of Wild Oats; Sexual Knowledge; Manual of Instruction in Sex Hygiene; Life Problems; The Doctor's Daughter; John's Vacation; Chums; Constructive Eugenics; A Physician's Counsel to Parents;* and he has made extensive contributions to medical and educational journals.

DOCTOR WILLIAM HEALY, Author of Chapter XII

Dr. Healy was born in England but came to America when he was a child. He secured his first degree at Harvard in 1899 and the degree of doctor of medicine from

Rush Medical College, University of Chicago, in 1900. He carried on his medical studies in Vienna, Berlin, and London during 1906 and 1907. He was assistant physician at the Wisconsin State Hospital for one year and instructor in the Northwestern University Medical School for two years. He was associate professor of nervous and mental diseases in Chicago Policlinic during 1903-16. He was director of the Psychopathic Institute of the Juvenile Court of Chicago for eight years, and in 1917 was made director of the Judge Baker Foundation, Boston, which position he now holds. He has been a lecturer in the psychological department of Harvard University Summer School. He is the pioneer in the United States in establishing the study of juvenile offenders in connection with the courts. His work in this field is epoch-making. He is a member and officer of many psycho-neurological, psychiatrical, and criminological associations. He is the author of the following works: *Case Studies of Mentally and Morally Abnormal Types; The Individual Delinquent—A Textbook of Diagnosis and Prognosis for All Concerned with Understanding Offenders;* (with Mary Tenney Healy) *Pathological Lying, Accusation, and Swindling—A Study in Forensic Psychology; Honesty; Mental Conflicts and Misconduct;* also monographs and numerous articles on psychological and medico-psychological subjects.

PROFESSOR EDWIN ASBURY KIRKPATRICK, Author of Chapter VII

Professor Kirkpatrick secured his first degree in science in Iowa State College and the master's degree in philosophy in 1899. He was awarded a scholarship and later a fellowship in Clark University. He taught mathematics and English in Iowa State College, and later in the Winona (Minn.) State Normal School. In 1898 he was made director of the Department of Child Study in the Massachusetts State Normal School at Fitchburg, which position he now holds. He has lectured on education at Smith College and in the summer sessions of various universities. He is a Fellow of the American Association for the Advancement of Science and a member of a number of psychological, educational, and child study associations. He received a gold medal as collaborator at the Child Study Exhibit at the St. Louis Exposition. He is author of the following works: *Inductive Psychology; Fundamentals of Child Study; Genetic Psychology; The Individual in the Making; The Use of Money; Fundamentals of Sociology; Studies in Psychology; Imagination: Its Place in Education.*

DR. HENRY NEUMANN, Author of Chapter V

Dr. Neumann secured his bachelor's degree from the College of the City of New York. He studied at Cornell and Columbia Universities, and secured his degree of doctor of philosophy from New York University in 1906. He was instructor in education and English in the College of the City of New York for eight years, and instructor in moral education in the summer session of the University of Wisconsin for several years. He has been a leader of the Brooklyn Society for Ethical Culture since 1911. He was secretary of the American Committee of the Second International Moral Education Congress held at The Hague. He is the author of *Moral Values and Secondary Education; Teaching American Ideals Through Literature; Education for Moral Growth.*

PROFESSOR M. V. O'SHEA, Editor of this volume and author of Chapters XVII, XVIII, XIX, XX and XXI

Professor O'Shea graduated in arts and philosophy from Cornell University. For three years he was professor of psychology and education at the State Normal School at Mankato, Minn., and for two years professor of Education at Teachers' College, Buffalo. In 1897 he was appointed to the professorship of education at the University of Wisconsin, which position he now holds. He has been identified with educational research and with university extension work. He has lectured extensively on education and related subjects in the United States, and in several foreign countries. He studied European education during 1906, and was chairman of the American Committee for the International Congress on Home Education, at Liége Belgium, in 1905, and at Brussels in 1910. He is a Fellow of the American Association for the

Advancement of Science, and is a member of the board of directors of various organizations devoted to the investigation and promotion of education and the well-being of childhood and youth. He is the author of the following works: *Suggestions for the Observation and Study of Children; Aspects of Mental Economy; Education as Adjustment; Dynamic Factors in Education; Linguistic Development and Education; Every-Day Problems in Teaching; Social Development and Education; Mental Development and Education; First Steps in Child-Training; Faults of Childhood and Youth; The Trend of the Teens; Every-Day Problems in Child Training*, and *Tobacco and Mental Efficiency*. He is joint author of *The Child and His Spelling; The Child and His Grammar;* and the *Macmillan Health Series* of six volumes. He collaborated with Professor Cook and Miss Holbrook in preparing *The Every-Day Spelling Series* of four volumes. He has served as editor of educational and home periodicals, and is now editor-in-chief of *Junior Home Magazine.* He is also editor-in-chief of *The World Book Encyclopedia; The Macmillan Experimental Education Series; The Childhood and Youth Series*, and *The Parent's Library.* He is editorial writer for *Normal Instructor—Primary Plans.*

HONORABLE JOHN JAMES TIGERT, Author of Chapter XVI

Dr. Tigert is the son of John James Tigert, sometime professor of mental and moral philosophy in Vanderbilt University and bishop of the Methodist Episcopal Church South. He was educated in the public schools of Kansas City, Mo., and Nashville, Tenn. He received his first degree from Vanderbilt University and his second and third degrees in the Honor School of Jurisprudence in Oxford, Eng. He was the first Rhodes scholar from the State of Tennessee. He did graduate work at the University of Minnesota, and holds honorary degrees from the University of Kentucky and from the Rhode Island State College. He has held the professorship of psychology and philosophy in Central College, Mo., and was president of the Kentucky Wesleyan College for two years. In 1911 he was appointed professor in the University of Kentucky, having charge of philosophy and psychology, which position he held until he was appointed United States Commissioner of Education in 1921, which position he still holds. During the War he did educational work in the American Expeditionary Forces in Scotland, England, and France. He was a member of the Army Educational Corps and extension lecturer in the University of Beaune, American Expeditionary Forces, France. He is the author of numerous monographs, articles, and reports on philosophical, psychological, and educational subjects in encyclopedias, periodicals, etc. He is a member of Phi Beta Kappa fraternity besides several social fraternities. He is an officer and member of various national organizations for the advancement of education and of child hygiene.

DOCTOR WILLIAM ALANSON WHITE, Author of Chapter X

Dr. White secured the degree of doctor of medicine at Long Island Medical College in 1891. He was assistant physician at the Binghamton (N. Y.) State Hospital for eleven years. Since 1903 he has been superintendent of St. Elizabeth's Hospital, Washington, D. C., a government institution in the Department of the Interior. He is professor of nervous and mental diseases in Georgetown University and also professor of nervous and mental diseases in George Washington University. He is lecturer on insanity in the U. S. Naval and Army Medical School. He is a member of the National Research Council and of many medical, psychiatrical, and psycho-pathological associations. He has been president of the American Psychoanalytical Association, and he has also been president of the Washington Academy of Sciences, and of the National Committee on Mental Hygiene. He is editor and translator (with Dr. Smith Ely Jelliffe) of *The Psychic Treatment of Nervous Disorders;* Editor (with Dr. Jelliffe) of *Nervous and Mental Disease Monograph Series* and *The Psychoanalytic Review;* also *Modern Treatment of Nervous and Mental Diseases.* He is the author of *Outlines of Psychiatry; Mental Mechanics; Mechanics of Character Formation; Principles of Mental Hygiene; Diseases of the Nervous System* (with Dr. Jelliffe); *Mental Hygiene of Childhood; Thoughts of a*

Psychiatrist on the War and After; Foundations of Psychiatry; Insanity and the Criminal Law; also various contributions to medical journals.

PROFESSOR MARY THEODORA WHITLEY, Author of Chapters II and III

Professor Whitley was born in London, England, and was educated at home and at boarding school. After travel and residence in Australia and Canada, Miss Whitley entered Teachers College, Columbia University, where she has taken the degrees B.S., A.M., Ph.D. In 1914 she became assistant professor of education in the department of educational psychology in that institution, which position she still holds. She was associated with Professor Norsworthy in the authorship of *The Psychology of Childhood*. She is author of *A Study of the Little Child; A Study of the Primary Child; A Study of the Junior Child*, three books used in the standard training course of the International Sunday School Council of Religious Education. She is a member of the American Psychological Association, the New York Society for Experimental Education, the American Association for the Advancement of Science, and the Federation for Child Study.

DOCTOR CHARLES-EDWARD AMORY WINSLOW, Author of Chapter XI

Dr. Winslow secured his bachelor and master of science degrees at the Massachusetts Institute of Technology, his master of arts degree at Yale University, and doctor of public health at New York University. He held a position for a time as professor of sanitary biology and biologist-in-charge of the Sanitary Research Laboratory of the Massachusetts Institute of Technology. He was assistant professor of bacteriology in the University of Chicago for a term, and associate professor of biology in the College of the City of New York. In 1910 he became curator of public health at the American Museum of Natural History, New York, which position he still holds. He was director of the Division of Public Health Education of the New York State Department of Health from

1914 to 1915. Since 1915 he has been Anna M. R. Lauder professor of public health in the Yale Medical School. He is a fellow of the American Association for the Advancement of Science, and is a member and officer of various scientific, biological, medical, and bacteriological associations. In 1921 he was general medical director of the League of Red Cross Societies in Geneva, Switzerland. He is author of *Elements of Water Bacteriology; Elements of Industrial Microscopy; Healthy Living;* and co-author of *Systematic Relationships of the Coccaceae; Sewage Disposal; Health Survey of New Haven.*

INDEX

based on imitation, 389–390; scientific basis of household arts, 390; usefulness of traditional education for girls, 390–393.

Glands, sexual, influence of, in human life, 305–307.

Goddard, Henry Herbert, contributor, biographical note on, 492–493.

Government, parallels educational system, 326–327; reality of, in teaching civics, 411–412; teaching of, 409–414; relation of, to rural people, 412–413.

Grace, development of, in drawing, 150–151.

Grammar, changing courses in, 384–385; dynamic principles applied to teaching of, 406–407.

Gregariousness, 108–111; among animals, 108–109; among primitive peoples, 109; in gangs, 109–110; in childhood, 110; in youth, 110–111; affiliation with societies a phase of, 111.

Group Games, 66–69.

Group Loyalty, learned through play. 68.

Growth, in relation to motor abilities, 54–55.

Growth Curves, of four girls (chart), 28; of three boys (chart), 28.

Guidance, of moral equipment and development, 90–106; of the sex instinct, 122–123.

Habitation, the, in play, 59–61.

Habits, health, teaching of, 414–415; value of, 415–416.

Hall, G. Stanley, on children's fears, 42; referred to, 91; on doll play, 120; on periodicity in human life, 318; on rôle of sexual glands, 306–307.

Hall, Winfield S., contributor, biographical note on, 494.

Happiness, objective of education, 364–367.

Harper, William R., on reorganization of curriculum, 339.

Hastings, W. W., on adolescent traits, 304.

Health and Physical Development of School Children, promoting the, 424–447; revelations concerning the health and physical development of our people, 424–425; our people becoming aroused, 426; hygiene of school buildings, 426–427; ventilation in school rooms, 427–428; posture in school rooms, 428–429; hygiene of the school program, 429–430; relieving young pupils of injurious school room tasks, 430–431; problem of malnourishment, 431–432; overstrain among school children, 432–434; cause of overstrain, 434–436; medical inspection in schools, 436–437; physical education, a regular part of school work, 436; playgrounds for children, 437–438; disad-

vantages of country children, 438–439; health and physical development of city children, 439–441; study of physiology and hygiene for promotion of health and physical development, 441; will knowledge influence conduct?, 441–442; value of study of physiology, 443; making study of hygiene effective, 444; aim in teaching hygiene, 444–445; instruction must be adapted to age and special needs, 445.

Health Habits, the teaching of, 444–445.

Health Inspection, in school, 182–183.

Health Services, in school, 229–230.

Health, safeguards of, 190; teaching habits of, 414–415; value of, 415–416.

Healy, William, contributor, biographical note on, 494.

Hearing, defects of, 220–221.

Height, individual growth curves in (chart), 26.

Herbart, in relation to science of education, 327; on memory work in teaching, 399.

Heredity, and physical development, 184–185; and mental hygiene, 196.

Hero-Worship, utilized in building character, 92.

Higher Education, in the United States, 341; public support of, 351–355.

High Schools, public support of, 351–353.

Historical Approach, in treatment of delinquency, 251–252.

History, dynamic principle applied to teaching of, 407–408; of the study of ability, 280–281.

Hofnungskinder, 295.

Hollingworth, Leta S., contributor, biographical note on, 493.

Home and the School, 170–171.

Home Control of Nutrition, 189.

Home-making, value of courses in, 390–393.

Hoover, Herbert, aiding in promotion of child health, 426.

Hormones, 306; in physical development of the boy, 307; in physical development of the girl, 309.

Horn, J. L., quoted, 335–366.

Household Arts, in girls' education, 388–389.

"Houses of Childhood," Montessori Schools, 403.

Howells, William Dean, on public opinion among children, 117; on hero-worship among children, 119; on love of approbation in children, 130.

Hygiene, the study of, for the promotion of health, 441–445; of the adolescent period, 300–321; of school buildings, 426–427.

Hygienic Program, of school work, 454–455.

Program, hygiene of, in school, 428–429.

Progress, in learning (charts), 135; of knowledge and of practice of education, 330; requires changing curricula, 376–377; and education, 449–450.

Promotion of Children, in school, application of principles of physical growth to, 29–30.

Protection against Evil Habits, secured by instruction regarding sex, 316–317.

Provisions for Intellectually Superior Children, 277–299; individual differences in children, 277; distribution of individuals in a group (chart), 279–281; history of the study of ability, 280–281; symptoms of ability in children, 281; segregation of able children, 282–283; character and temperament of superior children, 283–284; size and strength of superior children, 285–287; maturity of superior children (chart), 287–289; ancestry of gifted children, 289–293; individual cases of superior children, 292–294; experimental education of gifted children, 294–296; special talents, 296–297; present problems in the education of gifted children, 297–298.

Psychological Studies of Mental Deficiency, 264–267; Witmer's work, 265; Chicago Board of Education, 265; Faribault (Minn.) School for the Feeble-Minded, 265; Vineland (N. J.) Training School, 265; Binet's work, 265–266; World War, 266; Terman's work, 266; American investigations, 266.

Psychology, in the curriculum, 362–363.

Psychopathic Children, 169–170.

Puberty and Adolescence, distinguished, 301.

Public Opinion Among Children, 117; Howells' observations on, 117.

Puffer, on boys' gangs, 118.

Purpose of the School, 171–172.

Punishment Attitude, toward delinquency, 232–234.

Punishment and Discipline, in the treatment of delinquency, 257–259.

Race, on education of gifted children, 294.

Reading, dynamic principle in teaching, 418–420.

Reality, in the development of children, 196, when overwhelming, 197, when too easy, 197–198; of government, in teaching civics, 411–412.

Reason, a special not general power, 381.

Reasons why Practice Lags Behind Knowledge of Education, 331–339; conservatism in education, 332–333; popular control of education, 333–334; changing conditions outside the schools, 334–336; political rather than professional basis of educational control, 336–337; necessity of training teachers, 339.

Recency, law of, in learning, 132.

Reconstruction of Traditional Studies, 383–386.

Recuperation, lack of from effects of malnutrition, 185–186.

Regimen of the Adolescent Period, 300–321.

Rein laboratory school in Jena, 21.

Relative Progress, of knowledge and of practice of education, 330.

Religion in Children, impulses for, utilized in character building, 95; altruism as an aspect of religion, 123; religion in adolescence, 124; Starbuck on, 124.

Remediable Nature of Physical Defects, 216–217.

Repression, not enough in the guidance of children, 199–200.

Requirements, of nutrition, 228–229.

Research and Training, coöperative, 22.

Rest, as a cure of overstrain, 435–436.

Retardation in School Work, and underweight, 179.

Revelations, concerning the health and physical development of our people, 424–425; Fisher, 425; Life Extension Institute, 425.

Right Impulses, should be strengthened, 32.

Rights of Childhood, 210.

Riis, Mrs. J. A., on converting the gang, 120.

Rivalry, a sociable trait, 116; lying as a form of, 116; how utilized in education, 117–119; of the nations in education, 453–454.

Romanes, on ant life, 108.

Rousseau, on memory work in teaching, 399.

Rural People, relation of government to, 412–413.

Rural School, the problem of, 462–463.

Safeguards, of the child's health, 190.

Sage Foundation, investigation of compulsory education laws, 458–459.

San Francisco, medical inspection of schools in, 436.

Satisfaction, law of, in learning.

Schools, and character building, 97–99; as a cause of insanity, 169; and home, 170–171; the purpose of, 171–172; aims of, constantly changing, 325; must prepare for life, 377–378; dynamic principle in, of Winnebago County (Ill.), 405; hygiene of, 426–427; ventilation of, 427–428; posture in, 428–429; hygiene of program in, 429–430; injurious tasks in, 430; malnourishment in, 431–432; overstrain in, 432–434; cause of overstrain in, 436; medical inspection in, 437–438; the most imposing and conspicuous social institution, 448–449.

Classics In
Child Development

An Arno Press Collection

Baldwin, James Mark. **Thought and Things.** Four vols. in two. 1906-1915

Blatz, W[illiam] E[met], et al. **Collected Studies on the Dionne Quintuplets.** 1937

Bühler, Charlotte. **The First Year of Life.** 1930

Bühler, Karl. **The Mental Development of the Child.** 1930

Claparède, Ed[ouard]. **Experimental Pedagogy and the Psychology of the Child.** 1911

Factors Determining Intellectual Attainment. 1975

First Notes by Observant Parents. 1975

Freud, Anna. **Introduction to the Technic of Child Analysis.** 1928

Gesell, Arnold, et al. **Biographies of Child Development.** 1939

Goodenough, Florence L. **Measurement of Intelligence By Drawings.** 1926

Griffiths, Ruth. **A Study of Imagination in Early Childhood and Its Function in Mental Development.** 1918

Hall, G. Stanley and Some of His Pupils. **Aspects of Child Life and Education.** 1907

Hartshorne, Hugh and Mark May. **Studies in the Nature of Character. Vol. I: Studies in Deceit; Book One, General Methods and Results.** 1928

Hogan, Louise E. **A Study of a Child.** 1898

Hollingworth, Leta S. **Children Above 180 IQ, Stanford Binet:** Origins and Development. 1942

Kluver, Heinrich. **An Experimental Study of the Eidetic Type.** 1926

Lamson, Mary Swift. **Life and Education of Laura Dewey Bridgman, the Deaf, Dumb and Blind Girl.** 1881

Lewis, M[orris] M[ichael]. **Infant Speech:** A Study of the Beginnings of Language. 1936

McGraw, Myrtle B. **Growth: A Study of Johnny and Jimmy.** 1935

Monographs on Infancy. 1975

O'Shea, M. V., editor. **The Child: His Nature and His Needs.** 1925

Perez, Bernard. **The First Three Years of Childhood.** 1888

Romanes, George John. **Mental Evolution in Man:** Origin of Human Faculty. 1889

Shinn, Milicent Washburn. **The Biography of a Baby.** 1900

Stern, William. **Psychology of Early Childhood Up to the Sixth Year of Age.** 1924

Studies of Play. 1975

Terman, Lewis M. **Genius and Stupidity:** A Study of Some of the Intellectual Processes of Seven "Bright" and Seven "Stupid" Boys. 1906

Terman, Lewis M. **The Measurement of Intelligence.** 1916

Thorndike, Edward Leè. **Notes on Child Study.** 1901

Wilson, Louis N., compiler. **Bibliography of Child Study.** 1898-1912

[Witte, Karl Heinrich Gottfried]. **The Education of Karl Witte,** Or the Training of the Child. 1914